Anthropology of Health and Wellbeing

About the Editor

Prof. M.P. Sachdeva is presently the Head of Department and professor at Department of Anthropology, University of Delhi. He has received his M.Sc. training in Anthropology from Panjab University, Chandigarh where he was awarded the Panjab University Gold Medal and the Bureau of Police Research and Development, Ministry of Home Affairs Fellowship to pursue his doctoral research. He specializes in Human Population Genetics, Molecular Genetics and Forensic Anthropology and has been teaching papers on Population Genetics, Forensic Anthropology, Serology, Palaeoanthropology, Biochemical Genetics, Human Biological Diversity, Ethnic and Cultural Diversity since 1986 to both undergraduate and post-graduate students. He has completed and is pursuing several research projects in Population Genetics and Molecular Anthropology, funded by DBT, DST and UGC. He has successfully supervised 25 doctoral scholars in addition to several M.Phil. students and M.Sc. dissertations. He is a member of many academic bodies and in editorial board of national and international journals of repute.

Anthropology of Health and Wellbeing

Essays in Honour of Professor P.C. Joshi

Edited by

M.P. Sachdeva

CONCEPT PUBLISHING COMPANY PVT. LTD.
NEW DELHI-110059

ISBN: 978-93-5439-086-9

First Published 2022

Published and Printed by

Concept Publishing Company Pvt. Ltd.
A/15-16, Commercial Block, Mohan Garden,
New Delhi-110059 (India)
T: 91 11 41101460
E: publishing@conceptpub.com, *W*: www.conceptpub.com

Cataloging in Publication Data–Courtesy: D.K. Agencies (P) Ltd. <docinfo@dkagencies.com>

Anthropology of Health and Wellbeing
essays in Honour of Professor P.C. Joshi / edited by M.P. Sachdeva
pages cm
Contributed articles.
Includes bibliographical references and index.
ISBN 9789354390869

1. Medical anthropology--India. 2. Well-being--India. 3. Indigenous peoples--Health and hygiene--India. 4. Public health--Anthropological aspects--India. 5. Traditional medicine--India. I. Joshi, P. C., 1956- honouree. II. Sachdeva, M. P., editor.

LCC GN296.5.I4A58 2022 | DDC 306.4610954 23

Foreword

I feel honoured to write this foreword to a volume brought out in honour of Prof. P.C. Joshi, who has made significant contribution to Medical Anthropology during the last 45 years of his academic career. The papers included in the book clearly indicate the flowering of his teaching and research in the succeeding generations, under his promotion and guidance.

This book augurs well for Indian Medical Anthropology, since the teaching of Medical Anthropology as a course was first introduced in India, at Pune University in 1974. The International Congress of Anthropological and Ethnological Sciences (ICAES) was organized at Delhi in December 1978, under the leadership of Prof. L.P. Vidyarthi and Prof. I.P. Singh. Three day Post-Congress symposium on Medical Anthropology was organised at Pune University. It was attended by 50 anthropologists from Europe and North America. A special number of the international journal, 'Social Science and Medicine' was published with papers from the session on 'Medical Pluralism' in early 1980. Pandit Shiv Sharma, doyen of Ayurved, who rejuvenated Ayurved in Independent India chaired the whole day session on Ayurved at the instance of Prof. Charles Leslie. This paved the way for continuing interaction of Medical Anthropology with AYUSH. The symposium was also attended by Prof. P.C. Joshi and Prof. H.K. Bhat among the few delegates representing Indian anthropologists. They subsequently established 'Society for Indian Medical Anthropology' (SIMA), and continue to lead the organization. SIMA organises conferences very frequently. SIMA publications have made significant contributions to Indian Medical Anthropology.

The papers in this book in honour of Prof. P.C. Joshi cover wide areas in Medical Anthropology, such as socio-cultural and biological perspectives about health, disease, disability and disasters. The issues discussed relate to health system as provider system and access to health care; health attitudes and practices related to allopathic, Indian and folk medicine; public health and epidemiology connected to natural disasters and pandemics; bio-medical issues in the realm of genetics and molecular biology, and genetic disorders as challenge to community acceptance and management. Tribal health is a natural study area in Anthropology which generates significant ethnographic data about health care attitudes, practices and traditional health care professionals. Gender issues have become prominent in all social and behavioural disciplines, having policy and implementation related problems of mother and child health, neonatal and infant morbidity and mortality. Non-communicable disease management issues are branded as life-style problems correctable by emerging wellness industry. Yoga has assumed international credibility delinked from religion, by way of U.N. accredited 'International Yoga Day'. Sanitation as a health and stigma issue in Indian social organisation was brought in prominence by Mahatma Gandhi and is supposed to be monitored symbolically through his spectacles. Sanitation continues to be a major health and disease related issue in India. Vaccines have prompted us to rethink our biological relationship with other mammals and primates. Covid-19 has raised issues of bio-security with the risk of virus being used as a biological weapon. Mental health is coming into prominence due to uncertainties of living due to natural and pandemic disasters. Suicide which we discuss in the classroom while discussing Durkhiem is becoming a major issue. Farmer suicides have become endemic, but not yet attracting the attention of anthropologists. Suicides due to depression, isolation and helplessness in COVID-19 is no more a rear phenomenon. Several of these issues are addressed through the papers presented in this book.

Medicalisation of health is directly linked to pharma industry, as one of the most lucrative industry. As we experience, laboratory generated pathological reports have replaced clinical acumen and widen the distance between a physician and a reporting patient. Side effects of unnecessary over-use of antibiotics and now steroids, are giving rise to new disease symptoms, which tend to become fatal. In all disease control programmes, the emphasis has shifted to more potent drugs, while the side effects and resistance are discussed as major research areas in medical research institutes. Drug resistance, relapse and re-infection are the most commonly discussed research issues in leprosy research. TB continues to be a major national problem, despite available effective drugs. In leprosy, medical anthropological intervention has led to discussion about community, in preference to earlier exclusive focus on patients. Similarly, the objective of the programme, only to identify the patients and treat them with drugs, was extended to address community concerns due to problem of nerve damage consequences, leading to social exclusion and economic deprivation. Mere lip-sympathy is paid to these interventions, rather than becoming the priority interventions in the control strategies. In leprosy, nerve damage research is more important than research in chemotherapy.

Medical anthropology came into limelight since it was sought in public health programmes for addressing the community, to educate them to actively participate in the globally designed control programmes, which in plain terms meant compliance, to the advice about regular drug consumption. Creation of awareness in the community became the responsibility of field anthropologists designated as social scientists, mainly from the platform of NGOs. Health education programmes were designed for the people, to identify the disease symptoms, and to voluntarily report at the health centre. Health Education (H.E.) has been renamed as Information, Education and Communication (I.E.C.) and now rechristened as Behavioural Change Communication (B.C.C.). B.C.C. for whom: the people or health bureaucracy to engage in interactive dialogue with the people? We evaluated the Survey, Education, Treatment (SET) strategy of National Leprosy Control Programme (NLCP) for ICMR, in Odisha and Andhra Pradesh and found that 'E' was totally missing.

There is a conceptual paper on Gender, Sustainable Development and Environment in the book. This subject could additionally be subjected to analysis under 'Anthropology of Literature'. Irawati Karve analyzing Mahabharat from anthropological perspective, using the concepts of culture and personality, in her Sahitya Academy award-winning book, 'Yugant', discussed the role of 'seed' and 'field' in the practice of '*Niyog*'. Woman as 'field' was not considered significant and had no say in the selection of 'seed'. In Ramayan, Sita was found as an abandoned baby in the agricultural field. She decided to reject the patriarchal concept of suspecting woman's 'purity' to revert back to mother earth, not to heaven.

In fact, it is argued that women played major role in the domestication of plants and domestication of animals, in the economic and socio-cultural evolution of humankind. All Marathi plays on the stage continue to start with women from Brindavan going to Mathura market to sell milk products. Domestication led to surplus production which required muscle power for its protection. This evolved into kingship and militia, forcing 'extortion', institutionalized as taxes.

Now that Panchayati Raj Institutions have 50 per cent reservation for women, by statutory provisions, anthropologists could think of empowering them at least in areas of health. The ANM, Anganwadi worker,

ASHA who are health workers are all women. Dai as Traditional Birth Attendant (TBA) is an international health worker. Trained TBAs continue to perform delivery in modern hospitals, in several western countries, the obstetricians being called in case of complication. We in India are out to kill the institution of Dai, as a policy. How much do we interact with these health workers in our research process?

In tribal communities, which continue to be the special and exclusive preserve of anthropological studies, 'gender' is a non-issue. We have studied in HIV-AIDS research, that even college going tribal students in tribal towns, consider female breasts as mammary glands for feeding the babies, not as sex objects. Cows are not mulched with the analogy, that mother's milk is meant for the babies. Food and other supplies such as fuel wood is collected from the forests to satisfy the immediate needs and not for greed of markets. Cow can be used for ploughing, paired with a bull, since a woman also works on the field. A woman may be provided rest in a separate menstrual hut, not necessarily on grounds of ritual pollution alone, It is usually believed among the caste peasantry also, that body secretions could be easily used for black magic, and hence considered polluting. A tribal woman is never-ever molested by a tribal man. The custom of bride price as against our dowry in cash or kind, is a gender empowering custom. An infertile woman is likely to desert her husband and marry another, after a due and quick process of divorce, returning back a part of the bride price. We as field anthropologists know these practices but feel shy of saying it, in the absence of quantitative data. It has been observed that maternal mortality is low in tribal area, although neonatal, infant and child mortality is significantly high. During pregnancy, tribal women deliberately eat less, to have a low-weight baby for safe delivery. Tribal health need to be our priority research area not only in terms of access to health care facilities and its utilization. Paradoxically, malnutrition in the Naxal infested tribal area is relatively less, since the people have free access to forest resources of food, in the absence of regulatory forest rule presented in '*khaki*' uniform. Forest Department has been the creation of British Rule to exploit forest resources in market economy. Now, the corrections on paper, such as Forest Rights Act (FRA) are in place. We denigrate tribal herbalists who have expert knowledge of medicinal plants, but the pharma industry uses them and exploits them, for their herbal supplies to produce drugs.

Prof. P.C. Joshi has personally worked on several of the areas on which the papers have been included in the book. Working on government committees as experts, with multidisciplinary team and bureaucrats, is a learning process for everybody. We find the Higher Judiciary in India, becoming pro-active, responding to PILs and Suo Moto injunctions about public issues. But we academics do not want to take a stand based on research or to initiate research on public issues. We possess the expertise to win the confidence of the people in conducting our objective research among the communities.. Our qualitative methods are very useful to find the causation of issues and instinctive response of the people in the tribal and rural homogenous communities, as compared to urban communities. We have now learnt to quantify the qualitative data, since the administrative bureaucracy requires numbers for their planning and budget outlay. However, only the statistics of 'How Many' does not ensure success of planning or implementation at the micro level, or at the level of ethnic groups, unless we know the answer to 'Why' to ensure community participation.

One of the major issues is, who gives us research agenda? Like the judiciary, we have to be pro-active on public issues, form research teams to investigate various aspects since one researcher cannot deal with an issue holistically. Holistic understanding and analysis is our strength. If we go for vertical super-specialisations, we may be on the backseat with other disciplines, which have sophisticated laboratories, or statistical expertise with reductionist approach. We have to get the expertise of 'statistics of small numbers'. Our focus as spelt out in our UGC Anthropology curriculum (2001) is to develop 'Indian Anthropology' and not be content with 'Anthropology in India', which was a colonial hang-over, based on Lord Macaulay's strategy, spelt out in 1835, to break the nerve of India, through British education system. We are no more studying 'other people' as in the colonial days. We have to study ourselves, our own marginalized people, 'We, the People of India' taking the Constitution of India as the sacred document to preserve and promote the basic democratic and secular values of Indian Civilisation.

I am sure, this volume will further develop our research agenda for pro-people policy planning and effective implementation at the micro level. We are confident that Prof. P.C. Joshi will find more time to guide the colleagues and students to widen the horizons of anthropological approach and knowledge.

May 29, 2021 **R.K. Mutatkar**

Patron: United Indian Anthropology Forum (UIAF)
Patron, Society for Indian Medical Anthropology (SIMA)

Acknowledgements

This Festschrift has been developed out of the essays contributed by academicians, researchers and research fellows in honour of Prof. P.C. Joshi, a towering anthropologist, dear colleague and friend. First, at the very onset, I gratefully thank all the contributors for making this book a reality. I also owe thanks to many others who have assisted in the planning and preparation of this volume.

In the true sense, this book is an outcome of spirited and consistent efforts of Dr. Chakraverti Mahajan, Prof. K.N. Saraswathy, Prof. R.P. Mitra, and Prof. P.R. Mondal. Dr. Mahajan conceived the book's idea and remained a key contributor from its inception until the very end. It was Prof. Saraswathy who took this idea forward and worked for its realization. Prof. Mitra played a pivotal role in planning and drafting this volume through constructive ideas and discussions. I am deeply indebted to them. Special thanks are due to Prof. Mitra and Dr. Mahajan, who also contributed to shaping this book's introduction. They are masters of their craft. Apart from authoring a chapter and reviewing another, Prof. Mondal remained associated with the working group from the beginning and offered much-needed help from time to time.

I would particularly like to thank senior academicians and researchers, namely Prof. A.K. Sinha, Prof. Abhik Ghosh, Prof. Subho Roy, Prof. S. Sumathi, Prof. Roumi Deb and Dr. Sunita Reddy, for their contributions. Prof. Sinha was the first one to contribute a chapter for this volume. His submission served as a morale booster and brought positivity to our working group, and steered us to go ahead with the book. Prof. Sumathi, despite being busy with her son's wedding preparations, readily agreed to contribute a chapter for the book and did it well in time. Prof. Roumi Deb contributed a paper despite being unwell due to COVID-19 infection. They wrote essays for the book and helped in the review process. My special gratitude is due to Prof. R.K. Mutatkar for kindly and readily agreeing to write the foreword to the book at a terse notice. Erudite scholars and academicians like Dr. Venkatramana, and Dr. Ratika Samtani deserve special mention for extending their unrestricted support to the endeavour. Dr. Ratika, apart from co-authoring a chapter, also reviewed two of the chapters for the book. The book's publication has been greatly assisted by Dr. Gagandeep Kaur Walia and Priyanka Rani Garg by reviewing one chapter each. I am grateful to them.

Further, I would like to especially thank many of the former students of Prof. Joshi who were associated with this endeavour. They not only participated enthusiastically but also brought much-needed dynamism to the group. I would start by mentioning Dr. Urfat Anjem Mir, who was the first person to be contacted for his academic contribution. He was delighted to learn about the upcoming Festschrift. Dr. Mir put many of the former students of Prof. Joshi together on this task and followed up with them for their original contributions. Apart from this, he has also contributed a chapter for this volume and reviewed two of the chapters. Dr. Prashant Khatri also deserves a special mention for penning one and reviewing two chapters despite being unwell due to COVID-19 infection. I would also like to thank Dr. Oinam Hemlata Devi, Dr. Kalindi Sharma, Dr. Sonia Kaushal, Dr. B.S. Aribam and Dr. Minakshi contributed chapters and helped as reviewers. Their generosity is gratefully acknowledged.

Moving forward, I would also like to acknowledge a special debt to my dear colleagues, the other faculty members of the Department of Anthropology, University of Delhi, namely Prof. Manoj Kumar Singh, Prof. Benrithung Murry, Dr. Avitoli G. Zhimo, Dr. Vipin Gupta, Dr. Mitashree Srivastava, Dr. Shivani Chandel, Dr. Moiranthem Kennedy Singh, Dr. Naorem Kiranmala Devi and Dr. Suniti Yadav for their efforts, skills, unstinted support, and willing cooperation. They all have contributed one chapter for this volume and reviewed the chapters assigned to them.

I would also like to highlight the cooperation extended by Ms. Seema Sirpal of Delhi University Computer Center (DUCC). She shared the credentials of software to check plagiarism and answered our queries very patiently.

I would like to specially acknowledge the contribution of one of the research scholars of our Department, Mr. Imnameren Longkumer. Although he joined the working group when he was conducting his fieldwork, he fulfilled all the responsibility given to him impeccably. He pushed the group in the right direction at the right time. He has immensely contributed to the realization of this book. Another research scholar

Mr. Vineet Chaudhary assisted the group with handling the software to check for the plagiarism of all the chapters. God bless them both.

Further, I would like to thank Mr. Ashok Mittal, Managing Director, Concept Publishing Company (P) Ltd., to keep us bound to strict deadlines, sticking with a very tough timeline, and finally, publishing the book despite many hurdles, including the second wave of COVID-19 pandemic.

Finally, I would also wish to acknowledge someone who was not directly involved with either the planning or drafting of this volume; however, this book is seeing the light of the day only because of his towering personality and the respect that he commands, in the department, among his students, and in academic and research circles, Prof. P.C. Joshi. Every single person who was contacted for the book, from authoring a chapter to reviewing any chapter or draft, everyone contributed with utmost sincerity and willingness only because of Prof. Joshi. He is indeed the heart and the soul of this book.

Contents

PART II

Health, Disease and Health Seeking Behaviour

PART III

Physical Health and Wellbeing

List of Contributors

Abhik Ghosh is currently working as Professor of Social Anthropology at Department of Anthropology, Panjab University, Chandigarh.

Anand Kumar Gyanendra Singh Wahengbam recently completed his Ph.D. (2020) from Department of Anthropology, University of Delhi.

Angana Goswami is a Ph.D. Research Scholar in Department of Anthropology, University of Delhi.

Anil Kishore Sinha is a Professor of Social Anthropology at Department of Anthropology, Panjab University, Chandigarh.

Anushka Ghosh is pursuing Ph.D. from Biological Anthropology Unit, Indian Statistical Institute, Kolkata.

Anushka Singh is a Project Fellow in an ICSSR funded Project, School of Liberal Studies, Ambedkar University, Delhi.

Apoorva Sharma is an M.Phil. Research Scholar at Department of Anthropology, University of Delhi, Delhi.

Archita Tandon has completed M.Sc. from Department of Anthropology, University of Delhi, Delhi.

Avitoli G. Zhimo is currently an Associate Professor at Department of Anthropology, University of Delhi, where she has been teaching since January 2009. She received her Master's degree, M.Phil. and Ph.D. from Department of Anthropology, University of Delhi, Delhi.

B.S. Aribam is working as an Assistant Professor at Department of Anthropology, Dr. Harisingh Gour Vishwavidyalaya (A Central University), Sagar, Madhya Pradesh.

Benrithung Murry is Professor of Biological Anthropology at Department of Anthropology, University of Delhi. Prior to joining the department in 2004 as a lecturer, he worked in the capacity of Research Officer at Law Research Institute, Gauhati High Court and as Guest Lecturer in the Department of Anthropology, North Eastern Hill University, Shillong.

Chakraverti Mahajan is an Assistant Professor at Department of Anthropology, University of Delhi. He was trained in Social Anthropology at Panjab University, Chandigarh.

Chonsing Shimrah is pursuing Ph.D. from Department of Anthropology, University of Delhi, Delhi.

Imnameren Longkumer is a UGC-Senior Research Fellow and Ph.D. Research Scholar at Laboratory of Biochemical and Molecular Anthropology, Department of Anthropology, University of Delhi, Delhi.

Jagriti Mehta is a UGC-Senior Research Fellow and Ph.D. Research Scholar at Department of Anthropology, Panjab University, Chandigarh.

Jyoti Mishra is working as a Research Officer at Department of Obstetrics and Gynaecology, Lady Hardinge Medical College and Smt. Sucheta Kriplani Hospital, Delhi. She has completed her Ph.D. from Department of Anthropology, University of Delhi, Delhi.

Kallur Nava Saraswathy is currently working as a Professor of Biological Anthropology at Department of Anthropology, University of Delhi. She completed her post-doctoral research in Molecular Genetics from Albert Einstein College of Medicine, New York, USA. She completed more than 15 major/minor government funded projects and published more than 150 research papers in both national and international peer-reviewed journals.

Kalindi Sharma is working as an Assistant Professor at Amity Institute of Anthropology, Amity University, Noida.

Kiran Jyoti Kaur is a UGC Junior Research Fellows and Research Scholar at Department of Anthropology, Panjab University, Chandigarh.

M. Kennedy Singh is working as an Assistant Professor at Department of Anthropology, University of Delhi. He was educated in Manipur University and University of Hyderabad.

M.N. Nimal has completed M.Sc. from Department of Anthropology, University of Delhi. He is currently working as a Research Assistant in a research project 'The A. Aiyappan Omnibus'.

M.P. Sachdeva is the present Head of the Department and Professor at Department of Anthropology, University of Delhi. He has received his training in anthropology from Panjab University.

Manju Puri is a clinician and Professor at Department of Obstetrics and Gynaecology, Lady Hardinge Medical College & Smt. Sucheta Kriplani Hospital, Delhi.

Manoj Kumar Singh is a Professor of Archaeological Anthropology at Department of Anthropology, University of Delhi. He earned his doctorate in Archaeology from University of Delhi in 2002 and has subsequently been teaching Archaeological Anthropology and Palaeoanthropology in the Department.

Minakshi is a UGC Post-Doctorate Fellow at Department of Anthropology, University of Delhi, Delhi.

Mitashree Srivastava is an Assistant Professor of Social Anthropology at Department of Anthropology, University of Delhi. She was educated and trained in Social Anthropology at University of Allahabad, Allahabad.

Muniraj M. is a Ph.D. Research Scholar at Department of Anthropology, University of Madras, Chennai.

Naorem Kiranmala Devi is an Assistant Professor of Biological Anthropology at Department of Anthropology, University of Delhi. Prior to joining Department she worked as a research officer in INCLEN Trust International, New Delhi.

Nandita Babu is a Professor and a former Head of the Department of Psychology, University of Delhi, Delhi.

Naveen Kumar is a Ph.D. Research Scholar at Department of Anthropology, University of Delhi, Delhi.

Nivedita Som is affiliated to Department of Anthropology, Vivekananda College for Women, Barisha, Kolkata.

Nutan Kumari Jha is an ICMR-Senior Research Fellow at Department of Anthropology, Panjab University, Chandigarh.

Oinam Hemlata Devi is an Assistant Professor at School of Human Ecology, Ambedkar University, Delhi.

P. Annaiah is a doctorate in Anthropology from S.V. University, Tirupati and has published research papers on obesity and lipid profiles among different populations.

P. Venkatramana is currently working as an Assistant Professor in the Discipline of Anthropology, School of Social Sciences, IGNOU, New Delhi. He holds M.Phil. and Ph.D. in Biological Anthropology.

Prakash Ranjan Mondal is a Professor at Department of Anthropology, University of Delhi. He was trained in Anthropology in University of Kolkata and University of Delhi with a specialization in Biological Anthropology.

Prashant Khattri is working as an Assistant Professor at Department of Anthropology, University of Allahabad, Prayagraj, Uttar Pradesh. He is also a Charles Wallace Fellow in Social Anthropology, Queen's University, Belfast, United Kingdom. He has completed his Ph.D. from University of Delhi, Delhi.

Priyanka Kanrar is affiliated to the Department of Anthropology, University of Calcutta, Kolkata, West Bengal.

R.P. Mitra is currently working as Professor of Social Anthropology at Department of Anthropology, University of Delhi. He was trained in Social Anthropology at University of Delhi. Prior to joining the department as an Assistant Professor in 2003, he has worked as a research fellow in Institute of Human Behaviour and Allied Sciences (IHBAS), Delhi.

Rahul Kumar is working as Deputy Director at Centre for Cultural Resources and Training (CCRT), Ministry of Culture, Government of India.

Rajnish Kumar Singh is working as Guest Faculty, Department of Anthropology, University of Allahabad, Prayagraj. He has also served as ICSSR-Post Doctoral Fellow at Department of Anthropology, Panjab University, Chandigarh.

Ramandeep Kaur is a UGC Junior Research Fellow at Department of Anthropology, Panjab University, Chandigarh.

Ratika Samtani is an Assistant Professor at Amity Institute of Anthropology, Amity University, Noida. She has received her Ph.D. in Biological Anthropology from University of Delhi, Delhi.

Rita Kumari is an ICMR Senior Research Fellow at Department of Anthropology, Panjab University, Chandigarh.

Roumi Deb is a Professor of Biological Anthropology and Head of the Amity Institute of Anthropology, Amity University, Noida.

S. Sumathi is Emeritus Professor at Department of Anthropology, University of Madras, Chennai.

S.A.A. Latheef is presently working as a Visiting Scientist, Department of Genetics, Osmania University. He obtained his Ph.D. degree in Anthropology from S.V. University, Tirupati.

Sanjay Bhadada is working as a Professor at Department of Endocrinology, Post Graduate Institute of Medical Education and Research, Chandigarh.

Shalu is a Project Fellow at Department of Anthropology, Panjab University, Chandigarh.

Shivani Chandel is an Assistant Professor at Department of Anthropology, University of Delhi. After completing her Ph.D. in Anthropology from University of Delhi in 2012, she joined the department in 2013.

Shobana Sharma is a Ph.D. Research Scholar at Department of Anthropology, University of Madras, Chennai.

Shwetha Gopalakrishnan is a Project Fellow in ICSSR Project at School of Liberal Studies, Ambedkar University, Delhi.

Sonia Kaushal is working as an Assistant Professor in Department of Anthropology, School of Applied Sciences, Dr. Harisingh Gour Vishwavidyalaya (A Central University), Sagar.

Subho Roy is working as a Professor at Department of Anthropology, University of Calcutta, West Bengal. He has also served as the Head of this Department.

Sunita Reddy is currently working as an Associate Professor at the Centre of Social Medicine and Community Health, Jawaharlal Nehru University, New Delhi. She is also a founder member of Anthropos India Foundation.

Suniti Yadav is currently working as an Assistant Professor at Department of Anthropology, University of Delhi. Prior to joining the department she was working as a Scientist at ICMR, New Delhi.

Surendra Kumar Sagar is an Associate Professor at Department of Zoology, Swami Sharaddhanand College, University of Delhi, Delhi.

Swagato Pramanik is affiliated to Department of Anthropology, University of Calcutta, Kolkata, West Bengal.

Tajinder Kaur is a Ph.D. Research Scholar at Department of Anthropology, University of Delhi, Delhi.

Urfat Anjem Mir is an Assistant Professor at School of Liberal Studies, Ambedkar University, Delhi.

Vijay Hadda is a Clinician and an Associate Professor at Department of Pulmonary, Critical Care and Sleep Medicine, AIIMS, New Delhi.

Vineet Chaudhary is a UGC Junior Research Fellow and Ph.D. Research Scholar at Department of Anthropology, University of Delhi, Delhi.

Vipin Gupta is currently working as an Assistant Professor at Department of Anthropology, University of Delhi, Delhi. To date he has received research grant of INR 80 million from different funding agencies, like DBT, ICMR, UGC, SERB, and Wellcome Trust, UK.

1
Introduction

M.P. Sachdeva

This Festschrift is in honour of Professor P.C. Joshi and his seminal contributions to anthropology of health and wellbeing. He is one of the leading anthropologists of India, who has given a new direction to research by combining theory and application in the practice of medical anthropology. Born in a small village in Almora district of Uttarakhand, he had his later schooling in Delhi. He started his academic journey in 1972 as a student at Department of Anthropology, University of Delhi, and went on to do his graduation, post-graduation, M.Phil. and Ph.D. from the department. As an institutional builder and a visionary, he initiated and nurtured the teaching of medical anthropology in many institutions and is one of the founding members, and President since 2010, of the Society for Indian Medical Anthropologists. It all started with his doctoral research on the ethno-medical system of Jaunsaris, which was perhaps the first Ph.D. in medical anthropology at the Department of Anthropology, University of Delhi. What Malinowski was to Trobriand Islanders of Papua New Guinea, P.C. Joshi is to the Khasas of Jaunsar, Uttarakhand. He is the undisputed regional specialist of Jaunsar-Bawar. Any anthropologist coming to the area would visit him for academic guidance and seek his expert opinion on the subject and he is also quite generous in sharing his knowledge and time with them. This endeared him to leading anthropologists like William Sax and J.S. Alter, who all profited from his insights and understanding of the people and the region. 'Knowledge shared is knowledge gained', was one the academic values he always cherished and practiced throughout his academic career.

Prof. Joshi began his teaching career in 1985 at the Department of Anthropology, Hemvati Nandan Bahuguna Garhwal University, Srinagar where he not only expanded and nurtured the department of anthropology but also brought it to national limelight. He headed the department for 12 years from 1985 to 1997. Before returning back to his parent department at University of Delhi in 2003, he was an Associate Professor and Head, Department of Medical Anthropology, Institute of Human Behaviour and Allied Sciences, Delhi from 1997 to 2003. It is a well-accepted fact that one's academic journeys are greatly influenced by the nature of institutions one has been associated with. These three institutions have had a great bearing in shaping the academic trajectory of Prof. Joshi, his research and writings.

The impact of Garhwal University can be seen in the number of articles he wrote about the region Jaunsar-Bawar in the initial years. His publications were on medical anthropology and he touched upon topics like the traditional medical systems, health and healing in central Himalayas, with special reference to the Jaunsaris. One of the interesting articles he authored dealt with *Pursuit of Protein: On Meat Eating in Garhwal*, which was published in 1994 in the Indian Anthropologist. The article is an interesting account of how food, social institution, health and ecology are all linked together. It shows how a community judiciously manages the food resources with a spirit of cooperation and reciprocity which ensures an equitable distribution of animal protein in the community. Another article dealt with the issue of marital stability among the Khasa of Jaunsar-Bawar, which appeared in the journal *Spectra of Anthropological Progress*. The article examined the structure of family in relation to possibility of conflict and division of property and its role in marital stability and how in turn it leads to inter-generational and intra-generational unity. During this time, he also co-authored a book on medical anthropology which was published by Reliance Press, New Delhi. The book is a very good reference work and a must read for all those who are embarking on a career in medical anthropology. It is very lucidly written and explains the key concepts of medical anthropology like pluralism, ethno-medicine, meaning of the terms like illness and health and how all these have to be conceptualized in the socio-cultural context. These same ideas were re-examined in another article which was co-authored with another legend of the department late Professor Vinay Kumar Srivastava, *Dialogue and Interpretation of Illness* published in the Eastern Anthropologist in 1995. They made use of the illness narrative framework and explanatory model of Arthur Kleinman to understand how illness and disease model can be collated together to provide effective cure. Other than health, he also wrote an article on the issue of afforestation programme in the hill region and how they are important for maintaining the ecological stability of the region.

When he shifted to Delhi in 1997 as the Head of Medical Anthropology Division at the Institute of Human Behaviour and Allied Sciences, it was a major academic turn for him. Now one can discern a more clinical based and applied medical anthropological approach in his writings. This was an institution where he was working with psychiatrists and other mental health experts from hardcore biological sciences. They all viewed medical anthropology as an aid to solve their clinical problems. It was a medical institution with an attached hospital for people with psychiatric disorders. During this phase we see many cutting-edge researches by Prof. P.C. Joshi on issues like mental health, ageing, women's health and psychosocial consequences of traumatic events. This was a phase where he was looking at anthropology as a collaborative discipline working in conjunction with other behavioural sciences, focusing upon particular events. For instance, one of his earliest writings during this phase on women's health issues and how the involvement of traditional healers like priests can enable policy makers to improve the status of women's health, is a perfect example of use of anthropological knowledge for policy inputs. This article appeared in the prestigious medical journal, the *National Medical Journal of India*, 2000, and looked critically at the concept of 'targeted health care delivery strategies' and how medical anthropology can contribute towards it. He examined the role of traditional healers in an integrative template in conjunction with allopathic practitioners and health policy objectives. This idea was further examined by him in an article on 'Relevance and Utility of Traditional Medical Systems' which he wrote in 2000 for the Sage journal, *Psychology and Developing Societies*. This article again was a brilliant exposition of emic meanings of health, illness, body and healing in a traditional medical system and how they are all integrated in a quest for wellbeing in a partially isolated community. We also see him at this time, taking up new research topics. One of them was the study of aging and problems of elderly in India. The article which was published in the journal Seminar in 2001, addressed the psychosocial and somatic problems of elderly and ways to anthropologically address them. Elderly in India, the article says are plagued by multiple health problems including degenerative ailments like dementia, Alzheimer and musculoskeletal atrophies like arthritis, deterioration of vision and hearing capabilities. This is compounded by their increased vulnerabilities to infectious diseases due to weakening of their immune system. The article also draws attention to prevalence of well-known chronic health problems like diabetes, cardiovascular diseases and hypertension and lesser known but important health issues like the upper respiratory tract infection and urinary tract infections among the elderly in India. All these problems are compounded by mental health issues like depression, emotional disturbances and neurological problems among the elderly. Professor Joshi, tried to link up these problems to the changing value system and rapid social changes taking place in transformational India. He put forwarded the view that the changing family structures along with socio-economic driven migrations are leading to many 'lonely, solitary, forlorn, depressed and desolate' old people in India. He further elaborated on these issues in the review article, which was published in 1999 in the Sage journal: *Social Change*. In the same year, he wrote an interesting piece on 'Whose Forest is it Anyway?' in the well-known journal of Himalayan studies, *Mountain and People*. The article highlighted the significance of joint participatory forest management and community forestry in the context of mountain ecosystem in India. In the next couple of years, we see Prof. Joshi writing on anthropology of trauma and how trauma needs to be understood as a social suffering. He co-authored two very rich ethnographies in 2002, titled as 'Psychosocial consequences of traumatic events on adolescents: A study in context of Jammu and Kashmir' and 'Medical Anthropology and Traumatic Reactions: Emerging concerns in Medical Anthropology'. The first appeared in an edited book published by IHBAS and the second appeared in the *Eastern Anthropologist*.

In the year 2003, Prof. P.C. Joshi returned to his *alma mater*, the Department of Anthropology, University of Delhi. Here we see the emergence of the 'master medical anthropologist of India who combined the critical approach to applied aspects to produce a uniquely blended medical anthropology. The best way to look at this is through the lens of the research projects he undertook during this time. He got associated with important international and national projects during this time and his publications in top international journals were mostly related to research outcome of these projects. In 2005, he headed the EU funded project to determine the user's perception of health in collaboration with Catholic University of Louvain, Belgium and University of Heidelberg, Germany. He was also the India project leader, on mortality and injury risk factor in Tsunami, Tamil Nadu, India, sponsored by the UN in collaboration with CRED, Belgium. Then came the landmark projects on the integrated health, social and economic impacts of extreme events, as a part of MICRODIS, the European Union project consortium, and another project on indigenous knowledge in disaster management, funded by the Asian Disaster Reduction Centre, Kobe Japan and the SAARC, Disaster Management Centre, New Delhi. Both these projects were quite significant and led to the introduction of a new subdiscipline of 'Anthropology of Disaster' in the department. For a long time, disasters as distinct from accidents and tragedies, were seen as arbitrary, haphazard, unfortunate events which just seem to happen at a place and which tend to affect all. This fatalistic approach was changed by Prof. Joshi through the application of anthropology of disaster. With climate change and frequent extreme weather events happening all over the world, he relooked into the whole concept of 'haphazardness'. Prof. P.C. Joshi, through his research, has tried to provide a template for discerning the causes, variable impact, mitigation strategies and coping mechanisms of individuals and communities with respect to disaster. He redefined uncertainty and the critical concepts of risk vulnerability anthropologically and tried to show that cultural, social, ecological and political aspects are of crucial importance in the understanding of disasters and their long-term impacts. The phenomenological perspective towards disaster and its pre- and post-phases as cultural processes are clearly demonstrated in his work on Bahraich (a district in Uttar Pradesh) flood prone area and with the victims of super cyclone Aila in villages of Sunderbans (West Bengal). At the same time, he also developed interest in histories of institutions and discipline. He published articles on history of medical anthropology in India and an account of contributions of Hilda Raj, the first women faculty of the Anthropology Department at University of Delhi.

He has always remained very close to all the retired faculty of the department, especially his teachers welcoming them whole-heartedly by spending time and hosting them whenever they visit the department. He has an exceptional glint in his eyes whenever he happens to meet his teachers, who in turn, equally love and are proud of him.

He takes teaching and research very seriously and has taught all the branches of anthropology with ease. His varied experience in different settings and locales has made him a complete anthropologist. He is equally at ease with archaeology and biological anthropology, as he is with cultural anthropology. This kind of academic flair and span of issues he traversed and addresses through his writings are a clear reflection of his academic eclecticism and depth of understanding. On the one hand he has written on core social anthropological issues like caste, religion, witchcraft, family, fieldwork, sustainable development, disaster management, traditional and modern medical systems, and histories of disciplines and institutions, we also at the same time find him at ease in writing on archaeological issues like prehistory of Delhi and on topics like, human origin in India, stature estimation and somatometry, which are perhaps the sole preserves of biological anthropology. Not many may be aware that Prof. Joshi discovered a Palaeolithic site in Delhi, in 1983. However, it is in interdisciplinary topics like public health, aging, suicidal behaviour, impact of floods, antibiotic usages, and development anthropology where we find the real flavour of his writings. We can describe Prof. Joshi as a medical anthropologist, a specialist of anthropology of disaster and at the same time who is also a development anthropologist. He has been prolific in writing, and has authored about 130 articles in the leading journals of anthropology in India and abroad. He also has 56 sections and chapters etc. in books and his work figures in 14 national and international proceedings. He has been also associated as an author or co-author or as co-editor in ten popular medical anthropological books. He was instrumental in submitting 14 Reports to various national bodies and 6 Reports to the Government of India. Besides this, he has supervised and guided a large number of Ph.D. and M.Phil. students.

It is very difficult to summarize his laurels and achievements. As expected, he is a member of so many academic bodies, is holding and has been on the advisory panels of a large number of state and national level consultative bodies. He has organized a lot of seminars and conferences, presented papers and delivered keynote addresses in many national and international forums. Prof. P.C. Joshi delivered 1st Prof. S.R.K. Chopra memorial lecture at Department of Anthropology, Panjab University, Chandigarh in February 2019, where he also received Life Time Achievement Award. In INCAA Anthropological Congress 2020, he had the honour of delivering S.C. Dube Memorial Oration.

His international exposure and reach are second to none. He was a Visiting Lecturer, Department of Tropical Hygiene and Public Health, University of Heidelberg, Germany, 2000; Visiting Faculty, Global forum for Health, Geneva, 2001; Certificate of Honour, First France-India Meet on Psychiatry, Psychoanalysis and Psychotherapy, Delhi Psychiatry Society and Psychiatres—Du Monde, France, 2007; Asia Coordinator, European Union 6th Framework Micordis Integrated Project, 2007; awarded Plaque of Appreciation from Department of Sociology and Anthropology, Xavier University—Ateneo de Cagayan, Cagayan de Oro City, Philippines, 2008; Visited Hanoi, Vietnam to deliver lectures in Hanoi School of Public Health on Participatory and Qualitative Research Methods, 2008; Visited Pyeongtaek, Korea representing India to participate in the Asian Youth Leaders Forum, 2008; Visited Poznan, Poland and participated in United Nations framework Climate Change Conference (COP 14) as a delegate of European Union and presented a paper entitled "Health Impacts of Floods and Windstorms: The Microdis Experience in Asia" in the EU side event, 2008; Visited Healthnet TPO, Amsterdom, The Netherlands for consultations with regard to Microdis Project, Delhi University, 2008; Delivered Opening Speech in the Annual Meet of Microdis Integrated Project, Integrated Health, Social and Economic Impacts of Extreme Events: Evidence, Methods and Tools, Brussels, Belgium, 2009; Visited Lisbon, Portugal to participate in the European Sociological Association Conference, 2009; Visited University of Indonesia, Depok for participating in the Multi Meeting workshop and made presentation on Qualitative Research Analysis in the workshop, 2009; Delivered a talk entitled "Social Impact of floods in Bahraich, India" under seminar Series of the Institute of Public Health, Heidelberg University, Heidelberg, Germany, 2010; Visited Geneva, Switzerland to participate in the 20th IUHPE World Conference on Health Promotion, 2010; Prof. P.C. Joshi visited Hue University to participate in the International Asian Symposium on "Disaster Impact and its Assessment". Hue City, Vietnam, 2010; Visited Xavier University to participate in Scientific Conference on "Impact of Natural Disasters in Asia: Research Results, Methods and Tools". Cagayan de Oro, Philippines, 2010; Visited Citizens' Disaster Response Centre to Keynote Speech in a Conference on "Disaster and its Response", Tagayatey, Philippines, 2010; Visited Universitas Indonesia to participate in "Indonesian Workshop of Disaster Impact and Researches". Jakarta, Indonesia, 2010; Visited Heidelberg University to participate in International Symposium on "Health and Health Systems: Impacts of Natural Disasters", Heidelberg, Germany, 2010.

I know him from the last 30 years or so when he was at Garhwal University and I used to visit his department as an external examiner. Later, not only he is my colleague at the department, we have worked together in so many confidential assignments for the state and national level bodies. A simple and benevolent person at heart, a brilliant academician, a strict administrator, an institutional builder, he is all this and more rolled in a single personality. As a teacher he is very well liked by all his students. I have never seen him miss a class. His lectures were a unique mix of complex arguments as well earthly simplicity. This earthly simplicity has also been the hallmark of his persona. He always kept a firm and serious appearance but within he has always been a jovial, cheerful, good-humoured simple, generous and a kind individual. In June 2020, he took over as the acting Vice Chancellor of the University of Delhi. He has breathed new life to the university by resurrecting many of things, including the long due promotion process of the teaching and the non-teaching staff. He streamlined the functioning of many wings of the university which were mired in red tapism, tedious procedures and extreme delays. He is proving his mettle in the new administrative role as he did all through life as fearless, vocal academician and administrator.

Overview of the Book

This book is a collection of essays written by the leading anthropologists of India. These essays broadly engage with the Anthropology of Health and Wellbeing, which as a sub-discipline was carefully nurtured by Prof. Joshi during his illustrious career at the Department of Anthropology, University of Delhi. I have grouped the essays under the broader themes to provide a logical sequence. It is divided into six parts.

Part I : Indigenous Health and Medicine
Part II : Health, Disease and Health Seeking Behaviour
Part III : Physical Health and Wellbeing
Part IV : Psychological Health and Wellbeing
Part V : Women's Health and Wellbeing
Part VI : Reflections on Corona Virus Pandemic

Part I of the book examines the broad range of questions related to indigenous health and medicine. The papers in this section critically engage with the Prof. Joshi's abiding interest in the ethnomedical system of various Himalayan communities, ethnomedical systems of communities in North-East India and South India, the health status of PVTGs, ill-effects of Indian systems of medicine and empowerment of herbal healers. The essay by R.P. Mitra and Manoj K. Singh is an inimitable attempt to understand PCJ's contributions to the field of traditional ethnomedical systems. Mitra and Singh note that PCJ, through his writings, has argued that the traditional ethnomedical systems are an essential part of public health system and care in many of the tribal and rural communities of India. Building on PCJ's work that emphasised the physical body's relationship to the social, ecological and universal dimension of human existence, Mitra and Singh have critically explained PCJ's description of the concept of health and illness in Himalayan communities. Mitra and Singh argue that PCJ showed that the health care systems of Himalayan communities contain much wisdom and understanding, which we need to propagate and incorporate in our public health care systems, a prerequisite to achieving universal health and wellbeing for all.

PCJ, in his long career, has argued that tribal medicines are more acceptable to many people than other systems. Abhik Ghosh, in his article, argues that anthropologists should critically understand the harms of ISMs and tribal medicines using the same principles that we employ to critically analyse other biomedicines. He further argues that as anthropologists, we should also analyse biomedicine using the same principles adopted for ISMs. Abhik Ghosh believes that medical anthropologists should devise fresh paradigmatic approaches informed by current research on relevant issues rather than those that perpetuate our own biases and are subject to public whims and fancies. Health anthropologists should look within, forward and outward to newer regimes of healthcare that are not yet proposed and practiced today.

Based on empirical research conducted among the traditional healers in the state of Sikkim, Sunita Reddy argues that, on the one hand, there is a loss of traditional knowledge in healing due to the dwindling of the healers; at the same time, however, there is a renewed interest in herbal medicines world-over. In order to revive herbal medicine, there are renewed and vigorous efforts to recognize and document them, but, at the same time, the healers are anxious about their knowledge being taken away and not being acknowledged for their work. Sunita Reddy brings out the popularity of the healers and their narratives related to the challenges to their everyday practice and in getting herbal medicine. The paper argues that by recognising and supporting the healers, the primary level healthcare of the poor and marginalised communities should be ensured.

The traditional culture of communities views human health from its holistic perspective and practice medical pluralism. Avitoli G. Zhimo and M.N. Nimal, in their essay, describe the great wealth of ethnomedical knowledge among the Zeme, a Naga tribal group in Manipur. The essay details Zeme healing beliefs and practices, including their understanding of 'health', 'illness' and 'healing'. The authors note the existence of medical pluralism in the Zeme villages.

S. Sumathi, Shobana Sharma and Muniraj M., through a case study of the Devendrakula Velalar community, show that their cognitive ability and knowledge is far superior as far as agriculture, ecology, climate change are concerned and is instrumental in health and wellness of the society. The paper tries to substantiate that indigenous knowledge of local communities is sagacious when the advancement of technology is at its prudent best. Health and wellness for all is the motto that is the unwritten law. The paper argues that healthy relation with climate, environment, and land is the way for any community's future.

The tribal population, especially the Particularly Vulnerable Tribal Groups (PVTGs) in India, are endangered and marginalized and lag in all social, economic and health indicators. Sonia Kaushal, in her essay, notes that the vulnerability related to health becomes more pronounced among PVTGs due to the change and threat to the traditional means of livelihood, displacement, and that migration may place restrictions on the resources. Sonia Kaushal has tried to explore healthcare access concerning PVTGs livelihood insecurity by applying Health Access Livelihood Framework. The framework Kaushal argues pinpoints and highlights the factors that impact livelihood and influence resource mobilisation during critical health conditions. It can help to improve health care access in resource-poor PVT communities. It emphasizes the efforts to ensure universal access to health care and the availability of primary livelihood assets to encourage people to seek treatment.

The Part II of the book is titled 'Health, Disease and Health Seeking Behaviour'. The essays in this part of the book talk through multiple questions, including the bio-social understanding of diseases, behaviour concerning diabetes, acute respiratory tract infections and sanitation, and the medicalisation of health systems. Undoubtedly, the marvels of medical science and technology have come a long way from facelifts to transplants and with a thought of answer to almost all biological problems. By bringing the spotlight on the anthropologists' inherent ability to enable a bio-social purview, in terms of contextualisation of disease, illness, health, and wellbeing, M.P. Sachdeva and his co-authors explore the issues of Organ transplant, COVID-19 and AIDS.

Diabetes Mellitus is inheritable and lifestyle-related morbidity with additional risks of various associated comorbidities and complications. Based on a study to understand the prevailing myths and misconceptions about Type-2 diabetes mellitus (T2DM) in Chandigarh, A.K. Sinha and his co-authors argue that due to lack of awareness and adequate knowledge about the disease, most people harbour myths and misconceptions about diabetes. Especially, myths among non-diabetic individuals are more pervasive than among the diabetic patients and their attendants; females have more myths and misconceptions about T2DM than male individuals. These myths and misconceptions may have a potential impact on their health-seeking behaviour concerning diabetes, especially on the management of disease of patients living with diabetes. Hence, identifying and understanding the prevailing myths among people in any area will be helpful to create effective and correct awareness for better management of diabetes among patients and others.

Health seeking behaviour in developing countries is characterised mainly by the availability of multiple alternative treatment choices. The alternatives include applying a home remedy, self-medication with pharmaceuticals bought over-the-counter in the open market and from herbal medicine retailers. B.S. Aribam explores the health-seeking behaviour regarding Acute Respiratory-tract Infection (ARI) among the two slum colonies in Delhi. Aribum notes that the caretakers had a general curative attitude rather than a preventive outlook towards ARI. The considerable reliance of the caretakers on home remedies for treating ARI rather than seeking health care providers was profound among the two slums. Restricted autonomy of the mothers in seeking formal medical care or hospital care appeared to be one of the reasons for the delay in seeking prompt care for ARI.

Sanitation in rural India and its challenges are embedded in various domain areas. The constituent features are composite and contribute variably depending on the culture, geography, and economic condition of a community or society. Oinam Hemlata Devi attempts to understand the components of sanitation and its existential challenges. The focus is on the disposal of human excreta. Devi notes that different factors have influenced sanitation practices at Karang that have contributed to significant improvements in the hygiene and sanitation behaviour of the people.

M.P. Sachdeva and his co-authors in another essay explore the rapid insurgence of the health system's medicalisation through pertinent anthropological research. The article critically evaluates how childbirth and mental illness are among the most medicalised aspects of human life.

Part III of the book brings together essays on physical health and wellbeing. The study on ethnic variation in adult body composition and blood pressure levels has been recapitulated in anthropological research for decades. Citing three studies from Eastern India, Subho Roy and his co-authors attempt to delineate how culture influences the actual lifestyle pattern and eventually shapes body composition and blood pressure levels among the members of an ethnic group. The authors suggest that ethnic diversity remains embedded in cultural behaviour and practices regarding concerns over health and obesity, hypertension, and associated lifestyle pattern. Moreover, such practices rooted in the belief system of an ethnic group are likely to delineate the health condition of the group members.

Thalassemias are a group of anaemias resulting from inherited defects in the production of haemoglobin. Benrithung Murry and Anand Kumar Gyanendra Singh Wahengbam discuss the challenges and prospects of the screening programmes on β-thalassemia around the world with special focus on the Indian context as India is a multi-cultural and multi-ethnic nation. Roumi Deb and Ratika Samtani have reviewed and analysed the prevalence of Beta Thalassemia in the world and India and provide a road map for possible interventions that will help control the disorder in India.

Based on a detailed literature review Shivani Chandel and Chonsing Shimrah have tried to understand the association between psycho-social stress and musculoskeletal disorders (MSDs) among farmers. The authors argue that there is a need to develop ergonomic intervention and community-based awareness programmes among farmers to cope with high-stress levels. Future research should focus on understanding the etiological role of psycho-social stress in the development of chronic MSDs.

P. Venkatramana, S.A.A. Latheef and P. Annaiah, in their study, recruited a total of 900 subjects representing three endogamous populations: Reddy, Golla and Madiga of Chittoor district, Andhra Pradesh, to find out the effect of gender, ethnicity, and residence on 38 anthropometric variables/indices. They evaluated the effect of gender, ethnicity and residence on anthropometric parameters/indices using a two-way multivariate analysis of variance. The paper shows that gender, ethnicity and residence variables in combination also influence the anthropometric variables/indices contributing 0.9 per cent to 5.7 per cent variation in anthropometric variables/indices.

Over the years, psychological health and wellbeing have become an essential area in health anthropology studies. Part IV of the book deals with the psychological health and wellbeing among adolescents in conflict zones, infertile women and disabled children in an institutional setting. By reviewing recent literature on mental health of adolescents, caught amidst political conflict, Urfat Anjem Mir, Shwetha Gopalakrishnan and Anushka Singh critically discuss trauma experiences due to exposure to political conflict. Furthermore, by presenting research-based evidence, the authors highlight the need for an individual-centric, socially mediated and culturally applicable approach to studying trauma and mental health among adolescents.

Infertility affects millions of individuals and couples globally. Chakraverti Mahajan and his co-authors attempt to understand how infertility impacts North Indian women's psychological health and wellbeing. Based on a case-control study, the authors found a high prevalence of depression, anxiety, stress, and poor psychological and emotional wellbeing among females with infertility compared to females in the control group. The essay argues that healthcare professionals should also pay attention to this aspect and consider psychological counselling and psychiatric help for infertile women undergoing treatment.

Mitashree Srivastava and Tejinder Kaur, in their essay, explore the issue of adopting children with special needs in India and delve deeper into their mental health and wellbeing. The paper argues that laws governing the adoption of children with special needs are stringent and time-consuming, which often become an impediment in their timely adoption, affecting their mental health and wellbeing.

Part V contains essays on various other dimensions of women's health and wellbeing, including folate supplementation programme for women, social epidemiology of maternal health, quality of life of disaster struck women, menstruation issues and sustainability. The supplementation of folic acid, a synthetic form of folate, before and during pregnancy has long been recognised and practised. Kallur Nava Saraswathy, Imnameren Longkumer and Jyoti Mishra attempt to understand the importance of folic acid supplementation in the Indian context. Since supplementation is a foreign exposure to the fetus which governs the outcomes for the next two generations *via* genetic and epigenetic modulations, the authors argue that the nationwide evaluation of the effectiveness of this indiscriminate intervention is the need of the hour.

The pattern of health and disease in a community reflects the unequal distribution of benefits and risks. The analysis of social inequalities in terms of health is complicated by socio-cultural diversity within and between communities. Vipin Gupta and M.P. Sachdeva argue that social epidemiologists and medical anthropologists can disentangle these complexities in data collection by developing novel research methods and analytical strategies.

Minakshi and Rahul Kumar attempt to analyse the Quality of life (QoL) in physical health and mental health functioning among women in Kosi flood-affected Bihar, India. The authors found out that illiteracy and financial crisis in the form of loan burden were the predictors of poor Quality of Life in affected people.

There is a broad scope of improving menstrual hygiene and restoring a positive attitude towards menstruation. M. Kennedy Singh and Angana Goswami attempt to understand the practices related to menstruation in the state of Assam with particular reference to the puberty ritual called Tuloni Biya and its implication on young adolescent girls. The essay reveals that though the young girls are found to be well aware of the menstruation process due to the practice of Tuloni Biya yet misconceptions still prevail among them as people tend to avoid discussion on menstruation. Therefore, it demands more scientific discussion on this subject matter to remove misconceptions.

Within the discourse of environmental management, women have been considered *sine qua non* ingredient. Kalindi Sharma critically explores, through paradigms of ecofeminism, locations of gender *vis-à-vis* sustainable development focusing on women's health and wellbeing in India.

The work on this festschrift coincided with a critical event in world history. The corona virus pandemic has raised many questions for anthropologists interested in studying shared humanity and its welfare. Part VI of the book deals with some of the critical questions related to the pandemic and its implications for humans and other beings.

Prashant Khattri, in his essay, compares the pandemic with a disaster. He argues that disasters have been defined as events where the coping capacity of the affected population is challenged. The capacity to respond and overcome the event is seriously undermined, and thus external support and help is the only way out of the crisis. The COVID-19 pandemic, the essay argues, qualifies under this definition, and the management of a medical emergency is being done using the Disaster Management (DM) Act, 2005 at the national level. Khattri advocates that the field of disaster studies offers a wide range of concepts and theories to conceptualise the pandemic and provides a wide lens to comprehensively understand the pandemic, and opens up the scope for a critical understanding of the situation.

COVID-19 is a highly infectious disease. For studying the pathogenesis and medical biology of viral diseases, non-human primate models have been utilized. However, unlike in humans, no single non-human primate model can be sufficient to recognise the pathogenesis of this virus. So for this reason, several non-human primate models have been utilised to understand this virus' molecular mechanisms and pathogenesis. In their essay, Prakash Ranjan Mondal and Surendra Kumar Sagar argue that it is evident from studies that African and Asian monkeys and apes are much more susceptible to COVID-19 disease than American monkeys. Mondal and Sagar advocate that measures and precautions must be taken by the scientists dealing with these non-human primates for their survival or endurance during the times of COVID-19.

Naorem Kiranmala Devi and Vineet Chaudhary have tried to understand the direct and indirect risks posed by COVID-19 on maternal and child health in both the short and long term with the help of a detailed literature review. In their essay, the authors also compare the effect of SARS-CoV-2 with other corona viruses on pregnancy. They discover that the direct effect of the incidence of COVID-19 on pregnancy is not as severe as SARS (Severe acute respiratory syndrome) or MERS (Middle East respiratory syndrome). However, the indirect effect of the COVID-19 pandemic on maternal and child health is of socio-economic in nature. The COVID-19 has led to shortage of maternal and child health care, and unavailability of healthy food during lockdown and psychological turmoil can be far more critical. Naorem Kiranmala Devi and Vineet Chaudhary suggest that long term epigenetic implications cannot be ruled out.

The COVID-19 pandemic has also brought to light the public unpreparedness of the health systems. Suniti Yadav and Vijay Hadda, in their essay, argue that anthropologists have a significant role to play in the success of vaccination drives. The authors suggest an urgent need to understand the community behaviour towards vaccine acceptance and bridge the gap between the community and healthcare systems. They argue that social scientists, including anthropologists, should undertake rapid studies to understand individuals and communities' dilemmas, confusion, fears, and indecisiveness. Suniti Yadav and Vijay Hadda advocate a multipronged approach by augmenting the agendas from vaccine coverage for immunity to the end of the pandemic at this crucial juncture of human history.

PART I

Indigenous Health and Medicine

2
P.C. Joshi and the Study of Ethnomedical System of Khos

R.P. Mitra and Manoj K. Singh

One of the abiding interests in Professor P.C. Joshi's writings on medical anthropology has been with what is called as folk, indigenous or traditional, complementary or ethno-medicines and their role in promoting health and wellbeing among a large section of rural and tribal communities in India. In one of his seminal papers, titled as,'Relevance and Utility of Traditional Medical Systems in the Context of a Himalayan Tribe', published in the Sage Journal, *Psychology and Developing Society*,12,1 (2002), he gave a up, close and detailed account of healing practice of Khasa or Khos, a subgroup within Jaunsaris, a Scheduled Tribe community of Jaunsar region of Uttarakhand state. It is a vast hilly area, part of the Garhwal region of the state. The area remained semi-isolated for a number of years. The bounded and limited accessibility from other areas led to emergence of a unique cultural complex called as 'Jaunsaris', distinguishing the people here from the adjoining Garhwali culture. These 'cultural distinctions' led to recognition of the Jaunsaris as a Scheduled Tribe in 1967 (Berreman, 1997). Anthropological interests in the community have mostly focused upon presence of fraternal polyandry (Majumdar, 1955; Berreman, 1962); and later on in religion, politics and healing rituals (Sax, 2009; Utter, 2010; Ohri, 2019).

It has always been problematic how to define a *traditional* medical system. When we use the term tradition in anthropology, it involves two meanings. One reference to tradition is in terms of what Kroeber and Kluckhohn (1952) called as social heredity, implying thereby something which shows continuity from the past. Here the meaning of the term 'past' does not imply passivity and unchangeability, rather it implies its social, cultural and ecological embedded attribute. The second meaning comes from its binary opposition to modernity a vision of reality that emphasizes both the observable and a non-empirical world; intelligence as discovery of meaning rather logical consistency; facts laden with values and a connected vision of reality rather than a granular and atomistic understanding (Gellner, 2009; Gidden, 2013). In P.C. Joshi's (PCJ henceforth) usage, both these aspects of traditions are involved in understanding of traditional medicine (TM). PCJ conceptualizes health as a relational concept and the central idea of his article was to show health, illness and medicine were related to culture, tradition and ecology in an isolated tribal community (p. 1). Throughout the article, PCJ tried to show the 'deeply entrenched' notions of health with reference to 'morality, religion, economics and politics' among the Khos (p. 2). Other than the relational nature, TM also have to be seen as an 'episteme' with its distinctive epistemological and ontological concerns, which according to PCJ, needs to understood in its minute details (p. 3). The palpable contradictions of these epistemologies are significant and it is the job of a medical anthropologist to interpret them. Biomedicine has been dismissive and biased towards TM often calling it as superstitious and irrational, founded upon ignorance with no scientific evidence to support them. They looked at them as a hindrance in their treatment procedure and one of the main reasons for the patients delay in consulting a doctor or non-compliance with a treatment regime. The medical anthropology as a critical theory has often held a mirror to the biomedical systems by pointing at their hallowed claim of rationality and objectivity by showing the inherent biases and subjectivities in the practice of biomedicine. The very fact that TM continues to flourish and occupy an important place in delivering public health not only in rural and tribal areas but also in urban milieu is a testimony to the 'efficacy and functional' nature of TM systems. It is for this reason that WHO has referred to TM as a 'complimentary medicines' in promotion of public health. The PCJ's article is significant because it deals with this very axiology, the intrinsic and the extrinsic values of Khos TM systems in promotion of health and wellbeing. In this article, we would try to explain how PCJ:

(a) looks at the conception of health, illness, wellbeing and body among the Khos of Junsar-Bawar;
(b) looks at typology and variation of TM systems with reference to categories of ailments among the Khos community;
(c) interprets the healing rituals of *malis,* the tradition Khos diviners, shamans and medicine men; and

(d) a structural model of psychosomatic healing practice of *malis* can enable us to understand the efficacy of ritual healing practices.

Conception of Health, Illness and Wellbeing

The article begins with Khos' conception of health (PCJ, p. 8). According to PCJ the notion of health and illness among them needs to be located in the trilogy of indigenous conceptual categories, viz. the *pira-khora*, *bimari-dos* and *baghu-tokdeer* (pp. 8-9). *Pira-khora* is a concept of wellbeing, *bimari-dos* is Khos' conception of illness on the basis distinction between natural and supernatural causes of an ailment, and *baghu-tokdeer* is notion of destiny which predisposes one to any kind of ailment. In Khos conception, an individual is surrounded by natural and supernatural entities and is in a dynamic interaction with them. Any physical ailment can be attributed to the distortions or imbalance in this relationship. Here PCJ moves on from the WHO's definition of health as a 'state of' (physical, social and mental wellbeing) to a notion of health as a 'social and cultural process' that come to have a bearing on physical aspect of wellbeing. According to PCJ (p. 8), Khos considers illness as a misery but it is a 'functional suffering' as it resets the relationship of an individual with the natural and the supernatural world. This functionality is in sharp contradiction to the biological notion of disease, which is seen primarily in terms of morbidity. This shift from 'morbidity' to 'functionality' in conception of illness has a bearing on the notion of stigma or stigmatization. Disease as a morbid condition often lead to labelling of an individual as sick in certain categories of ailment even while when a patient is cured (Srivastava, 2020). Even after being cured people may not be healed, as the stigma of the disease continues to bother them. But Khos does not look at illness as a 'suffering' it is also a 'social experience' for an individual. PCJ uses three key concepts as discussed below to explain Khos etic understanding of health, wellbeing, ailment and suffering.

Wellbeing as pira-khora

The meaning of the term illness becomes clear in their concept of *pira-khora,* the first of our concept in understanding of health among the Khos. The literal meaning of the term *pira-khora* is 'disturbed state of affairs'. It is a state of misery caused due to accidents, illness or any unfortunate events that takes away the wellbeing of an individual or a group. The Khos thus relate health of an individual to the health of his surroundings.

There can be *no healthy individual in an unhealthy society*. Health has to be seen as *'web of health'* (human, animal, non-animate and supernatural)' in which health of individual is merely a connecting node.

Supernatural and Natural (dos-bimari) Axis

The second axis of health for the Khos according to PCJ (p. 8) is the distinction between *dos* and *bimari.* The term *dos* symbolizes imbalance in individual's relationships with others, their natural world and the supernatural world. In Khos, cognitive classification, supernatural world is home to malevolent and benevolent spirits, who at times can afflict an individual or cause accident or misfortune to a group. All these afflictions caused by the 'culturally postulated supernatural entities' are termed as *dos* (p. 9). On the other hand, cause of *bimari* is the naturalistic imbalance of three humors, which constitute the human body. *Bimari* is mainly treated through naturalistic medicines derived from herbs and other plant-based products or through eating a specific diet, which helps the body to rectify the imbalance of the humours (p. 9). One's own action is an important causative factor for *bimari*, symptomised as cold, cough, fever, skin eruption, pain and swelling. *Dos* can aggravate a *bimari* but reverse is not true, a *bimari* cannot increase one's susceptibility to acquire a *dos*.

Time Space Dimension (bhaghu-tokdeer)

The third and the most crucial axis of Khos' conception of health is *bhaghu-tokdeer* roughly translated as destiny (PCJ, p. 10). This is an independent cause as well as predisposing condition for an ailment. As an independent cause it acts like a residual causative factor. When one cannot attribute an ailment to any of the known causes, it is supposed to have been caused by destiny. Khos believe that one is born with a preordained stock of destiny (PCJ, p. 17). There are a number of contributing factors that influence one's fate which include the time of birth, positions of constellation and other planetary bodies including the sun, the moon and stars and the complex matrix of family and kin relationships in which one is born. The specialist who deals with this is locally called as *bahaman* (See Fig. 2.1).

Each of these spheres is well defined in terms of what constitutes them and the specialist healer to be consulted for them. Table 2.1 explains the various types of ailments, religious specialist involved and the nature of healing popular with the people. Khos have their cognitive map based upon classification of symptoms and different categories of

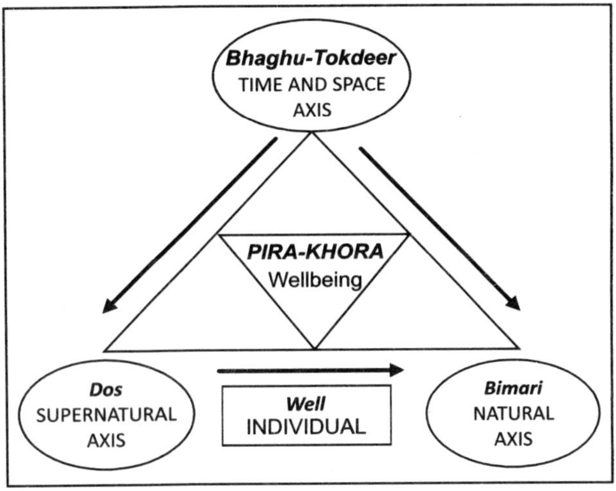

Fig. 2.1: Model of health and illness among Khos

healer who would deal with the problem at hand. As mentioned simplest and the most elementary classification would divide an ailment as a *bimari* or *a dos. Bimari* is symptomised as cold, cough, fever, pain, indigestion and skin eruptions. As mentioned earlier these categories are not exclusive in the sense that it may be possible that an ailment can have multiple causative agents. There are certain ailments where the causal relationship is not understood. For example, people are aware that if they move out in the cold there is a possibility of 'catching cold' cough and fever. Such well-established causes of ill health are dealt through naturalistic healing techniques. However, if someone does not get relief even after following a prescribed treatment than the same ailment may require a super-naturalistic diagnosis and cure. Similarly, when one happens to get frequently struck down by cold than it requires a consultation with a supernatural healer. Table 2.1 looks at the cognitive map of classification of ailments and the healers among the Khos.

According to PCJ supernatural healing by the *mali* forms numerically the most predominant form of healing among the Khos (p. 16). A *mali* is essentially a shaman who can communicate between the supernatural and the natural world (p. 16). Khos, according to PCJ, explains the existence of supernatural entities like *devtas* with the analogy of air (p. 17). As air is everywhere, unseen similarly *devtas* are omnipresent but cannot be seen. Khos conceptualize of *devtas* as a *moralistic guardian force*. They are

Table 2.1: Khos Classification of Ailments and Healers

Category of Ailment	*Causative Agent*	*Healer*	*Technique of Healing*
Supernatural *Dos* *Paap* *Dag* (Witch craft)	*Devtas:* Mahasu, Silgur, Pandava and Kedarnath *Devis*: Durga, Kangra and Jwala Fierce Spirits: Kali, Narasingh, Kalua, Pokhu and Bhairo *Maitri* or *Pari*: Succi, Masan, Sukka and 61 others *Bhut-Pret*: Unidentified Spirits	Mall	Divination based Shamanistic and Magico-Religious healing
Dunkin (Evil Eye)	Dunkin malevolent Person Centric malevolent force	Mali/Other Magico-ritual Specialists	Magico-rituals
Dose Astrological governed destiny	Time, space, location at the time of Birth. Location of Astronomical bodies, Relational position like family of birth	Bahaman	Textual Religious Supernatural Healings Multiple Techniques including at times Supernaturalised empowered Herbs
Naturalist *Bimari*	Humoral/Energy imbalance *Vata, Pitta* and *Kapha* disorders	Jariyas	Herbal Specialists Pulse reading Dietary restrictions Supernatural healings
Naturalist Traditional Masseurs and Birth attendant	Anatomical Displacement Especially of the abdomen / *Pet tolla*	Female Specialists *Dais*	Massaging Stroking Pressing Kneading

the keeper of conscience and protector of *Dharma*, righteous conduct and performance of one's duty. Anyone who would digress from the path of righteous conduct or conduct a sin, he or she would be punished by *devtas* by inflicting *dos*. Not only one has to perform virtuous actions, one's thinking and intentions also needs be pure and free from any malice (p. 16). The second reason for being struck down with a *dos* is *transgressions*. These transgressions relate to either disturbing, or interfering in the work of natural or supernatural agents. There are definite resting places, mostly associated with specific trees or geographical spaces. If one were to soil, pollute or contaminate such a place in any manner than he or she will be punished for the transgression through godly infliction of *dos*.

Concept of Biological Body

PCJ on the basis of surveying 371 villages, covering a population of 25,000 found that out of 397 traditional healers, 222 (55.4 %), practice divination healing (p. 16). PCJ throughout the article used the term healing to describe the outcome of the divination processes as distinct from curing, a concept which is employed for describing the outcome of biomedical treatment. Thus, we can say traditional medicines produce healing and biomedicine only cures (Waldram, 2000:164). The primary focus of biomedicine is on the *body as a physiological and biological entity.* But, PCJ in the article clearly showed that Khos do not look at body in terms of its physiology only. A body is simultaneously located in social, natural, supernatural and cosmic spaces (see Fig. 2.2). Therapeutic healing involves correcting not just the physiological anomalies but it also involves reconfiguring the relationship of body with other spaces also. Physiological or biological problems may be the 'effect' of an actual cause, located at some other place. For example, it may be in the social location of the body. Therefore, any process of healing must touch upon these spaces. Traditional medicine and biomedicine approach a therapeutic treatment from different directions. While biomedicine focuses upon the physical or the biological body and once the biological body is cured process of treatment is seen as complete. In the epistemology of bio-medicine there are no concept such as supernatural or cosmic entities. On the other hand, traditional medicine begins with cosmic, social or supernatural connections of the body. *Healing in traditional medicine is more holistic than curing in Biomedicine.* In traditional healing, body is an embodiment of five spaces as shown in Figure 2.2. Csordas (2000) in his article on ritual healing among Catholic Pentecostalism looked at this in terms of body, mind and spirit distinction and how it is related to health (p. 91). In the entire process, the personality of the healers also play an important role. Thus, he referred to it as charismatic healing. PCJ also talks of charisma of the *mali* among the Khos and how it plays an important role in healing (p. 19).

Healing of Mali: A Therapeutic Process

According to PCJ the central method of *mali* healing involves divination (*devta ka anna)* (p. 16). The literal meaning of divination is visitation of a supernatural entity in the body of the *mali.* PCJ in his article looked at these divination rituals as *therapeutic processes.* Taking a cue from the framework provided by Csordas (2000), we can divide a healing ritual into following sections:

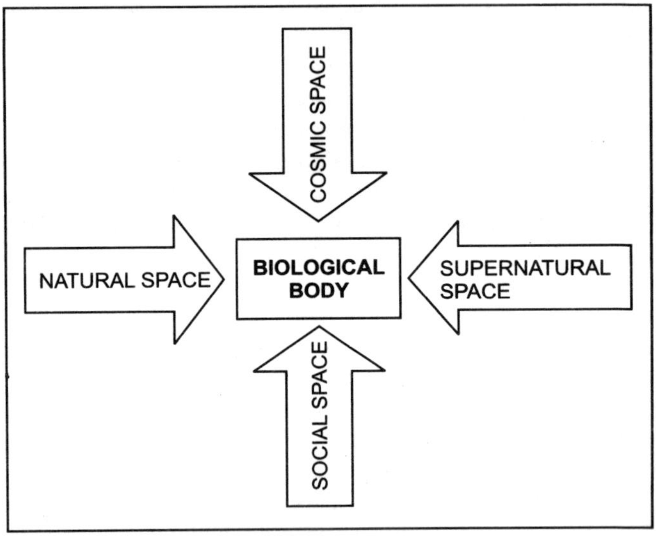

Fig. 2.2: Biological Body and Its Social, Natural, Supernatural and Cosmic Extensions

(a) Invocation of the Sacred: This involves how the supernatural and the natural world are brought together. The supernatural is evoked or brought about by establishing a communication with the supernatural forces. Any therapeutic session of the divination according to PCJ (p. 17), begins with a formal request by a patient's relative, which is called as *oraj lagana*. The first step in the ritual is to determine the specific supernatural force involved in the causation of an ailment. This is called as *channt lagana*, i.e. the process of locating or isolating the cause of ailment (PCJ, p. 16). A therapeutic session is called as *puja*. Once an *oraj* is received from a patient's family an auspicious date is chosen by the *mali* to perform the session. It is generally held in the household of the client. Divination is a learnt art. A *mali* has to undergo a rigorous apprenticeship under a established *Mali* to learn how to do it. PCJ (p. 17) made a distinction between an expert and a neophyte diviner. An expert is called as *bochawan, boidori* or *dor,* literally meaning one who knows the language or is an expert in supernatural communication (p. 18). An apprentice is called as *noitre,* one whose tongue is still tied and yet to learn the language of communication. A *noitre* has to attend many sessions of divination under a *bochawan,* before he can aspire to 'open his mouth' or *bhak kulna* (p. 18). According to PCJ, an important part of the training period is what is called as *bawaal*, a phase during which a *noitre* has learnt to induce a *devta,* but has no control over the altered state of consciousness. During this time a neophyte *mali* behavioural anomalies and psychosomatic disturbances. He may not eat for days or may wander about completely lost, with no consciousness. This is a period of great pain, suffering and tribulation. Duration of *bawaal* varies depending upon how powerful is the *devta,* a *noitre* is trying to control. Thus, the whole training is a participant experiential learning to become a *mali.*

(b) Theorizing the ailment: Every symbolic healing system is based upon a set of theoretical propositions and concepts. These propositions not only define the concept of health, illness and disease. They also connect to the wider concept of existence, wellbeing and after life. Most importantly they place these concepts in the context of 'norms of living i.e. 'living well' and 'living right'. It operates through marking the cognitive limits of what can be imagined, the behavioural boundaries of moralities and boundaries of actions and practices. It comes as an 'arrangement of a set of narratives', we often called as cultural myths (Dow, 1988:59). Historically speaking the region Jaunsar-Bawar, has had a strong presence of religion in the form of religious cults of Mahasu and other deities and their economic and political roles (Ohri, 2019:4). In fact, the area is referred to as the Kingdom of Mahasu, attested by the fact it does not have a ruler or king as it existed in the neighbouring regions of Garhwal and Kumaon. The politics and economy of Jaunsar-Bawar was carried out at the local village level assisted by the tutelary 'speaking *devtas*'. These speaking gods create the fulcrum around which the mythical world of the Khasas revolves. A *mali* actualizes the reality of the myth through various material and linguistic utterance during a therapeutic episode. This symbolization of the theoretical proposition into actual reality is what constitute the 'paraphernalia of a ritual'.

(c) Giving meaning to the affliction: A set of narratives often occurs in a generalized framework. This has to be particularize during a therapeutic healing session to the problem of the patient. This projection of the mythical world to the problem of an individual sufferer is the *'art of healing'*. This projection is not a singular creation by the *mali.* It is a joint creation and this is especially seen in those 'sessions of healing' where participants (sick persons) are also induced into an 'altered sense of consciousness'. The whole process is based on the same principle of 'psychotherapy' wherein the analyst help a patient to look back at the 'unconcious' mind to discover the hidden events in the past causing emotional upheaval in the present. The difference is instead of looking within, the *mali* attempts to look outside to discover meanings. The final cause of the ailment has to come from the patient. The role of diviner here is opposite to the psychoanalyst. In psychotherapy, the psychoanalyst does the diagnosis, but in a divination session the real cause is pinpointed by the patient himself/herself. The point of 'self-introspection' leading to 'self-identification' is high point of a therapeutic session. But this is not possible every time a patient may be able to identify the cause of the ailment. A *mali* may use other methods wherein a ritual is setup which symbolically represents the mythical world. The patient may identify the cause in the mythical model of the ritual which then is interpreted by the *mali* as the cause of the ailment. The idea is to get the patient involved as mere sufferer to an active participant in the process in healing. To undergo transformation from the *physical world to a physiological universe.* Csordas (2000) referred to it as *'creation of disposition'*. According to him, this creation of disposition has two references (p. 101). The first step is the psychological reference, which involves creation of state of mind wherein a person finds hope and conviction that he can change the existing state of affairs. The second meaning of disposition is in Durkheimian reference to the social network who rally round the sick individual in a transformative mood that he/she would be healed.

(d) Transition of the *mali* to medium of *devta*: One of the reasons a *mali* can induce disposition is the belief of the patient that the *mali* is representing the *devta* during the evocation of healing ritual. Often a *mali* may be tested through a ritual called as a *gatti* to establish his credential as someone who is authentic. In this ritual, a client would bring different heaps of rice and present it to him. Each of the heaps would represent a specific sphere like health, misfortune, domestic conflicts, employment etc. A *mali* has to select the correct heap which stands for the problem the client has come for an audience. A correct selection enables a *mali* to establish his credentials as someone who can really talk to the supernatural. Transition to medium happens through attaining an altered state of consciousness, which is generally induced through rhythmic beating of drums.

Process Involved in Healing

The fundamental process involved in healing ritual is a *therapeutic suggestibility* or *persuasion* whereby the patient is persuaded to change the existing routine of activities and try up an alternative pathways. There are different techniques used by *malis* in a divination ritual. This include:

(a) Infused abreaction: Abrecation in psychotherapy implies relieving or becoming aware of a repressed painful, thought, incident or action which may be affecting the present behaviour. According to Levi Strauss (1967), many shamans are expert abrecators, while doing a session of divination they offer a performance (p. 181). This performance constitute a vivid portrayal of the crisis of *bawal* (a phase of his own psychosomatic disturbance and mental turmoil) in all minute details and violence which initiated him into his calling. At the end of the performance he returns to the normalcy after re-enacting ontogenically his own past mental turmoil. This abreaction also induces the patient to symbolically follow the shaman and to abreacts his/her own disturbances. Other than this Dow (1986), proposed three possible methods which we can apply to understand efficacy of *malis* in solving the psychosomatic problems of the people (pp. 58-59). They are:

Catharsis: According to Dow (1986) quoting Sheff (1977), large number of mental ailments are because of repression of one's emotions (p. 60). His theory which is called as, 'hydraulic' theory of mental ailment, posits that many mental illnesses involve damming of emotions. Most of them can be healed if one let the emotions flow. This process of giving vent to ones pent up emotion is called as catharsis. A *mali* through his ritual performance enable a sick person to 'loosen up' wherein he or she is encouraged to release the suppressed feeling by joining the ritual. What would have been an abnormal behaviour become normal and expected way of behaving for the patients. This induces a catharsis therapy for the patient which allows transaction of the emotion during a ritual and contribute to healing of a patient.

Social Restructuring: This is another mechanism used by *malis* to bring about relief to a disturbed individual. Any *puja* necessitates the participation of all family members and other near relatives of the family (PCJ, p. 18). In the Khos understanding of body, it is not just a biological it is also a social body. An individual is located in a web of social relationship. The stress and strains of the social relationship are reflected on the mind and the body of an individual. The *mali's* healing ritual happens in a social setting wherein the entire kindred of a sick individual participate in the healing. This participation enables rejuvenation of the social ties and restructuring of the relationship. A *mali* draws upon the social resources of the sick individual and thus activates them as a therapeutic management group to induce a *social cathartic* effect on him or her. This restructuring of social ties enable a successful healing for a disturbed individual.

Psychochemical action: According to Dow (1988) quoting Prince (1982), the psychological state which is induced in a patient during a healing ritual leads to release of many neuro-chemicals like endorphins (p. 59). A recent study by Charles *et al.* (2020) reported that religious rituals contain many elements like synchronized movements, dancing and singing which lead to release of mu-opoid endorphins which creates a positivity and motivation for social bonding in the participants. Similar studies linking spirituality and neurobiology indicate increased blood flow to the parietal and occipital part of the brain during rituals (Mohandas, 2008). All these studies suggest that rituals can induce psychochemical activations which in turn can have therapeutic value for the patient (p. 69).

Conclusion

The article by PCJ suggests that the traditional ethno-medical systems are an important part of public health care in many of the tribal and rural communities of India. The WHO in its recent Thirteenth General Programme of Work (GPW), Report 2019 to 2023, clearly states that the *Sustainable Development Goal 3*, which aims for universal health coverage for 3 billion population, the tradition and complementary medicine has to play an important role. They preferred to call the traditional medical systems as integrative system of medicines thereby attesting to their role alongside the biomedicine in providing affordable and assessable health services to all. The challenges of climate change and recent global pandemic crisis have pushed us to rethink the way we look at health and wellbeing. The Lancet (2009), in its editorial, what is health, stated that we need to move beyond the WHO's traditional conceptualization of health as a state of physical, social and psychological wellbeing, to a more comprehensive conception of health as *a process of adaptation* (p. 781). Considering the variable impact of Covid we need to closely examine the interplay of biology, body, culture and ecology and how it is all going to affect our health and wellbeing. In this regard, the PCJ's article was quite futuristic and relevant with respect to how we need to revise our understanding of concept of health. PCJ's article emphasized the relationship of the physical body to social, ecological and universal dimensions of human existence when describing the Khos' concept of health and illness. Therefore, we do not have to only talk of a health *body* we also have talk about a health society, a health eco-diversity and a health planet when we are referring to health. Only then, we can ensure a health for all. *Malis*, the traditional healers in Khos society play a very important role as indigenous mental health care provider to the community. The modern psychiatry can incorporate many of their practices like their understanding of social suffering, abnormality, stigma, patient-healer-society relationship to rethink the concept of wellbeing. They clearly showed the untapped potential of cultural healing and its bearing on the relationship between self, social and somatic processes. PCJ in this article on a traditional medical system of the Khos showed that the health care systems of these communities contains many wisdoms which we need to understand and incorporate in our public health care systems. It is only then we can achieve the goal of universal health and wellbeing for all.

REFERENCES

Berreman, Gerald D. (1997). *Hindus of the Himalayas* (2nd Edition). New Delhi: Oxford University Press.

Berreman, Gerald D. (1962). "Pahari Polyandry: A Comparison". *American Anthropologist, 64,* 1, 60-75.

Charles, S.J. *et al.* (2020). "Blocking mu-opioid receptors inhibits social bonding in rituals". *Biol. Lett. 16*(20), 1-5.

Csordas, Thomas J. (2010). "Elements of charismatic persuasion and healing". In Good, B.J. *et al.* (eds.). *A reader in medical anthropology: Theoretical trajectories, emergent realities*. Malden Mass: Wiley-Blackwell.

Dow, J.(1986). "Universal aspects of symbolic healing: A theoretical synthesis". *American Anthropologist*, 88, 56-69.

Gellner, E. (1994). *Reason and culture: The historic role of rationality and rationalism*. Oxford: Blackwell.

Giddens, A. (2013). *Social theory and modern sociology*. New York: John Wiley and Sons.

Joshi, P.C. (2012). "Relevance and utility of traditional medical systems in the context of a Himalayan tribe". *Psychology and Developing Society, 12*(1), 1-25.

Kroeber, A.L. and Kluckhohn, C. (1952). *Culture: A critical review of concepts and definitions*. Peabody Museum, Cambridge: MA, 181.

Lévi-Strauss, C. (2009). *Structural anthropology*. New York: Basic Books.

Mondas, E. (2008). "Spirituality and neurobiology". *Mens Sana Monogr. 6*(1): 63–80.

Ohri, L. (2019). *Till kingdom come: Medieval Hinduism in the modern Himalaya*. Albany: State University of New York Press.

Prince, R. (1982). "Introduction to shamans and endorphins". *Ethos 10*(4):299-302.

Sax, W.S. (2009). *God of justice: Ritual healing and social justice in the central Himalayas*. Oxford: Oxford University Press.

Srivastava, V.K. (2020). "Anatomy of stigma: Understanding COVID-19". *Social Change*. *50*(3) 385–398.

Sheff Thomas, J. (1977). "The distancing of emotion in rituals". *Current Anthropology 18*(3), 483-505.

The Lancet Editorial (2009). "What is health? The ability to adapt". *The Lancet*. 373, 781.

Utter, H. (2010). *Trance, Ritual, and Rhythm: The cult of Mahasu Deota in the Western Himalayas*. Delhi: B.R. Rhythms.

Waldram, J.B. (2000). "The efficacy of traditional medicine: Current theoretical and methodological issues". *Medical Anthropology Quarterly, 14* (4) 603-625.

World Health Organization. (2019). *WHO global report on traditional and complementary medicine 2019*. World Health Organization. https://apps.who.int/iris/handle/10665/312342.

3
The Dark Side of Indigenous Medicines
Adverse Effects and ISMs

Abhik Ghosh

Introduction

The ISM (Indian Systems of Medicine) industry and the attendant pharma companies are one of the really large businesses in the world. As the recent assessments show, according to the report *Ayurveda Market in India 2021-2024*, the Indian market of this sector showed a value of 300 billion in Indian Rupees in 2018 and was expected to gross a value of 710.87 billion by 2024, increasing at a compound annual growth rate of 16.06 per cent.

According to this report, the key drivers of the growth of this market include:

- Maintenance of a healthy lifestyle, increase in the consumers preference for food products like herbal tea, cornflakes, oats, cookies, biscuits, jam, spices, and almond oil made with natural ingredients. A shift of preference of consumers for herbal personal care products, with the increase in awareness of the harmful effects of chemicals on health, used in the production of popular conventional skin, hair, body and other beauty care products, has become the driving force behind the growth of the market.
- The traditional practices of herbal and Ayurveda treatments has found global acceptance, thereby broadening the prospects of 'Ayurveda Tourism' in India. As a consequence of which many Ayurveda rejuvenation and therapeutic centres have been established in states like Kerala, Uttarakhand, Goa and Odisha.

There are also some problems that hamper this growth. They include:

- There is low yield of high quality herbal and medicinal plants in India, due to adverse weather conditions. Besides, the large scale use of insecticides and pesticides causes degradation of the quality of herbs with medicinal properties. These two factors lead to shortage of high quality plants lead to deteriorating quality of these products and services.
- Quality certifications in India are carried out by several players. They include FPS (Finished Product Specifications), GMP (Good Manufacturing Practice) and ISO (International Organization for Standardization). Often, they do not adhere to the quality standards for the products and services offered, so regular tests to check whether manufacturing guidelines are met or are not carried out. The lack of proper scientific documentation of traditional Ayurveda practices, is also a major problem.

Some estimates put the total number of formulations in the market relating to herbal medicines at about 1289 botanicals from 2,400 plant species in 960 plant taxa.

On the 17th of March, 2020, the Rajya Sabha tabled two bills for consideration. The first was the National Commission for Indian System of Medicine Bill, 2019 and the second, the National Commission for Homoeopathy Bill, 2019.The purpose of these bills was to repeal the Indian Medicine Central Council Act, 1970 and create a regulated medical education system to ensure the availability of quality medical professionals practising the Indian System of Medicine such as Ayurveda. This, along with providing quality medical education for Homoeopathy and adopting the latest medical research are the primary objectives of these Bills. Some of the others are to include a periodic assessment of medical institutions and an effective grievance redressal mechanism. The Minister of State for AYUSH, Mr. Shripad Yesso Naik introduced the Institute of Teaching and Research in Ayurveda Bill, 2020 on February 10, 2020. This Bill seeks to merge the three Ayurveda institutes into one institution under the name of Institute of Teaching and Research in Ayurveda.

The National Commission for Indian System of Medicine Bill, 2019 provides for the establishment of the National Commission for Indian System of Medicine (NCISM). It consists of 29 members appointed by the Central Government. The NCISM will serve a number of functions. These include:

1. Framing policies for regulating medical institutions and medical professionals of Indian System of Medicine.
2. Assessing the requirements of healthcare-related human resources and infrastructure.
3. Ensuring compliance by the State Medical Councils of Indian System of Medicine of the regulations made under the Bill.
4. Ensuring coordination among the autonomous boards set up under the Bill.

In the year 2016, the Confederation of Indian Industry (CII),estimated the total market size of Indian Ayurveda industry at 3 billion USD. This includes the Ayurveda products and services including classical, ethical, over the counter (OTC), personal care and beauty products; as well as medical, wellbeing, payor and medical tourism services. The product market of USD 2.27 billion (75 per cent of the total market compared to the services market (USD 0.75 billion) is obviously larger and the industry is envisioned to grow to USD 9 billion by the year 2022. According to another estimate, the Ayurveda market is expected to go from USD 2.5 billion to USD 8 billion by 2022.

Table 3.1: Registered Medical Practitioners in ISM&H (as of 2001)

Ayurveda	4,27,504
Unani	42,445
Siddha	16,599
Naturopathy	429
Homoeopathy	1,94,147
Total	**6,81,124**

Source: Department of ISM&H, 2001.

ISMs and the Pressure of Business: A Nexus of Practices

Thus, we can see that many kinds of plant-based treatments are often clubbed under Ayurveda (see, for instance, Ravishankar and Shukla; 2007). Also, they are very important to the business practices in India where they seem to have one of the largest roles to play in International trade. Having said that, it is also true that ISMs are being clubbed together since they can be a part of a larger sales unit without an overall definition and also being checked out as being a part of an overall trend towards a better and healthier lifestyle (Kuruvilla, 2002; Gupta *et al.*, 2006; Zheng *et al.*, 2011; Nirmal *et al.*, 2013; Pandey *et al.*, 2013). In fact a resurgence of herbal medicines was felt by some authors (Jawla *et al.*, 2009).

Table 3.2: Market Size and Growth Across Select Sub-sectors — CII Survey of Private Sector

Select Segments	*Market Size in 2017-18*	*Growth Projections for Next Five Years (CAGR in percentage)*
Manufacturing (75 per cent of the total Ayurveda market)	Around INR 22,500 crore (for top 50 companies)	16
Ayurveda Veterinary Medicines and Feed Supplements (which is a sub-component of manufacturing)	Around INR 700 crore	12-14 (10-12 in domestic market and 20 in exports)
Wellness Sector	Not Available	Products - 50 Services – 30
Hospitals	Around INR 1000 crore	Over 50
Day-Care Treatment Centre, Clinics, Dispensaries, etc.	Around INR 5000 crore	Over 50

This is part of a subtext where Western or Allopathic medicines are considered to be hegemonic and having major side-effects. They are supposed to subvert the body's systems, use excessive force and medicinal power to deal with the supposed disease and also damage the body in their rush to get at the root or cause of the illness. One narrative in Western treatment of illness has often been that the 'bad' cells are killed with a few 'good' cells in the body by the treatment but the 'good' cells grow back while the 'bad' cells do not.

On the other hand, ISMs, as well as indigenous medical systems in other countries did not have such bad adverse reactions or harmful side-effects on the body. In a perfect world, then, herbal, organic medicines were the good guys and allopathic medicines became the bad guys. This led to a massive increase in sales in health and wellness products, with India being a major player.

The Politics of Medical Systems and the Hegemony of Healing Practices

This injustice has been meted out through a policy of business practices and a set of lobby enthusiasts who have ensured that regulations in such areas prefer the business practices that have given large profits. Over the years the pharma lobby has had tremendous influence until they were brought down through a set of litigations and rules that curtailed their power to some extent.

The power then went to the next layer in the echelon. Herbal medicines were then marketed, researched and appropriated using the same unethical practices used by the Allopathic lobby. This has become the second layer, neither giving up on these issues. Sometimes the same company sold both kinds of products, tested and conducted in the same way.

Anthropologists have always been with the underdog in most cases. In this case, in their theory as well as in their practice, they turned out to be naïve. The first thing they were wrong about was in dealing with medical practices in Allopathic work as being monolithic and having a set of practices that could be labelled as being 'one system'. This was definitely not true.

Having dealt with the enemy as if it was one thing, it continued to see the alternative as being a large and inchoate mass of products having certain common ideas that linked them up:

1. Each set of herbal practices was linked to a well thought out logical system linked to a culture. It was thus impossible for a particular herbal medicine to exist without having its own attendant belief system and worldview. The fact that even ethnographically, many practices could not be linked to such ethnographic practices or be seen as part of the system did not deter anthropologists. They kept feeling this was only a result of a lack of data. For instance, it has often been stated that each practice is part of a system of belief and thought where ideas of classification of symptoms and their types and as well as food and medicines to be used in each case go hand in hand. Authors go so far as to create elaborate flow diagrams to illustrate this or create tabular formats to show the linkages. Perhaps, this was unwarranted.
2. Each medical system was associated with a cultural system, belief, worldview and often linguistic system. It was immaterial to the idea of how such medical practices borrowed or acted across cultural barriers.
3. Within this methodology was hidden the idea that each method was sacrosanct. Borrowing, leakage or sharing was limited or of no account. It was a matter of shock that such medical systems were crossing cultural borders but also that they used

raw materials from far off regions and ideas and concepts from other cultures to recreate their way of life.

4. It was also a matter of note that Ayurveda and other practices were touted as one systemic set of practices that enveloped other systems of health and herbal medicines under one set of principles and rubric. Its own history belied this hegemonic practice.
5. Finally, ISMs and indigenous medical practices were treated as if they had all a set of active principles and methods of action. Eventually, Western rationality and science would uncover these practices and the logic underlying them, thus opening them to be marketed under a system very much like the Allopathic one. Homoeopathic practices were denied and then brought under chemical principles in the same manner. Tribal medicines were recorded independent of the other and any linkages between different medical practices used by different tribes was seen to be rare and coincidental.

Thus, in this kind of a logical system, the idea that a very systemic wrong was being committed and that adverse reactions were as much present in other systems of medicine, was something that got pushed under the carpet.

Adverse Reactions and Alternative Systems

Adverse reactions to various kinds of herbal medicines were being published in different journals for a long time. For instance, it was known that drugs containing licorice were contra-indicated with aged, hypertensive or patients with inflammation (Yasue *et al.*: 2007). Aristolochic acid (AA) containing herbs have regularly been used for making herbal formulations of varying kinds in South Asia and South East Asia. They are strongly indicative of a variety of cancers in human beings according to papers in *Science Translational Medicine* (Mole, 2017).

By 1990 (Mitchell-Heggs, *et al.*, 1990, Smithermann and Herber, 1991, Dunbabin *et al.*, 1992, Keen *et al.*, 1994, Hasegawa *et al.*, 1997, Ernst, 2002, Ibrahim and Latif 2002, Sood *et al.*, 2003, Weide *et al.*, 2003, Schilling *et al.*, 2004, Roche *et al.*, 2005, Kirchgatterer, 2005, Kanen and Perenboom, 2005, Levit *et al.*, 2007), it was clear that lead was often an element of herbal medicines that caused adverse reactions in herbal treatment formulations. Americans were warned against using such formulations (Pierce, 2012). By 2004, herbal medicines from India sold in America were found to have not only Lead but a host of other heavy metals including Mercury and Arsenic that poisoned Americans, Europeans and those from other countries who used such formulations (Saper *et al.*, 2004, Wood *et al.,* 2004, Dargan *et al.*, 2008). Such herbal remedies also affected genetic conditions like G6PD (Lee *et al.*, 2017). Though, it may be stated that parallel medicines or foods were needed to be taken alongside these medicines to avoid such cases, it must be pointed out that certified Ayurvedic and other practitioners of ISM had used such drugs or prescribed them (according to data collected by the author) which eventually caused such reactions. This did not just happen in one case but in a whole class of cases after which such cautionary bans came into effect in other countries. It is also true that medicines banned in other countries have been seen to be regularly used in India across different systems of medicine.

It was also clear that plant products themselves could have some toxicity and cause adverse effects, though they were often used in regular herbal medicines. One such example is that of *Adhatoda vasica* (Claeson *et al.*, 2000).A review of adverse drug reactions and other issues were put together by some researchers (Ajanal *et al.,* 2013). It was made clear eventually that adverse drug reactions in herbal medicines were caused not only through impurities but also by the components inherent within them. Examples of such items included, Gold (*Swarnabhasma*), Reserpine and steroids (Paudyal *et al.*, 2019).

There are reports from homoeopathic medicines of toxic effects that are life-threatening as part of adverse reactions also (Kirby, 2002, Dantas and Rampes, 2002, Dantas *et al.*, 2007, Posadzky *et al.*, 2012, Dantas, 2017). These are often ignored by aficionados and practitioners.

Similar issues have also been found in products related to Tibetan medicine also (Sallon *et al.*, 2017, Liu *et al.*, 2019).

Conclusion

It is time, perhaps, for Anthropologists in India to rethink their biomedical and other paradigms relating to Medical Anthropology. Joshi (2019) has given a host of commendable reasons why tribal medicines are more acceptable to many people than other systems. Having said that, there are many reasons why we should be wary in promoting and supporting systems of medicines that have a potential to harm others.

In my opinion, then, ISMs, herbal, tribal and Ayurvedic medicines (including Unani, Siddha, Tibetan and Homeopathy) need to be analysed critically by Anthropologists using the same principles that we use to analyse Allopathic and other systems of medicine. Further, as anthropologists one should analyse Allopathic systems using the same principles used for ISMs.

Looking for systems of belief and logic within medical practices may be a good goal. However, they should not be a hindrance in looking for actual truth practices. Our basic guiding principles should not blind us to inconsistencies and issues where a holistic system may be interrupted by actual practices at the ground level.

The Medical Anthropology that we practise today is urgently in need of fresh paradigmatic approaches that are informed by current researches on the topic rather than those that perpetuate our own biases and are subject to public whims and fancies. It should look within, forward and outward to newer regimes of healthcare that are not yet proposed through the practices of today. We really urgently need these today as we look through a Covid-infested world where our current healthcare systems show signs of stress, wear and tear. A predictive science of health-practices is the only suitable goal for an Anthropology of human behaviour that intends to use its knowledge for the good of humankind.

Acknowledgements

My knowledge of Medical Anthropology has been informed by the writings and lectures of Prof. V.K. Srivastava and Prof. P.C. Joshi. I am most grateful for the baseline that they helped me form. I am also grateful to the facilities extended to me by the CAS-II Programme and the Department of Anthropology, Panjab University, Chandigarh for the research work that I was able to conduct within its premises.

REFERENCES

Ajanal, Manjunath, Shradda Nayak, Buduru Sreenivasa Prasad and Avinash Kadam. (2013). "Adverse Drug Reaction and Concepts of Drug Safety in Ayurveda: An Overview", In *Journal of Young Pharmacists*, Vol. 5, pp. 116-120.

Claeson, Ubonwan Pongprayoon, Torbjorn Malmfors, Georg Wikman and Jan G. Bruhn (2000). "*Adhatoda vasica*: A Critical Review of Ethnopharmacological and Toxicological Data", In *Journal of Ethnopharmacology*, Vol. 72, pp. 1–20.

Dargan, Paul I., Indika B. Gawarammana, John R.H. Archer, Ivan M. House, Debbie Shaw and David M. Wood (2008). "Heavy Metal Poisoning from Ayurvedic Traditional Medicines: An Emerging Problem?" In *International Journal of Environment and Health*, Vol. 2, Nos. 3-4, pp. 463-474.

Dantas, F. and H. Rampes (2000). "Do Homeopathic Medicines Provoke Adverse Effects?" In *Br. Hom. J.*, Vol. 89, pp. 35–38.

Dantas, F., P. Fisher, H. Walach, F. Wieland, D.P. Rastogi, H. Teixeira, D. Koster, J.P. Jansen, J. Eizayaga, M.E.P. Alvarez, M. Marim, P. Belon and L.L.M. Weckx (2007). "A Systematic Review of the Quality of Homeopathic Pathogenetic Trials Published from 1945 to 1995", In *Homeopathy*, Vol. 96, pp. 4–16.

Dantas, Flavio (2017). "Do Homeopathic Medicines Cause Drug-dependent Adverse Effects or Aggravations?", In *Revista de Homeopatia*, Vol. 80, Nos. 3-4, pp. 142-150.

Dunbabin, D.W., G.A. Tallis, P.Y. Popplewell and R.A. Lee. (1992). "Lead Poisoning from Indian Herbal Medicine (Ayurveda)", In *Medical Journal of Australia*, 7-21 December, Vol. 157, Numbers 11-12, pp. 835-836.

Ernst, E. (2002). "Heavy Metals in Traditional Indian Remedies" in *European Journal of Clinical Pharmacology*, February, Vol. 57, No. 12, pp. 891-896.

Gupta, R., D.K. Dubey, G.M. Kannan and S.J. Flora (2006). "Concomitant Administration of Moringa oleifera Seed Powder in the Remediation of Arsenic-induced Oxidative Stress in Mouse" in *Cell Biology International*, Vol. 31, No. 1, January, pp. 44-56.

Hasegawa, Setsuo, Kazutaga Nakayama, Katsuhiko Iwakiri, Emi An, Seiji Gomi, Kazuo Dan, Masao Katsumata and Ichiji Wakabayashi (1997). "Herbal Medicine-Associated Lead Intoxication" In *Internal Medicine*, Vol. 36, No. 1, pp. 56-58.

Ibrahim, A.S. and A.H. Latif (2002). "Adult Lead Poisoning from a Herbal Medicine", In *Saudi Medical Journal*, May, Vol. 23, No. 5, pp. 591-593.

Jawla, Sunil, A.K. Gupta, Rachit Singla and Varun Gupta (2009). "General Awareness and Relative Popularity of Allopathic, Ayurvedic and Homeopathic Systems", In *Journal of Chemical and Pharmaceutical Research*, Vol. 1, No. 1, pp. 105-112.

Joshi, P.C. (2019). "Ethnomedical Practices and Indian Scheduled Tribes", In *Rom. Jour. of Sociological Studies*, New Series, No. 2, pp. 111–124.

Kanen, B.L. and R.M. Perenboom (2005). "Chronic Lead Intoxication Associated with Ayurvedic Medication", In *Ned. Tijdschr. Geneeskd.*, 24 December, Vol. 149, No. 52, pp. 2893-2896.

Keen, R.W., A.C. Deacon, H.T. Delves, J.A. Moreton and P.G. Frost (1994). "Indian Herbal Remedies for Diabetes as a Cause of Lead Poisoning", In *Postgraduate Medical Journal*, February, Vol. 70, No. 820, pp. 113-114.

Kirby, Brian J. (2002). "Editorial: Safety of Homeopathic Products", In *Journal of the Royal Society of Medicine*, Vol. 95, No. 5, pp. 221-222.

Kirchgatterer, A., M. Rammer and P. Knoflach (2005). "Weight Loss, Abdominal Pain and Anemia After a Holiday Abroad – Case Report of Lead Poisoning", In *Deutsch Med. Wochenschr.*, 7 October, Vol. 130, No. 40, pp. 2253-2256.

Kuruvilla, A. (2002). "Herbal Formulations as Pharmacotherapeutic Agents", In *Indian Journal of Experimental Biology*, Vol. 40, No. 1, January, pp. 7-11.

Lee, Shaun Wen Huey Lee, Nai Ming Lai, Nathorn Chaiyakunapruk and David Weng Kwai Chong (2017). "Adverse Effects of Herbal or Dietary Supplements in G6PD Deficiency: A Systematic Review", In *British Journal of Clinical Pharmacology*, Vol. 83, pp. 172-179.

Levit, T., J. Ablin, A. Agbaria, J. Veinberg, Y. Goor and O. Elkayam (2007). "An Unlikely Cause of Anemia and Abdominal Pain", In *Israel Medical Association Journal*, May, Vol. 9, No. 5, pp. 408-409.

Liu, Jie, Feng Zhang, Velagapudi Ravikanth, Olumayokun A. Olajide, Cen Li, and Li-XinWei (2019). "Chemical Compositions of Metals in Bhasmas and Tibetan Zuotai Are a Major Determinant of Their Therapeutic Effects and Toxicity", In *Evidence-Based Complementary and Alternative Medicine*, Vol. 2019, pp. 1-14.

Mitchell-Heggs, C.A., M. Conway and J. Cassar (1990). "Herbal Medicine as a Cause of Combined Lead and Arsenic Poisoning", In *Hum. Exp. Toxicol.*, May, Vol. 9, No. 3, pp. 195-196.

Mole, Beth (2017). "Herbal Remedies Embraced by Naturopaths, Alt Med Widely Linked to Liver Cancers", In *Ars Technica* Blog, 17 October.

Nirmal, S.A., S.C. Pal, S.O. Otimenyin, Aye Thanda, Elachouri Mostafa, Sukalyan Kumar Kundu, Rajarajan Amirthalingam Thandavarayan and Subhash C. Mandal (2013). "Contribution of Herbal Products in Global Market", In *The Pharma Review*, November-December, pp. 95-104.

Pandey, M.M., Subha Rastogi and A.K.S. Rawat (2013). "Indian Traditional Ayurvedic System of Medicine and Nutritional Supplementation", In *Evidence-Based Complementary and Alternative Medicine*, Vol. 2013, pp. 1-12.

Paudyal, Buddhi, Astha Thapa, Keshav Raj Sigdel, Sudeep Adhikari and Buddha Basnyat (2019). "Adverse Events with Ayurvedic Medicines — Possible Adulteration and Some Inherent Toxicities", In *Wellcome Open Research*, Vol. 4, pp. 1-15.

Pierce, J., Matthew R., Carlos A. Estrada and Ronnie E. Mathews, Jr. (2012). "Buyers Beware: Lead Poisoning Due to Ayurvedic Medicine", In *J. Gen. Intern. Med.*, Vol. 27, No. 10, pp. 1384-1386.

Posadzki, P., A. Alotaibi and E. Ernst (2012). "Adverse Effects of Homeopathy: A Systematic Review of Published Case Reports and Case Series", In *Int. J. Clin. Pract.*, December, Vol. 66, No. 12, pp. 1178–1188.

Ravishankar, B. and V.J. Shukla (2007). "Indian Systems of Medicine: A Brief Profile", In *African Journal of Traditional, Complementary and Alternative Medicines*, Vol. 4, No. 3, pp. 319-337.

Roche, A., C. Florkowski and T. Walmsley (2005). "Lead Poisoning Due to Ingestion of Indian Herbal Remedies", In *New Zealand Medical Journal*, 29 July, Vol. 118, p. U1587.

Sallon, Sarah, Yahav Dory, Yazeed Barghouthy, Tsewang Tamdin, Rigzin Sangmo, Jamyang Tashi, Sonam Yangdon, Tenzin Yeshi, Tsetan Sadutshang, Michal Rotenberg, Elinor Cohen, Yehudit Harlavan, Galit Sharabi and Tali Bolah-Abram (2017). "Is Mercury in Tibetan Medicine Toxic? Clinical,

Neurocognitive and Biochemical Results of an Initial Cross-sectional Study", In *Experimental Biology and Medicine*, Vol. 242, pp. 316–332.

Saper, Robert B., Stefanos N. Kales, Janet Paquin, Michael J. Burns, David M. Eisenberg, Roger B. Davis and Russell S. Phillips (2004). "Heavy Metal Content of Ayurvedic Herbal Medicine Products", In *JAMA*, Vol. 292, No. 23, 15 December, pp. 2868-2873.

Schilling, U., R. Muck and E. Heidemann (2004). "Lead Poisoning after Ingestion of Ayurvedic Drugs", In *Med. Klin. (Munich)*, 15 August, Vol. 99, No. 8, pp. 476-480.

Smitherman, J. and P. Harber (1991). "A Case of Mistaken Identity: Herbal Medicine as a Cause of Lead Toxicity", In *American Journal of Ind. Med.*, Vol. 20, No. 6, pp. 795-798.

Sood, A., V. Midha and N. Sood (2003). "Pain in Abdomen — Do Not Forget Lead Poisoning", In *Indian Journal of Gastroenterology*, November-December, Vol. 21, No. 6, pp. 225-226.

Weide, R., S. Engelhart, H. Farber, F. Kaufmann, J. Heymanns and H. Koppler (2003). "Severe Lead Poisoning Due to Ayurvedic Indian Plant Medicine", In *Deutsche Med. Wochenschr*, 14 November, Vol. 128, Number 46, pp. 2418-2420.

Wood, D.M., S. Athwal and A. Panahloo (2004). "The Advantages and Disadvantages of a 'Herbal' Medicine in a Patient with Diabetes Mellitus: A Case Report" in *Diabetic Medicine*, Vol. 21, pp. 625-627.

Yasue, Hirofumi, TeruhikoItoh, Yuji Mizuno and Eisaku Harada (2007). "Severe Hypokalemia, Rhabdomyolysis, Muscle Paralysis, and Respiratory Impairment in a Hypertensive Patient Taking Herbal Medicines Containing Licorice", In *Internal Medicine*, Vol. 46, pp. 575-578.

Zheng, X.X., Y.L. Xu, S.H. Li, X.X. Liu, R. Hui and X.H. Huang (2011). "Green Tea Intake Lowers Fasting Serum Total and LDL Cholesterol in Adults: A Meta-Analysis of 14 Randomized Controlled Trials", In *American Journal of Clinical Nutrition*, August, Vol. 94, No. 2, pp. 601-610.

4

Healers' Hut

Action Plan to Recognize and Revive Herbal Healing Practices in Sikkim, Northeast India

Sunita Reddy

Introduction

The plurality of healing systems is universal, but the expansion of professionalized, State-patronized biomedical systems, with ever-expanding biomedical markets, dominates the capitalist world (Stoner, B.P., 1986). Only recently has there been an effort to document, preserve, conserve, and integrate indigenous healing systems like Ayurveda into mainstream clinical practice (Sen, S., & Chakraborty, R., 2017). But the 'non-codified systems' have not yet found any place in mainstream healthcare in India. With increasing outbreaks of diseases and the financial burden that comes with treating chronic ailments, there is a renewed interest in herbal practices (Pan, S.Y., *et al.*, 2014)—especially the codified systems of healing, like Ayurveda, Yoga, Unani, Siddha, and Homoeopathy (AYUSH), which were integrated into the mainstream in 2005. Codified systems like AYUSH are recognized and put together under the AYUSH Ministry to promote, but non-codified systems like folk healing and tribal healing, also called traditional healing, are not yet recognized and brought into the mainstream.

Traditional systems, which the tribal populations practice, receive little attention. So far, it has been well established (by anthropological, ethno -botanical, and ethno-pharmacological studies) that tribal communities have been utilizing various flora, fauna, and natural/mineral substances for therapeutic uses (Jugli, S., *et al.*, 2020; Uniyal, S.K., *et al.*, 2006). Studies have shown that there are numerous local health traditions and two million local herbal healers serving a large section of the population, not just the indigenous population but also rural and urban populations, both in developing and developed countries (Hamilton, A.C., 2004). There is a growing interest in natural and herbal medicine in contemporary times. When the cost of healthcare is soaring, and the consumer expectations for care are rising, the role of traditional medicine is being recognized more and more (WHO, 2019). In 2018, 98 member-states developed national policies on Traditional and Complementary Medicine (T & CM), 109 launched national laws, and 124 implemented regulations for herbal medicines. The WHO is halfway through implementing the WHO traditional medicine strategy, 2014–2023. The focus is to develop documents with reliable information, support member-states, and appropriately integrate traditional healing into health systems for universal health coverage and attaining sustainable development goals (WHO, 2019).

However, the tribal population, who holds the knowledge and know-how of nature, has been left behind. The growing concern is that the number of practitioners is dwindling, with the younger generation not willing to learn due to non-recognition by the State, and the non-availability of herbs owing to deforestation, displacement, development, and migration of the indigenous people (Vijayagiri, R.C. & Mamidala, 2012; Mohanty, R., 2011).

In most of the low and middle-income countries, there exists a variety of traditional healers—shamans, magico-religious healers, faith healers, herbalists, bonesetters, snakebite healers, jaundice healers, poison healers, midwives, masseurs, and other practitioners (Ember & Ember, 2004; Pratt, C., 2007).

Traditional/folk healing practices are largely unregulated, informal, and unorganized, with the healers possessing no formal education and training, and the practice itself being non-commercial and yet popular in the community. These are the most affordable services available with easy access to the communities, especially in low and middle income countries, where a sizeable section of the population live in far-fetched and remote areas. These traditional healing practices are non-codified systems and the healing knowledge is handed down from one generation to the next, usually through oral traditions. There is a plethora of writings about the important role played by these folk and traditional healers (Taid, T.C., *et al.*, 2014; Muthu, C., *et al.*, 2006; Yabesh, J.M., *et al.*, 2014; Suwankhong, D., *et al.*, 2011).

There is a renewed interest in knowing these traditional healers' knowledge base, especially the herbal healers, in the past few years. Various institutions, like the Foundation for Revitalization of Local Health

Traditions (FRLHT[1]) and AYUSH[2] are documenting folk healing practices, validating them, and exploring possibilities of patenting new formulations. However, given the elderly age group of the healers, the disappearance of traditional knowledge systems is a grave concern. Further, there are hardly any effort to recognize and support them to revive their traditional healing practices.

This chapter is based on qualitative empirical research conducted in 2019 with selected healers in three states of the Northeast: Arunachal Pradesh, Sikkim, and Manipur. The study was supported by the Indira Gandhi National Centre for the Arts (IGNCA) and carried out by the Anthropos India Foundation. Focusing on Sikkim, this paper addresses the importance of healers in the community who cater to primary level care and their issues, concerns, and challenges in practising herbal healing, given various kinds of constraints they face. Further, the paper looks at the efforts made by the State and some key institutions to revive these healings systems. In the conclusion, the paper gives recommendations by healers and key personnel in State institutions to recognize, revive, and support the traditional healers.

Methods

It was decided to select a few major ethnic communities in Sikkim and find herbal healers from the Lepcha, Bhutia, and Nepali communities. In-depth interviews with 20 well-known healers, predominantly herbal healers, were carried out for a whole month in February 2019. A team of three people carried out the research. Two research scholars, Dr. Tshering Lepcha and Sehfali Bharati accompanied the author. Some of the healers were able to speak in Hindi, where the author could interview. In most other cases, however, the healers spoke Nepali, and a student researcher who spoke Nepali was accompanying to translate. The other researcher took audio-visual documentation. Initial contacts were made through phone, and permissions were taken from the key informant. The written research permission and pass were also taken from the Sikkim State Biodiversity Board to carry out the study. Finding the healers was easier due to Tshering Lepcha earlier study in the region. In-depth interviews were also conducted with health professionals, members of the biodiversity board, the state plant medicinal boards, AYUSH, and other officials. Literature review was done along with observations, group discussions, case studies, and photo documentation. Further, narratives of the healers were collected through the 'emic' perspective. Ethical clearance was taken from the Ethics Review

Board of the Anthropos India Foundation; the names of the healers have been used after taking their oral/written permission. The study was carried out under the aegis of the Anthropos India Foundation, with the funding and collaboration with Dr. Sachindanand Joshi and Dr. Ramesh Gaur of the Indira Gandhi National Centre for the Arts.

Findings

Folk Healers of Sikkim

The main communities of Sikkim are the Lepchas, Bhutias, and Nepalese. Lepchas are the original inhabitants of the state, concentrated in Dzongu Valley (Lama, 2001; Tamsang, K.P., 1983). The tribal population of Sikkim comprises 55.8 per cent of the total 6.8 lakh population of the state. Most of its population resides in the rural areas (74.8%), practising Hinduism (57.7%), Buddhism (27.5%), and Christianity (9.9%) (Census, 2011).

The Scheduled Tribes (ST) population are the *Lepchas* and *Bhutia* including *Chumbipa*, *Dopthapa*, *Dukpa*, *Kagatey*, *Sherpa*, *Tibetan*, *Tromopa*, and *Yolmo*, constituting over 22 per cent of the population. The Scheduled Caste (SC) population are the *Kami*, *Damai*, *Lobar*, *Sarki*, and *Majhi*, constituting 5.95 per cent. The Backward Castes include *Tamang*, *Gurung*, *Rai*, *Limbu*, and *Sunwar*, which also constitute a significant section of the population (Das, 2015:12).

Various anthropological studies show that there are a large number of traditional healers across the North-Eastern states. All the states in the Northeast consist of diverse ethnic communities and tribes with their own unique culture, language, and healing practices (Ningombam *et al.*, 2014).

The folk healers are the primary healthcare providers for the local communities, especially in the rural areas. The folk practitioners carry out their art of healing in various ways. Each healer practices their distinct methodology, such as herbal healing, spiritual healing or a combination of both, along with massage and acupressure.

Sikkim is the land of faith healers along with herbal healers. There is a large number of healers in Sikkim, such as the *Dhami*, *Jhakris*, *Phendongba*, and *Bonbo* in Nepali communities; *Pow* and *Nejum* in Bhutia community; *Bongthing* in Lepcha; *Bijwa* (Rai), *Baidang* and *Phedagma* in Limboo; *Joghi*, *Baidya* (folk healer), *Sodhini* (massagers) and so on (Das, N.K., 2015; Lepcha, T., 2018; Sharma, A., 2015).

There are various estimates of the number of healers in the state. According to a healer, Lila Ram Dhakal, there are about 400–500 healers in all districts of Sikkim. Among the healers too, there are specialists, like poison healer, bonesetter etc. Some healers treat one to two illnesses. Every healer does not treat all diseases.

Estimate Medicinal Plants

There are different estimations on the number of medicinal plants by the healers and the State Biodiversity Board. According to 64 year old Mangal Bir Subba from Yaksum, Sikkim has more than 14,000 medicinal plants, whereas The Mountain Institute (TMI[3]) estimates around 700 medicinal plants. Another estimate is 488 species of aromatic and medicinal plants used by the indigenous communities (Sharma & Sharma, 2010). It is claimed that more than 95 per cent of Sikkim plant diversity is medicinal. Not all plants can be cultivated since they require varied altitudes, temperature, and geographical location.

Divine Powers and Oral Traditions of Learning

All the healers shared that they had learned the art of healing from their forefathers or fathers, and very few were first-generation learners. Some of them said that they consider it as a divine power, so not everyone can become a healer. Titit Gatsya said,

> "*My grandfather used to practice, though my father did not learn and carry these healing practices. After that, I learned the art of healing (Bongthing). In the field practice of Bongthing, no one can learn from a text or any guru. It will come automatically or through lineage. I have learned through my dreams. In my dreams, my ancestors or grandfather's spirits guide me to do this healing. I do not have any guru. I do pujas in the villages and other places. I practice this healing since I was 14 years old. My whole family has this knowledge through dreams.*"

Whereas Titit Tashi Tshering Lepcha, who is a bonesetter, also learnt modern ways of diagnosing and is cautious not to treat complicated cases but to refer them. He said,

> "*I started this healing practices since I was 40 years old. I did not learn the healing practices from anyone. One or two treatment methods and the medicine I have learned from my father. Other*

than that, I have learned myself. Slowly I have learned the treatment for cut, wounds etc. and also, I searched for some medicine in surrounding areas and the jungle. Sometimes, I use mantras and do rituals, but mostly I use herbal medicine. I can see the X-ray reports of the patients. I do not treat multiple fracture or complications."

Diagnosis and the Process of Healing Rituals

Healers have their ways and methods of diagnosis and aetiology of illnesses and sickness.

Titit Gatsyo narrates how he diagnoses:

"First, I see jokhana and then if it is confirmed of that patient is having kapat, I use the root of the medicinal plant to treat the case. I also see the eyes and nails of the patient. If half of the nail portion is yellow, the body of the patient looks swollen, and in some case, the body starts becoming thin and looks like TB patients, I diagnosis accordingly."

Fifty seven year old Titit Gatsyo from Lingthem Dzongu, North Sikkim, described the healing rituals thus:

"I use puffed rice, local egg, rice, organic chi, dry fish, dry birds, fruits, ginger, flower, and do not sacrifice animals. I use the flower according to the condition of the patient. My grandfather told me to use items carefully in the rituals, according to the suffering from house deity or dewta or spirits, I use chi[4] for the healing rituals. If the patients are suffering from jungle dewta or spirits, then I do rituals in banana leaf. I must praise the dewta. He asks the patients to bring coins for rituals, bird, fish, egg, which is boiled and kept for the rituals."

He further identifies biological causative agents to be referred to the medical doctor,

"If I conduct the ritual for the members of my own house and it is due to the cause of own ancestral deities, then I will use chi. If the rituals are being conducted for other people, then it will be conducted by using the bark of banana, old home-grown tea

> *leaves, and flour. All the items are burnt while doing the rituals. I would be going to the houses, wherever there is a sick patient. If it is identified that the sickness is due to the biological cause, then the patients are told to seek treatment from the hospital."*

The healers have the good sense to refer to doctors, in case of complications, multiple fracture, trauma, or emergency.

Treating Patients

Healers shared the places from where the patients come for treatment. Their healing is marketed all through word of mouth. They even send the medicines to their patients in other states and personally visit if the patient stays close by. The volume of patients coming for treatment from other regions indirectly shows the efficacy of the treatment, faith, and trust in the healings of the healer.

Bhim Bhadur Neopani has treated more than 50,000 patients in his entire life, some of whom have returned from the hospital after unsuccessful treatment. They come from Gangtok, Mangan, Gazing, Kaluk, Soreng, Nepal, and Darjeeling.

Another healer, Nar Bahadur, said patients, come from Siliguri, Gangtok, Yaksum, Darap, Gazing, and Nepal. Some patients demand medicine through the phone. "*I also visit the patient's house who live nearby. I prepare and keep the medicine at home, and sometimes, I get it from the market. Sometimes, patients stay one or two days at my house and go back after their bandage's changed and come again to get the medicine.*"

Lila Ram Dhakal said his patients come from the West Bengal districts of Kalimpong and Darjeeling also, apart from local surrounding areas.

> "*I have sent medicine to Kashmir, Delhi, Tamil Nadu etc. Once I had sent 7 kg of medicine to Tamil Nadu for gastritis, cancer, hair growth etc. The medicine cannot be kept for long after preparation. Therefore, it is prepared only when it is required.*"

Nandalal Subba, 44 years old, has treated nearly 1,200 patients in his lifetime. They come from Namchi, Jorethang and nearby places. "*I go to the patient's house for the treatment if they are with serious injuries or fractures and in a critical situation and not able to move. The plaster is changed in 10 days or 15 days or 22 days or 50 days, or sometimes it is changed every week if the bone is not in its proper alignment. I treat the patients only after seeing the X-ray report of the patients. There are patients who come to me when they do not get successful treatment from the doctor. Whereas some patients come directly and some after taking 2–5 months of treatment from the hospital.*"

Some healers like Nandalal are integrating modern methods of diagnosis like X-rays by self-learning to read the reports.

Forty eight year old Gopal Sharma from Daramdin, West Sikkim, treats snakebite; around 2–3 patients come every month for the treatment, and for jaundice, about 20–25 patients come in a year. *"I have treated more than a thousand patients who have come from different parts of Sikkim as well as Darjeeling and Kalimpong in West Bengal."* Sixty four year old Mangal Bir Subba from Yaksum, West Sikkim, said he has treated more than 1,000 cases for fractures, gastritis etc.

After the training by the State Biodiversity Board and FRLHT, they have started keeping a record of the patients visiting them, with details like name, age, place, phone number, and the problem treated. This helps them to show their popularity and acceptance far and wide. They have also started collecting testimonials from the patients written in their own handwriting. The author was shown all these certificates and testimonials with a lot of pride for the good work they are doing. The testimonials were also proof of their popularity. They also shared with pride that educated people, officers, doctors, and scientists too have taken medicine from them.

Vanishing Traditional Healing Knowledge and Practices

Across the healers, the narrative was that they are keen to teach their knowledge to the next generation, but there are not many takers as they don't see any future of it. Healer Gopal Sharma said, *"My children are not interested in learning, and all are studying. If anybody wants to learn the mantras, I am ready to teach but only for healing and not for commercial purpose. This is a service for the community; if this becomes commercial, then poor people cannot afford it. If any patient gives me money, I accept that money and use it to support poor or deserving students in school.*"

With a concern of losing the valuable knowledge, Lila Ram Dhakal, 73 years old from Gangchung, Sikkim started self-documenting his knowledge. He said, *"When I die, my skills and knowledge of traditional healing practices will not perish with me. Many old people who were healers in the community died, and their skills and practices have vanished."* The efforts of the FRLHT have also been to motivate healers at least to write down in their diaries the names of the herbal plants, their medicinal value, and how to use it, leaving for the future generations to learn. Apart from that, AYUSH, under a project, also documented the herbal healing practices.

Demand and Access of Herbal Medicine

Sixty four year old Mangal Bir Subba from Yaksum, West Sikkim, said, "*I practice only herbal healing, and I realize there is a high demand for herbal medicine in Sikkim. About 10 per cent of people still demand herbal medicine. There is a sale of up to 1 lakh rupees of herbal medicine in Sikkim, and I sell herbs worth rupees 40 thousand per day during the workshops.*"

Bhim Bahadur Neopani shared that there are difficulties in collecting medicine as one must climb the mountains, which can take up to three days, for medicine just enough to treat one patient. "*I go to the mountain every 15 days for the collection of medicine. To access and collect the plants, I need to pay Rs. 500 per month as a fee to the Forest Department. I treat my patients at my own house, and sometimes, I go to the patient's house.*"

Almost ten healers shared that they are maintaining a herbal garden in their backyard. Though other healers too expressed their wish to have a herbal garden and demanded that the government should provide land and some funds to maintain the medicinal herbal gardens.

Bhim Bahadur Neopani said, he prepares the medicine at home and has bought some land for 5 lakh rupees to build a herbal garden at his home. At the same time, Mangal Bir Subha started farming in 1992 and built a nursery of herbal medicine in 1995, which is spread across 15 acres, though he reported that he did not get any support to build the garden from the government. The medicinal plants grow in their own specific local areas and cannot be replicated in other geographical areas.

Preparing Medicine

Preparing a herbal medicine is a tedious job, where the healers pluck various parts of the trees and plants—it can be root, leaf, seed, bark, or fruit—and then they dry it under sunlight. Then they grind or pound it to make medicine. One healer said, '*Sometimes, 108 medicines are used and mixed for the treatment.*' Titit Tashi Tshering Lepcha said, '*I collect medicine when the patients come for the treatment. I do not prepare and keep the medicine. I use traditional bamboo support or tree barks (mawa and wild avocado tree barks) in the fracture cases and apply medicine, which is prepared by herbs.'*

He continued to explain the process of treatment, '*I give treatment for the first seven days; after that, if the patients are not showing improvement, I extend the treatment to seven more days. I give both oral powder medicine and external medicine. All the medicines are prepared from medicinal plants' leaf, roots, seeds, fruits, minerals, and animal products pounded in a traditional wooden grinder.*'

Krishna Prasad Pyakurel, 73 years old, who died just a few months back, reported that for treating patients, only one medicinal plant is not enough; to make a single medicine, one must combine 8–10 medicinal plants. He first tries the medicine on himself and then gives it to his patients for treatment.

Nar Bahadur Limbu, said, "*I have medicinal plants for hepatitis, sugar. Three medicines together are used for preparing medicines for cancer malabas (bamboo), jatimaingo, Kala haldhi.*"

Lila Ram Dhakal, shared that he has some 55 varieties of medicines for problems like the removal of poison, bone-setting, hepatitis, sugar, cataract, menorrhagia, postpartum haemorrhage, fever, burns etc. "*I used to treat 8–15 cases per day. Once, I managed 50 cases in my workplace.*" Lila Ram proudly compared his work and the accolades he gets from the patients with that of a doctor, saying, "*Patients get a certificate from the doctor during discharge, but when I treat the patient, I get certificates, testimonials, and appreciations from the patients after successful treatment.*"

Traditional Healing is a Gift (*pai rashi*)

It is ironic that almost all the healers are poor and come under the low-income category, with the few exceptions of those who have made some permanent bone-setting clinics. Despite their divine powers, magic in their hands, and treating thousands of patients in their lifetimes, they continue to be poor as they barely charge for their treatment and their practice is altruistic in nature. The healers are aware that when the same patients go to doctors, they incur high costs, but when they come to the healers, they don't shell out much.

Krishana Prasad Pyakurel, living in a small hut, shared, "*I once treated a lady doctor with haemorrhoids who had spent around Rs. 18,000 in the hospital. However, my charges were just a fraction of that. At another workshop in Assam, I gave my medicine to two doctors, one for the treatment of tumour and haemorrhoids for his wife and the other for gout to his mother. Both of whom were successfully treated.*"

He further said, "*Ironically, patients come to me for treatment, thinking that the services are free of cost or affordable since the knowledge is gifted to the healers by God. But at the same time, when they go to the hospital for treatment, they agree to pay a huge amount of money.*"

Another strong reason for not charging from the patients was shared by Satal Singh Limboo, "*I believe healing and doing the traditional treatment is gifted (pai rashi). If I reveal things about my treatment to the others, it would not be effective.*" Titit Gatsyo never asks cash for the treatment but receives whatever amount the patients give after healing. He said it is a sin for them to demand cash from the patients.

The commercialization and overcharging from the patient in the biomedicine system pushes patients to herbal medicine, which have further won their trust and helped to relieve their pain. The nominal cost, which is not asked for and depends on the patient's own choice and capacity, have earned the respect of people and is one of the reasons it has become the popular choice among the people. The visitor's book with the healers had many words of appreciation from various patients, scholars, doctors, and scientists from both India and in one case from outside, applauding the good work of the Baidya and the efficacy of his treatments.

Permits and Restrictions in Collecting Herbal Medicinal Plants

Nar Bahadur Limbu shared the challenges in collecting medicinal plants. They are very particular about conserving the plants. He said, "*I have the permit of collecting medicinal plants from the forest, but the Forest Department will not allow collecting the medicinal plants from the mountains. However, royalty must be given for the collection of medicinal plants to the Forest Department. Therefore, I collect the medicinal plants from the nearby jungles and the local surroundings. I make sure when I collect the plants from the jungle; I do not plough the whole plant. If I plough the whole plant, then it disappears completely.*"

Healers shared that the medicinal plants cannot be regrown in new and exotic places; they have to be native to be potent. They are mostly found in cold areas like the Himalayas and the mountains. At present, the availability of some medicinal plants, like *bikuma, kurki, sharmaguru, panch amli, mahaguru, shamguru, humguru, lappaguru*, is less. When I tried planting medicinal plants in a cold area, they did not survive.

Bhim Bahadur Neopani shared, "*I had requested from the government a provision to build a herbal garden and own an X-ray machine in the year 2008. To date, I have not received any response or support from the government. The AYUSH department has never contacted me either."*

Many healers reported that the AYUSH department had come and taken the details of their medicinal plants. Though Titit Tashi Tshering said, "*Till date, I have not had any problem in collecting medicine. I have a government certificate to collect it.*"

Certificates, Testimonial, and Training

The North East Christian University partnered with the North East Institute of Folk Medicine (NEIFM), Quality Council of India (QCI), and FRLHT, to recognize and certify the traditional healers. It is a voluntary certification in two stages, where the healers can fill to get certified. Though it is voluntary, not many have been registered, as many healers are not even aware of such certification. There is a need for a proactive approach to identify healers and certify them.

For the past few years, there have been some efforts to document the traditional knowledge on health and healing by various agencies like FRLHT and AYUSH. Few training programmes were also conducted to make the healers understand the vast knowledge they have, the need to document it, and keep a record of patients visiting. The healers were also given certificates of participation. Most of the herbal healers had a bag full of appreciation letters and certificates of participation in various training programmes. These trainings are conducted by the Sikkim Medicinal Plant Board, Sikkim Biodiversity Board, TMI, FRLHT in Bangalore, North East Institute of Folk Medicine in Pasighat, and Regional Research Institute (Ayurveda), Sikkim. Some of the healers also showed group photographs taken during the trainings and some of them had detailed letters of appreciation from the Forest Department. However, all the healers were of the opinion that even though they were called for training, they did not gain much; in turn, they shared their knowledge, which was documented by the departments.

Except for two healers, Yamuna Prasad Bastola and Nar Bahadur Limbu, who shared their positive experience and said they had gained out of all the training experience, no other healer was satisfied. Yamuna Prasad shared, "*I went to Bangalore for a meeting and learned about Serpagandha. I got a certificate from the FRLHT Research Centre for 15 days and got training on medicinal plants. I have also attended training with the biodiversity board and got a certificate. I have been practising for two years. I am also involved in research projects with Sikkim University on Maize. I am now preparing 'Organic Bering Herbals' and selling them in different markets.*"

Nar Bhadur Limbu shared that he attended workshops in Jaipur, Chandigarh, Guwahati, Delhi, and Dehradun. "*Two army officials also took my medicines in Chandigarh and in Dehradun; there were many army people who have purchased my medicines. In Gangtok, my medicines were sold for 5 lakhs in a workshop. I prepare the medicine in powder form and supply it to both the Forest Department and local people.*" Though the two healers who mentioned of making good money during workshops/ fairs, their living conditions did not reflect their earning, and it may not be sustainable.

Others' experiences were limited. Nandlal Subba received 3–4 certificates from the panchayat, AYUSH, and the Forest Department. He was also taken for a tour by the Forest Department in Darjeeling. Nar Bahadur Limbu from West Sikkim shared that "*The state departments of Sikkim started connecting with me. They provided training and gave certificates for my traditional healing practices. I have received over 15 certificates and two awards.*" Interestingly, the departments are learning from the healers. Nar Bahadur said, "*I am connected to all the departments of Sikkim, and they all come and take the medicinal plants from me. I give all the details of the medicinal plants, their local and botanical name. I also told all the details of all the herbs. Teachers also come and ask the details of various plants and herbs to teach their students in the school. In most training, the department learns from me. They also make videos of me preparing medicines from the medicinal plants. Department such as AYUSH or pharma companies come once a year and take all the knowledge of the medicinal plants, in exchange for some compensation. AYUSH Department (Rs. 500), Zhandu (Rs. 1,000–1,200) Horticulture Department (None).*"

In training, all the healers were sent to the forest with the permit from the Forest Department and collected all the medicinal plants they knew. The collected plants were then taken back to the training, and the healers were told to share the details about the plant medicines. They were also packed and taken by the trainers. The shared anxiety by the healers was very palpable. They were complaining that their knowledge is being taken away and they are not getting any benefit out of it, except for a certificate of participation in the training programmes. This raises ethical and moral issues and questions related to intellectual property rights and Access and Benefit Sharing (ABS).

The Indian Biological Diversity Act, 2002

On the law front, the Indian Biological Diversity Act, 2002 and Indian Biological Diversity Rule, 2004 include provisions for ABS, that essentially regulate access to genetic resources and ensure equitable benefits. This initiative aims to maintain a fair trade-off between providers and users. The knowledge and understanding of these genetic resources are owed to indigenous communities and their inter-generational experience and learning. However, in practice, this was not happening, as all the healers were unaware of any such law and the provisions it offers.

The official from the Sikkim Biodiversity Board shared that the main mandate of the Board is to implement the Biodiversity Act, 2002. The Act has three main objectives: (1) Conservation of biodiversity, (2) Sustainable use, (3) Exercising benefit sharing. In order to function well, Biodiversity Management Committees (BMCs) are constituted at the Gram Panchayat Unit (GPU) level. At the current date, April 2021, they completed the constitution of BMCs in 187 GPUs, 7 municipal areas, and 4 districts. In total, they have 198 BMCs. Further, the People's Biodiversity Register (PBR) has been prepared for all the BMCs under different funding provisions like United Nations Development Programme (UNDP), Global Environment Facility (GEF), State Grant in Aid, National Biodiversity Authority (NBA) funding, and State Compensatory Afforestation Fund Management and Planning Authority (CAMPA). The rule or law does not prohibit the healers from collecting medicinal plants for their use. Only commercial collection is banned in Sikkim.

> "It is essential that the value of traditional knowledge is understood and valued appropriately by those who use it, and that the rights of Indigenous and Local Communities (ILCs) are considered during negotiations over access and use of genetic resources. Failing to do this can put the knowledge, the resources and the communities at risk."
> (Secretariat of the Convention on Biological Diversity, 2010, p. 5)

However, some claim that the stricter rules set by the government to collect medicinal plants goes against the healers, and thus they remain at a loss (Lepcha, 2018; Pradhan & Badola, 2008; Chhetri *et al.*, 2005). Across Sikkim, the healers practice herbal medicines and now find it difficult to obtain rare plants, which they claim are vanishing. At the same time, the state is promoting medicinal plants, leading to the commercial growth of only certain herbs that have a demand in the markets. The State Medicinal Plant Board promoted the commercial growth of the medicinal plant, which led to a monoculture of only growing Chiraita under the scheme on a national mission on medicinal plants. But, it turned out to be expensive, and marketing was a problem. Often, companies approach the Medicinal Plant Board, but the supply of these medicinal plants is not meeting the demands. Thus, people are losing their interest in harvesting these medicinal plants.

The officials also share the illegal sale of few traditional medicinal plants like the Ophiocordyceps, supplied by the local traders to Nepal, and from there, the supplies reach China. Later on, an official reported that it was difficult to stop the illegal supplies; therefore, the Government of Sikkim passed a notification and legalized the sale of Ophiocordyceps in 2002. As per the notification, the Ophiocordyceps is being collected by the members of the Joint Forest Committee. Once the collection is done, it has to be sold through auction. After selling, 75 per cent of the profit would be taken by the collector, and 25 per cent would be given to the government as royalty.

Concerns of Healers

Most of the healers were of the opinion that though there have been many meetings, and they have been called for training and given certificates, they are not really recognized for their knowledge. Most often, their knowledge is being documented—audio, video, pictures—and then they never hear back from them. However, some of them are able to sell their herbal products and herbal medicine at different fairs when they are invited, but it is purely their own initiative to collect and sell. There are no incentives given to them. They are not supported by the government. However, the officials said they are given a small amount as incentive to continue with their vocation.

Krishna Prasad Pakhurel expressed his concerns relating to the State's indifference, *"There has been no integration of knowledge of traditional healing in Sikkim. The government always talks about integration, but it has not come into existence. I have attended many workshops across the country, but they usually are of no benefit. We are asked to show the herbs we use, which they note down, but all interactions are casual and are not documented. For a workshop in Guwahati, we were promised Ayurvedic training for 6 days but none of that actually happened. On the other hand, we were told to bring the herbal medicines we use for treatment and the documents of having treated patients."*

Yamuna Prasad Bastola shared his disappointment with the outside people who do not even acknowledge them, "*Researchers come and collect details from us and later, once the work is done, they never acknowledge us. That is why we are cautious in giving out information about our herbal medicine. The least we expect is recognition and credit for sharing our time, expertise, and knowledge.*"

Nar Bahadur Limboo shared, "*The Government of Sikkim is taking us to various workshops and training. This is great, but they should aim to impart more knowledge about medicinal plants in their workshops. There is so much to learn.*" Nar Bahadur also suggested that perhaps, the government can provide them with grinding machines which cost Rs. 50,000–60,000.

Nanda Lal Subba suggested that there should be training for the healers. She said, "*I have the skills in treating the patients, but if I get the proper training, I could do it in a better way. I have continued my practices and treated many patients successfully even after the government has not supported me. Every time we are told of the arrangement of proper training, but till date, it is not done.*"

Dileep Sharma mentioned that there is a healer's association of the North East Traditional Treatment Welfare Association. It is not functional as the government does not support healers. Some incentives should be given to them in order to make sure they continue their practice. Whereas Nar Bahadur Limboo said, "*The government has given us certificates but never supported us to open and run a small hut or clinic. I was a member of the healer's association, and we consulted with AYUSH department and placed our proposal, but the government did not respond.*"

Dr. Ghanashyam, who works at TMI, Sikkim Division, since March 2009, shared that a project on ABS to create awareness among people and document the strength of healers and their knowledge was conducted. Almost 500 healers were mapped in the year 2008, but not in the whole of Sikkim. The list of healers' names and details were submitted to the Cultural Affairs Department, Government of Sikkim. They organized a healers' workshop at Jorethang, South Sikkim, inviting the healers and practitioners from different areas of the practice. After the workshop, many healers started getting recognition from the Cultural Department and are still getting a nominal amount to encourage them. However, this was not confirmed by any healer.

Since 2008, TMI is also working with the healers and community members to prepare the Peoples' Biodiversity Register (PBR) and creating awareness on the Biodiversity Act and its rules and regulations. They also work with various government bodies like the State Medicinal Plant Board, State Biodiversity Board, Sikkim University etc. The governmental department has even started working with healers, meeting them, travelling to villages and identifying the healers, documenting their knowledge and healing practices. At present, they are in the process of digitizing the People Biodiversity Register. In 2018, the Zoology Department of Sikkim University also contributed by forming 4 BMCs and helping them to prepare PBR through their university fund.

Challenges

One of the reasons for the fading away of traditional knowledge is the degradation of biodiversity. An official from the Biodiversity Board, said when people continuously use the resources of herbal plants from the forests, it is a kind of conservation. At present, the traditional healers are not given recognition for their practices, due to which they have stopped practicing traditional healing, therefore, leading to loss of knowledge of biodiversity. Therefore, the species can also get extinct from the wild, and it is also difficult for *ex-situ* conservation. Further, once the older generation, who are aware of the medicinal value, is gone, despite having the trees around, their value will not be appreciated for they won't be in use.

In many cases, healers do not form a priority issue for the government. One of the healers (name withheld) said that the State Biodiversity Board does not recognize the healers, although they are documenting the knowledge. But recently, the Government of Sikkim constituted a committee called Traditional Knowledge Committee. Departments like the Forest Department, Biodiversity Board, Sikkim Medicinal Plant Board, Horticulture Department, and Agriculture Department exist, but they are also engaged in their own work, and there is no intra-sectoral coordination among the departments. An official from the Biodiversity Board further added that in Sikkim, there is no policy for traditional healers; though now the state government has taken the initiative to form the policy for the traditional knowledge and practices along with protection of knowledge and recognizing healers.

The researcher from AYUSH shared how the Sikkim Regional Ayurveda Research Institute is working with folk practitioners through documentation of healers and validation of new plant species but raised doubts about how the healers would benefit from this. These doubts were also raised by most of the healers. He further said, 'the other challenge for disappearing traditional knowledge base is due to the fragmentation of the family. The knowledge is not being transferred to the new generation since everybody is going to English schools and do not want to work in the villages. The government wants to promote organic agriculture, but none of the students wanted to go to the farm and do agriculture. The paradigm shift that is happening from one generation to the next generation is that the knowledge and the resources will be depleted in due course of time. The documentation being done by AYUSH is excellent, and we will have that knowledge with us, but then 'who is going to practice?' The biggest loss will be the poor, marginalized sections, which will be losing even access to primary level care if we lose these healers and the biodiversity.

Recommendations

Through this study, the recommendations were gathered from the stakeholders themselves. Some of the practical and pragmatic suggestions are given below, which the State, NGOs, and other relevant boards can take up in order to promote traditional healing and conserve biodiversity. On an urgent basis, these recommendations have to be taken up.

- It is important to sensitize the younger generation regarding their culture and traditions. There are many things to learn and know about one's history that the education system does not talk about, and a gap has been created in the cultural phase (Minket Lepcha).
- Many healers suggested that they should be given a small plot of land on which they could build a small kitchen garden and grow at least 15 varieties of medicinal plants.
- The government should take the initiative to prevent the loss of medicinal plants by establishing nurseries and growing and preserving various types of medicinal plants (Dileep Sharma).
- It would be good if the government supports the healers with infrastructure (build healers' huts) where the healers could assemble, and patients can reach them easily (Mangal Bir Subba).
- A proposal can be sent to the Chief Minister or the concerned departments through the panchayat to make them aware of the consequences of loss of traditional knowledge, and a signature campaign should be done to promote the healers (Laxman Karki).
- It gets difficult for healers as old as me to do the labour work in the field for planting medicines. The government should bear the labour charges so that we can employ people to plant the herbs and medicine (Krishna Prasad).

- We are criticized by doctors and not permitted to establish a clinic. We should be able to set up a small room in the market/ town area and do an advertisement of our treatment. I would benefit from an X-ray machine to treat the patients. Other small resources such as cotton and bandages should be provided free of cost by the government (Nanda Lal Subba).
- There is a high need for reorganization of healers and collaboration between the government and faith healers (excerpts from group discussion).
- There has to be coordination between the different departments, like tourism, forest, horticulture, agriculture, and culture, to promote traditional healing.
- The officials also wanted to promote, conserve, and propagate medicinal plants at a commercial level and use the bioreserve, which is otherwise going to waste. Also involve technology, universities of repute, and commercial industries. But these suggestions need to be critically evaluated; otherwise, they may lead to exploitation.
- The Traditional Knowledge Digital Library (TKDL) should include the names of the healers and geographical location and give them due credits.
- The study concludes that if the healers are given recognition by QCI proactively and allowed to establish their healing centres by providing licence, then it would act as motivation for the younger generation to have an interest in learning the traditional healing systems.
- The study found that at every panchayat level, there are few healers who treat different ailments can be brought together and the State can help in construction of healers' huts or community healing centres at the panchayat level, where they can practice and also have few beds for inpatients. This will encourage the younger generation to learn traditional healing and continue to serve the marginalized communities at the grassroots level for primary level care.

Acknowledgements

The author is grateful to the IGNCA for funding and collaborating with Anthropos India Foundation to carry out this research. Special thanks to Dr. Sachidanand Joshi, Dr. Ramesh Gaur, Prof. Sanghmitra Acharya, and other experts for their valuable suggestions. The author is also thankful to Dr. Tshering Lepcha and Ms. Shefali for their research and audio-visual documentation and Uma Shankar for administrative support.

NOTES

1. http://envis.frlht.org/bot_search
2. https://main.ayush.gov.in/sites/default/files/Introduction_2.pdf
3. The Mountain Institute, founded in 1972, is an NGO based in Gangtok which seeks to preserve mountain environments and advance mountain cultures.
4. Chi is the locally brewed fresh rice beer.

REFERENCES

Ember, C.A., and Ember, M. (2004). *Encyclopedia of Medical Anthropology: Health and Illness in the World's Culture.* Carol R. Ember and Melvin Ember, eds. (Vols. 1–2). New York: Springer Science and Business Media.

R. Hamilton, A.C. (2004). "Medicinal plants, conservation and livelihoods." *Biodivers Conserv.* 13:1477–1517. doi: 10.1023/B:BIOC.0000021333.23413.42.

Jugli, S., Chakravorty, J., and Meyer-Rochow, V.B. (2020). "Zootherapeutic uses of animals and their parts: an important element of the traditional knowledge of the Tangsa and Wancho of eastern Arunachal Pradesh, North-East India", *Environ. Dev. Sustain. 22*, 4699–4734. https://doi.org/10.1007/s10668-019-00404-6

Lepcha, T. (2018). "Traditional Healing Practices and the Role of Traditional Health Practitioners in Primary Health Care: A Medical Heritage of Sikkim", In *The Cultural Heritage of Sikkim*. Sarit K. Chaudhuri, Sameera Maiti, and Carisma K. Lepcha, eds. (Chapter 6). New Delhi: Manohar Publishers and Distributors.

Marshall, G. (1998). "Ethnomedicine." *Oxford Dictionary of Sociology* (Second Edition). Oxford: Oxford University Press.

Ministry of Tribal Affairs, Government of India (2010). "Statistical Profile of Scheduled Tribes in India 2010." New Delhi: Ministry of Tribal Affairs.

Mohanty, R. (2011). "Impact of development project on the displaced tribals: a case study of a development project in Eastern India", *Orissa Review*, *48*(2–3), 67–73.

Muthu, C., Ayyanar, M., Raja, N., and Ignacimuthu, S. (2006). "Medicinal plants used by traditional healers in Kancheepuram District of Tamil Nadu, India", *Journal of Ethnobiology and Ethnomedicine*, *2*(1), 1–10.

Pan, S.Y., *et al.* (2014). "Historical perspective of traditional indigenous medical practices: the current renaissance and conservation of herbal resources." *Evidence-Based Complementary and Alternative Medicine, 2014.*

Pratt, C. (2007). *An Encyclopedia of Shamanism*. New York: The Rosen Publishing Group, Inc.

Sen, S., and Chakraborty, R. (2017). "Revival, modernization and integration of Indian traditional herbal medicine in clinical practice: Importance, challenges and future", *Journal of Traditional and Complementary Medicine*, *7*(2), 234–244.

Sharma, A. (2015). *The Lepchas of Dzongu Region in Sikkim: A Narrative of Cultural Heritage and Folklore*. New Delhi: INTACH.

Stoner, B.P. (1986). "Understanding Medical Systems: Traditional, Modern and Syncretic Health Care Alternatives in Medically Pluralistic Societies", *Medical Anthropology Quarterly*, *17*(2), 44–48.

Suwankhong, D., Liamputtong, P., and Rumbold, B. (2011). Existing roles of traditional healers (*mor baan*) in southern Thailand. *Journal of Community health*, *36*(3), 438–445.

Taid, T.C., Rajkhowa, R.C., and Kalita, J.C. (2014). "A study on the medicinal plants used by the local traditional healers of Dhemaji district, Assam, India for curing reproductive health related disorders", *Adv. Appl. Sci. Res.*, *5*(1), 296–301.

Tamsang, K.P. (1983). *The Unknown and Untold Reality about the Lepchas*. Kalimpong: Mani Print Press, p. 61.

Uniyal, S.K., Singh, K., Jamwal, P. *et al.* (2006). "Traditional use of medicinal plants among the tribal communities of Chhota Bhangal, Western Himalaya", *J. Ethnobiology Ethnomedicine* 2, 14. https://doi.org/10.1186/1746-4269-2-*144*(34), 2012, 13–17, ISSN 0975-3575.

Vijayagiri, R.C., and Mamidala, E. (2012, December). "Ethnobotanical investigations among traditional healers in Warangal district of Andhra Pradesh, India", *Pharmacognosy Journal*, *4*(34).

WHO (2019). *WHO Global Report on Traditional and Complementary Medicine*.

Yabesh, J.M., Prabhu, S., and Vijayakumar, S. (2014). "An ethnobotanical study of medicinal plants used by traditional healers in silent valley of Kerala, India", *Journal of Ethnopharmacology*, *154*(3), 774–789.

5

Zoopharmacognosy, Dreams and Incantation

Indigenous Healing Practices among the Zeme Naga

Avitoli G. Zhimo and *M.N. Nimal*

Margaret Mead was once asked what she considered the earliest evidence of civilization, she answered that it was a human thigh bone with a healed fracture excavated from a fifteen thousand year old site (Byock, 2012). To survive, the person should have been cared for — sheltered, protected, brought food and drink. Mead's reply emphasises the role played by healing in defining human civilization, which in turn serves as the basis for anthropological interest in the same. Health and healing are important concerns of human beings ever since the time we began living in social groups. Medical anthropology has time and again emphasized the need to recognize the cultural dimension of illness and healing. It has succeeded in directing attention to diverse ways in which health is harmed and restored among different cultures. The cross-cultural focus of medical anthropology is best reflected in ethnomedical studies. They help in understanding a variety of diagnostic and therapeutic aspects rooted in indigenous knowledge systems practised by different cultures. Ethnomedicine deals with concepts of disease and illness, disease causation principles or aetiology, deviant behaviour, magico-religious and preventive medicine, healing practices and the role of different medical practitioners (Lieben, 1973; Fabrega, 1975). Although ethnomedicine is often referred to as 'folk medicine', 'primitive medicine' or 'ethnoiatric', they all commonly convey systems of medical knowledge that are primarily transmitted orally across generations.

The use of plants as medicine for various ailments is not new to the tribes of Northeast India (Rout, 2010). Before the advent of modern allopathy, various tribes in North East India depended on traditional healers who knew medicinal plants, and the ability to fix fractured bones. The forces of globalization have been instrumental in ushering changes in many tribal communities and Zeme Naga is no exception. The traditional lifestyle including consumption and healing practices is undergoing a transition; but sometimes in conundrum, as the traditional beliefs clashes with modern ideas or new religious principles.

Locating the Zeme Naga

The Zeme are one of the Naga tribes living in Nagaland, Manipur and Assam in the Northeastern region of India. Since India's Independence in 1947 and the creation of different states subsequently, the Zeme people, despite living in one contiguous area, have been divided into three different states. This division of their population has affected the Zeme tribe politically and socially. They are known as Zeliang in Nagaland, Zeme (erstwhile Kacha Naga) in Manipur and Zemi or Zeme in Assam. Although there are about 214 Zeme villages and towns across these three states, they are still at the periphery and being marginalized on all fronts due to inadequate political representation. There are about one hundred thousand population of the Zeme in total. Just like any other tribes in transition, they practice different religions like Christianity, *Papau Renet*[1] or *Poupaise* and *Heraka*[2], of which, Christians are in majority. The Zeme speak their dialect, also called, Zeme which belongs to the Sino-Tibetan language group. There are some variations between the northern and the southern Zeme. This has become a challenge to some extent, as communication between the Zeme living in the extreme north and the extreme south becomes problematic.

The history of *Ze-Mnui* village could be described as a never-ending struggle against the challenges posed by various demographic, livelihood, topographic and climatic factors. Moreover, according to their cultural system, there are supernatural beings like spirits who freely roam around the village and interfere in the everyday life of people. Their forefathers, who had to confront the extreme difficulties posed by nature, come across many manifestations like the perennial pond or the thirty roots tree (*Ngahpei-chamrei*) which despite being boons bewildered their reasoning capacities. Hence attributed with sacredness, these marvels acted as revelations that encouraged them to seek the secret of survival within nature. The thick blanket of miraculous efforts put by their ancestors still guards the villagers against all these odds. Thus, *paupairenet* (translated as forefathers' religion), a belief system that manifests reverence and worship for their forefathers developed amongst them. The ancient wisdom, which is orally transferred across generations and proved to be pivotal for survival, intensified their faith in the past. The influence of this animistic religion could be noticed in almost all aspects of their social life.

Similar to other Naga tribes, group participation is a significant feature of Zeme social life. Be it a collection of firewood and wild fruits from the forest or agricultural activities in the fields, they depart and return in groups. This sense of togetherness influences value systems related to different social institutions thereby manifesting in decision making, norms, laws, distribution of resources, acquisition of knowledge, healing etc. By locating the traditional system of healing in the network of other social institutions, we set out to understand the cultural conception of health within the Zeme society. Unlike Ze-mnui, Impa village has abandoned the forefathers' religion. The entire village has converted to Christianity. It was learned that Christianity emerged in Impa village way back in 1947.

It was William H.R. Rivers (1924) who first described indigenous medical systems as social institutions and argued that they should be studied in the same way as social institutions in general; and that indigenous medical practices are rational actions when viewed in the light of respective causation beliefs. Leonard B. Glick (1967) later confirmed that "in many cultures, ideas and practices relating to illness are for the most part inseparable from the domain of religious beliefs and practices" (Glick, *c.f.* Foster, 1976:777). The coexistence of diverse cultural practices, traditional knowledge and social organizations within tribal systems of medicine has been emphasized. Therefore, it is not a single system but "systems of medicines, knowledge of herbs, ritualistic practices, explanatory models, amulets and charms, humoral ideology, bonesetters, midwives and myriad other ecologically meaningful and culturally appropriate ideas, beliefs, practices and personnel" (Joshi, 2004:403).

Fieldwork in Zeme Villages

The present work is an outcome of fieldwork conducted in Zeme villages on two occasions. In January 2020, as part of the curriculum, the M.Sc. Anthropology final year students at University of Delhi embarked on anthropological fieldwork led by the first author. The fieldwork was conducted in Ze-mnui also known as Yangkhullen in Manipur. The village is located on a very steep mountain in the district of Senapati, Manipur. To reach the village, the team carried their bags and climbed the steep mountain. The fieldwork was very challenging; the team had to sleep on a cold hard floor and share one common toilet. The harsh weather and discomfort did not hamper the spirit of the team. Fieldwork at Ze-mnui was full of spirit-filled stories, making us jump to every slight odd sound. On the other hand, the other village—Impa was a different experience. In the year 2015, the first author conducted fieldwork in Impa village which is in the remote part of India's northeast. The village comes under the Tousem sub-division of Tamenglong district, Manipur. It is geographically located between the states of Nagaland and Manipur. Below is the first author's account of the journey and experiences as a female researcher-cum-mother.

To reach the study village, was not a matter of a single day. It was in December 2015; the flight from Delhi to Imphal (capital city of Manipur state) took just four hours only but I had to rest at one small town Noney which is located 41 km away from Imphal. I had no option but to avail myself constant rest as I was bringing along my one-year-old daughter. After resting at Noney, I resumed my journey towards Tamenglong district headquarters, the next day. The road condition was at a deplorable stage and the journey was full of bumps and turns. In the evening, we rested at Tamenglong town. It took another day to reach Impa village. The village is located only 60 km away from Tamenglong but the difficult terrain which had remained inaccessible till 2014, prolonged the journey to a whole day. The people of Impa village had never seen a vehicle coming to their village till 2014. The road was freshly cut across rocky mountains and dense forest. Although it was just a single lane with no metal road, it was better than no road at all. My journey was disrupted when a woodcutter from a neighbouring village chopped down a huge tree thereby blocking the narrow road. It was difficult for the vehicle which I was travelling to pass through. We had to wait for reinforcement from the neighbouring village to come and cut the tree to pave the way for the vehicle. It took around four hours to clear the road, by the time it was already dark, and the winter short day had bid farewell. The nocturnal noise of the jungle was deafening. Some of the passengers I was travelling with gathered dry twigs and sticks to light a fire. It was a cold winter night and my daughter started having a runny nose. I carried my daughter on my back, covered her with a thick shawl and tried to lull her to sleep. I was reminded of the stories which I have heard during my earlier fieldworks. According to some Naga tribes' sayings, one should not call out the real names of children at night especially when you are in a thick jungle. The jungle spirits are supposed to be roaming around only in the dark. If the spirits hear the name of a child, they may be tempted to take away the child. That is why children were given names that sounded bitter for example, among the Sumi Naga, most of the boys were named 'akhakhu' (bitter eggplant) and the girls were named 'akishi' (another bitter vegetable). I never believed this concept of giving bitter names to children for fear of evil spirits but when I was situated in a space surrounded by thick jungle from all sides and nocturnal noise became too loud, I inadvertently start calling my daughter 'akhishi'. We resumed the journey to Impa village after the road was cleared of the tree debris. It was almost midnight when we reached the village. The villagers were waiting at the village council hall. They had already prepared a scrumptious dinner for us. It was too overwhelming. The absence of shared language remained a constrain.

Concepts of Illness and Health

Matei and *Manei* are the two terms that connote different types of bodily afflictions for *Zeme*. They indicate mild and severe conditions of illness respectively. A person is described as *matei* when he/she has feelings of pain or discomfort, i.e. there can be multiple factors or symptoms responsible for this condition. Appetite is often considered as an indicator of *matei*; some experience a reduced appetite while for others it is enhanced. Being in the state of *matei* does not necessarily restrain one from carrying out activities related to their everyday life. In most cases, it is the persistence of *matei* condition that leads to the confirmation of *manei* or the departure from the mind-body equilibrium. *Manei* denotes the inability to take part in everyday activities and the person is confined within the walls of the house. This involves changes in social roles, therefore, entry into the 'sick role' (Parsons, 1975).

Unlike many of the informants, who described health as a condition where one can take part in the livelihood activities normally without any hindrances, Tingnnapei, a centenarian suggested a perspective acquired from the forefathers. According to him, health is a peaceful atmosphere achieved by pleasing the spirits thanks to blessings from *Tingrangfui* (God). This hints at the logic behind their different causation beliefs and healing techniques.

Illness Aetiology

Among Zeme, both naturalistic and personalistic agents cause diseases. Naturalistic agents affect the body while later affect the soul. The *Hechuinehiak* is an example of illness caused by naturalistic factors. The black bark of *Hechui* trees, if touched, causes pox like blisters all over the body. The affected person may experience severe itching. There are two varieties of *Hechui* trees found in the forest (*Hoi Hechui* and *Hou Hechui*) among which *Hou Hechui* has more potential for causing *hechuinehiak*. The extremity of the infection may vary from person to person. Tingnnapei (chief priest), was affected some years ago. He had swollen eyes which affected his vision for more than two weeks. Personalistic causation is largely due to the intervention of spirits. There are benevolent and malevolent spirits who roam around the village and interfere in the life of humans. *Ntungbe* is a benevolent spirit who guards the village while *Radea,* a malevolent spirit, consumes the soul of a person. Diseases that affect the soul of a person can only be healed by pleasing the spirit/s. Soul loss is considered both a sickness in itself, as well as a contributing factor in other illnesses.

An equilibrium model based on the hot and cold theory of illness comprises an important aspect of disease aetiology. The roots of this theory which is based on the concept of bodily humors can be traced to the ancient Greek belief of four fundamental elements (earth, water, air and fire) and their qualities (hot, cold, dry and moist). The Greek theory ascribes personality characteristics to the four bodily fluids which are: blood (hot and moist), phlegm (cold and moist), black bile (cold and dry) and yellow bile (hot and dry). As per this tradition, an illness is believed to occur from a humoral imbalance which causes the body to become excessively dry, cold, hot, wet or a combination of these states. Food, fluids and herbs are classified under hot and cold categories which are suitably used therapeutically to restore the equilibrium. According to *Tingnnapei* (chief priest), many illnesses are said to be seasonal and associated with temperature. Meat is considered a hot object and hence restrained for people suffering from fever. At the same time, a diet with more meat is preferred during winters.

Healing Practices

Apart from causative factors, symptoms comprise important criteria for the diagnosis and healing of diseases. Symptoms like reduced or increased appetite, lethargy, tiredness etc. may be associated with multiple diseases. Usually, the elder family members suggest respective home remedies when a person exhibits symptoms related to common ailments. This may include staples like eggs, lemons, garlic, rice soup etc. In addition, herbal medicinal gardens are maintained in most households. If symptoms persist, the patient is taken to the village shaman (*Kemimeime*) for expert opinion. There are few persons specialized in massaging and bone setting. They can fix dislocated bones and minor fractures by massaging. They locate the nerves and gently massage with oil. Some traditional healers learned the craft from their father or mother, however, there are some exceptions like Raje Pame, who learned the art of setting bone by observing a raven.

Learning from Raven: The Case of a Bonesetter

The Zeme of Impa village is dependent on local healers and divine healers for immediate relief from their ailments. A case study of a local bonesetter revealed how he learnt the art of making medicine using locally available herbs and plants from a raven. Raje Pame (50M) is a bone setter in Impa village. He gets patients from all over the neighbouring villages. How he came to master the bone setting is intriguing. One fine day, he came across the nest of *Nggak* (raven) with young ones in the jungle. He broke the leg of one of the young chicks and hid behind the bushes. When the mother raven saw that her young one's leg is broken, she flew away and brought varieties of herbs and plant leaves. Everyday the man observed the mother nursing back her young one to health. Eventually, the young chick recovered and flew away. After observing for many days, the man collected all the leftover herbs and start searching for the same in the jungle. He collected the herbs used by the mother raven and experimented with them on a human being. It worked. These locally available herbs could fix broken bones. The man was unable to identify the names of the herbs. He had no idea what they were called in his dialect. This is understandable as the village Impa is very rich in vegetation. Hundreds of species do not even have names in their dialect. Learning from animal's self-medication has been reported in scientific papers too.

The science of animal self-medication is called Zoopharmacognosy. The word is derived from the roots zoo (animal), pharma (drug), and gnosy (knowing). As per Shurkin (2014), it is not clear how much knowing or learning is involved, but many animals seem to have evolved an inherent ability to sense the medicinal constituents in plants. The evidence may be circumstantial, but the examples are plenteous like Pame's findings. Shurkin (2014), a Science writer reported that many animal species have their own medicine from ingredients that are commonly available in nature. Michael Huffman (1997), a biologist argued the chimps were self-medicating. He observed how a parasite-ridden chimpanzee in Tanzania chewed the leaves of a toxic plant that has rough leaves. That plant is not a part of a regular diet. By the next day, the chimpanzee was completely recovered. Huffman theorized the chimps were consuming the plants to burnish their intestines and relieve themselves of parasites. The scientists researching zoopharmacognosy perceive that humans can learn from animals, especially in identifying new medications. Shurkin (2014) argued that folk medicine in small scale societies might have come from medicine men observing animals self-medicate. Likewise, Raje Pame's ingredients for setting bones are identified based on observation of the mother raven in action.

Dreams and Shamans

Generalist and specialist practitioners can be found in almost all folk medical systems. They may be working full-time or part-time administering folk medicines and remedies to clients regularly. In return, they may or may not receive some form of direct or indirect remuneration (Das, 2004). Some of them have been found to practice both supernatural and natural means of treatment (Kar, 2004). Shamans are distinguished from ordinary people as they possess the power to intermediate between supernatural and human to perform certain actions which can bring about changes in the real world. Ethnomedical healing practices in the village can be broadly divided into two types: those practices for healing mild ailments which could be performed by anyone for others or themselves (e.g. use of medicinal plants or animal body parts); and those meant for severe cases and epidemics which require the involvement of a specialized person who possesses exclusive knowledge and skills. *Kemimeime* or the traditional healer of *Zeme* is a hereditary status whose special powers of healing are said to be a gift from the *Tingrangfui* (God). He possesses exclusive knowledge about a wide variety of medicinal plants as well as the power to appease both malevolent and benevolent spirits through prayer. *Kemimeime* is a visionary for whom, the information about causative agents and methods of treatment were revealed in his dreams. Currently, there is no practising *Kemimeime* in Ze-mnui village as the last one died a few years ago and his son, who was supposed to take up his father's role, migrated to a nearby village.

In Impa village, there is a female shaman, who inherited healing abilities from her deceased father through her dreams. Manailiu Pame (25 F) was eleven years old when her father passed away. He was a renowned man in the hills of Manipur, Nagaland and Assam. He could heal people using indigenous herbs and plants. He was never trained by anybody; he just knew it. She recollected how his death left a big void in her life. When she attained the age of 18 years, she had a dream. Her father appeared to her in a dream and told her that he will reveal his secret of healing. He made her promise never to disclose the secret to anybody, not even her mother. She received instruction from him in her dream and obeyed his instructions when she woke up. She was able to heal people using prescribed herbs and plants. She said that it has been more than seven years that she has been healing people. She claimed that many patients from Impa and surrounding villages have been cured of kidney stones, cancer, spinal pains etc. In her village, there was no medical dispensary or hospital till 2014. For hundreds of neighbouring villagers, she was their immediate source of getting help. She said that she does what she can to help relieve and cure people. She attributed her gift of healing to God. Manailiu also added that she never disclose the ingredients she used for healing as promised to her deceased father. Manailiu as a shaman was created in her dreams of her father. Becoming a shaman in this way has been reported among the Parintintin Indians of Brazil too; they believed that dreaming is the special domain of shamans for they were created in the dreams of older shamans (Kracke, 2006).

Incantation

The chanting of series of words to cast a spell or to heal an ailment is not new to the Zeme. In fact in Ze-mnui village, it is still practised. The healing process of *Hechuinehiak* (illness caused by naturalistic factors) involves a ritual performed by the friends or relatives of the patient. Usually, two men accompany the patient to a *Tengta* tree carrying bamboo spears. From a distance (less than ten metres) the companions chant the following verses and throw bamboo spears aiming at the tree.

> *Ine qui* (poked by me)
> *Ine hei* (hit by me)
> *Ine dang* (cut by me)

A spear is thrown at the tree after each chanting. The branches of the *Dekie* tree are hanged in the *rehangki* (male dormitory) after this.

In Impa village, the incantation is not encouraged anymore due to Church's intervention. Those who were familiar with incantation voluntarily gave up so as not to antagonize the Church. There is a tendency for the converts to look at incantation as something evil or oppose to Christian beliefs. However, certain illnesses can only be cured by incantation as believed by the people in Impa. Simeon Pame (26 M) narrated how he got stung by a bee during a hunting spree. He thought that it was just a bee sting but when he reached home he was in so much pain. His relatives who saw him remarked that it was not a simple bee sting but the evil has entered into his bloodstream *via* a bee sting and hence the unbearable pain. In circumstances like this, incantation was usually sought in pre-Christian days. Hailei Pame (80 M) used to be specialised in incantation but he voluntarily gave up after converting to Christianity. He was requested by Simeon's relatives to perform incantation. He reluctantly agreed just because he did not wish to see a young man of his grandson's age withering in pain. The pain went away and Simeon was up and well the next morning. When it comes to healing, the Church has its prayer warriors and counsellors who claim to heal people through their prayers. The practices of previous faith might have discontinued but in a given circumstance, they have been sought again for immediate relief. In Impa village, the co-existence of both traditional and spiritual healing practices is evident.

Ethical Question

In Impa village, Raje Pame the bone-setter voluntarily went to the deep jungle and brought eleven unnamed herbs for us to take photographs. He obtained those herbs from the cliff. We were excited about the mysterious plants but when we asked him if other people knew about these herbs; he said he had not disclosed to anybody yet. We took photographs of the herbs but did not bother to identify their scientific names. Our stance is, if the herbs are so difficult to get and he intends to keep it secret, we should let them be. He was obliged to show his herbs because of the presence of the first author's husband who happened to be from the same village, but we decided not to betray his trust by exposing it to the outside world. Perhaps scientific intervention may be sought when the time is right and falls in favour of the original custodians like Raje Pame.

Manailiu, a young woman who has the gift of healing many serious illnesses in Impa village refused to reveal the types of herbs used for healing. She said that her deceased father made her promise never to reveal the secret to anyone. She intends to honour her father's will, and for that reason, we also need to honour the same. Most of the healers we talked to are not after material things; they did not ask for anything in return. They believed that they are doing service to society by helping and curing the sick. None of them feels that they should be rehabilitated by the government.

The Intervention of Western Biomedicine

Impa village had no road and no primary health centre. In 2014, a small hospital was established in the village. It goes by the name of Haitung Memorial Hospital and is being run with the help of Karuna Trust. Some philanthropists donated building materials and even an ambulance. The village hospital has one full-time doctor and two nurses. The nurses revealed that despite the presence of an allopathic system, the villagers hardly visit. They prefer to stick to their traditional methods of healing. Only in cases of life and death situation, they come to the hospital.

The situation in Ze-mnui is different. The government established a Primary Health Sub-centre in Bendramei[3] (5 km away from Ze-mnui) in 1981. But the people of Ze-mnui had limited access to it until the national highway connecting the village with Imphal was constructed in 1996. This marked the arrival of western biomedicine in an institutionalised form. In 2008, it attained the status of a Primary Health Centre (PHC hereafter). Currently, there are 13 staffs in the PHC including 4 doctors. The single storied building has separate rooms for labour, ward, immunization, dispensary, laboratory, OPD and storage of medicines. All medicines and 14 different laboratory services are provided free of cost.

The Accredited Social Health Activist (ASHA) programme introduced by the Government of India under the National Rural Health Mission plays a crucial role in ensuring health care services to the villagers. There are three ASHA workers in the village, who were the first batch recruited when the programme was launched in 2007. The ASHA workers directly provide health services through home visits, first-aid and immunization sessions. They pay special attention to maternal and newborn health care, along with encouraging institutional delivery at the hospitals under the supervision of health personnel. Now-a-days, the majority of pregnant women go to hospitals in Senapati town, which is 80 kilometres away from Ze-mnui, before their due date of delivery so that they are eligible for Janani Suraksha Yojana[4].

The reception of biomedicine in the village occurred in phases. In the beginning, natives were apprehensive about the new medicine as it introduced methods and concepts of aetiology alien to them. People doubted the effectiveness of biomedicine and chose not to avail services provided by the Primary Health Sub-centre. Both denominations of Christianity encouraged villagers to utilise biomedical services especially promoting childbirth under clinical care. The advocates of biomedicine argued that traditional medicine is not capable of curing new diseases introduced into the village as a result of increased interaction with the outside world. The minorities who began using biomedicine were either Christians or people who had travelled to other parts of the country. They were often ridiculed, especially by the elderly, as biomedicine was thought to be useless by the majority in the village. Many saw it as a threat to the traditions of the village. However, the minority found the new medicine efficacious and capable of faster recovery. As they began testifying in favour of biomedicine, more people began availing health services provided by the government as well as Christian agencies. 'Modern' Education played a crucial role in the spread of biomedicine. The Ze-mnui Youth Club, established by a group of educated youngsters in 1988, spread awareness among villagers about the need to use biomedicine and the importance of healthy sanitation.

Concluding Remarks

The current status of health care in both Zeme villages can be described under the rubric of medical pluralism. Although biomedical dependence has enhanced over the years, they still utilize ethnomedicinal knowledge for a variety of ailments. The villagers, especially women and the elderly, know many of the plants with medicinal values. They collect it from the village surroundings and forest. Most of the people in both Zeme villages, consider traditional bone setting practices to be more effective than biomedical treatment. Recently, a man in his middle ages met with an accident during hunting and broke a few of his ribs. He sought biomedical treatment in a hospital situated at Senapati. It took him nearly a year for complete recovery. Many of the villagers opined that traditional bone setters in the village could have healed him much faster, maybe within months. Another important factor that sustains the use of ethnomedicine is the unavailability and practical difficulties in getting biomedical services. When they get sick at night or inside the forest, they often resort to their traditional methods of healing. In such cases, they often consult the Doctors for further treatnent. Thus, ethnomedicine has now become an expedient arrangement for them.

The present chapter does not intend to counter the efforts made by government and religious agencies to provide medical healthcare service to the people of Impa and Ze-mnui. Rather, an attempt has been made to emphasize the need to recognize the cultural implications of medicine. The Zeme ethnomedical knowledge comprises key insights specific to their ecology and culture, which cannot be ignored while planning healthcare strategies for the village. The ethnomedical claims need to be scientifically verified to assess the contribution of the Zeme community to the world of healing. In that case, the intellectual property rights should remain with the actual custodians. We suggest the establishment of a combined therapeutic system capable of healing both illnesses and diseases.

NOTES

1. *Papau Renet* is the name of forefathers' religion which is still practiced by one-third of people in Ze-mnui. This term is commonly used in Ze-mnui village. However, the Zeme in Impa village refer to their traditional religion as *Poupaise.*
2. *Heraka* is a religious reform movement started by Jadonang, a Rongmei Naga in Manipur in the late 1920s. After he was hanged to death, his niece Gaidinliu led the movement in the political background of post-Independence India in North Cachar Hills district, Assam. At present, the majority of the Heraka followers are found in Assam and are mainly the Zeme Naga (Roy, 2013).
3. Development programmes that involve building of infrastructure like schools or health centre are being diverted to Bendramei village which is around 5 km away from Ze-mnui. The fact is that Ze-mnui is on a steep mountain and there is hardly any empty plot of land to build houses. The younger generation are shifting to Bendramei as it is in plain area and connected to state highway. Ze-mnui on the other hand is ecologically sensitive; it has frequent landslides.
4. A Central Government sponsored scheme implemented with the objective of reducing maternal and infant mortality rate and motivating mothers to have institutional births whereby they are paid Rs. 700 per delivery.

REFERENCES

Byock, I. (2012). *The Best Care Possible: A physician's quest to transform care through the end of life.* USA: Avery (Penguin).

Das, M. (2004). "Disease and illness and their ethno-medical treatment among Rathwas of Suskal, Gujarat". In A.K., Kalla and P.C. Joshi (Eds.), *Tribal health and medicines* (pp. 283-300). New Delhi: Concept Publishing Company Pvt. Ltd.

Fabrega, H. (1975). "The need for an Ethnomedical science". *Science, 189*(4207), 969-975.

Foster, G.M. (1976). "Disease etiologies in non-western medical systems". *American anthropologist, 78*(4), 773-782.

Huffman, M. (1997). "Current evidence for self-medication in primates: A multidisciplinary perspective". *Am. J. Phys. Anthropol.,* volume 104, issue S25, pp. 171-200.

Joshi, P.C. (2004). "The world of tribal healers". In A.K. Kalla and P.C. Joshi (Eds.), *Tribal health and medicines* (pp. 202-241). New Delhi: Concept Publishing Company Pvt. Ltd.

Kar, R.K. (2004). "Ethnomedicine and tribal health: An illustrative appraisal". In A.K. Kalla and P.C. Joshi (Eds.), *Tribal health and medicines* (pp. 376-390). New Delhi: Concept Publishing Company Pvt. Ltd.

Kracke, W.H. (2006). "To Dream, Perchance to Cure: Dreaming and Shamanism in a Brazilian Indigenous Society". *Social Analysis: The International Journal of Anthropology. 50*(2): 106-120.

Lieban, R.W. (1973). "Medical anthropology". In J.J. Honigmann and A. Alland (Eds.), *Handbook of social and cultural anthropology* (pp. 1031-1072). Chicago: Rand Mcnally Company.

Parsons, T. (1975). "The sick role and the role of the physician reconsidered". *The Milbank Memorial Fund Quarterly. Health and Society, 53*(3), 257–278.

Rivers, W.H.R. (1924). *Medicine, Magic and Religion.* New York: Harcourt.

Rout, J., A.L. Sajem, M. Nath. (2010). "Traditional Medicinal Knowledge of the Zeme (Naga) of North Cachar Hills district, Assam, on the treatment of Diarrhoea". *Assam University Journal of Science and Technology: Biological and Environmental Sciences. 5*(1): 63-69.

Roy, B. (2013). "Mapping the Heraka Identity: Are We Engaged Truly?" *Economic and Political Weekly, 48*(40): 76-78.

Shurkin, J. (2014). "News Feature: Animals that self-medicate: Many animal species have created their pharmacies from ingredients that commonly occur in nature". *Proceedings of the National Academy of Sciences of the United States of America,* Vol. 111, No. 49, pp. 17339-17341.

6
'Health and Wellness' A Perspective
A Case Study of the Devendrakula Velalar Community, Tamil Nadu

S. Sumathi, Shobana Sharma, and *Muniraj M.*

Health, Wellness and Illness Discourses

Concerns with wellness and health are universal in human life and present in all societies. Each community organises itself collectively through material means, and intangible cultural elements, to comprehend and develop techniques in response to experiences of illness and misfortune, whether individual or collective. As a consequence, each and every society develops knowledge, practices and specific institutions that may be called the health care system. Ideas of health and wellness can be found in deep history, thousands of years ago. Traditional cultures had sophisticated health care systems, aimed for balance of human body, mind and spirit and perceived human health from its holistic perspective (Cohen, 2010; Strohecker, 2010). The concept of wellness is an application of the positive definition of health; it extends beyond prevention and health promotion. The main goal of prevention is to avoid illnesses, but wellness aims for a happy, balanced, quality and fulfilled life (Donald Ardell, 1997).

The traditional health care systems across nations had many aspects in common. Besides curing a disease, their focus included religious and philosophical systems, which fused with the societal context. Traditionally the individual approach to the patient was practiced, which is so different from contemporary medicine. These traditional healthcare systems emphasised one's lifestyle, nutrition, physical activity, quality sleep, moderation, ethical behaviour, development of positive thoughts and emotions through prayer, meditation which are simple tools to keep balance in one's life (Strohecker, 2010). In scientific literature the term health and wellness is used in the same context as well-being and those terms are being used interchangeably (Miller and Foster, 2010).

Contemporary scholars who laid its foundation, while establishing the subject matter felt that achieving universal definition of wellness was not successful and explained its multiple perspectives (Corbin & Pangrazi, 2001). In practice, wellness is often simplified and becomes a synonym of everything that makes one "well and healthy". A more deep distinction between various interpretations of wellness concept has been established by Don Ardell. He talks about two concepts of wellness they are quasi/ spiritual wellness and secular wellness. The former is based on faith, emotions and spirituality and the latter is based on science, self-ethos, logical thought flow, body awareness and a deliberate search for added meaning and purpose in life. Such taxonomy brought out the integration of health and wellness at all times.

Halbert L. Dunn (1961) pioneered and used the term health and wellness in modern context and he was expert in the field of vital statistics. The quantitative interpretations proposed health and wellness as an absolute opposite of illness. Travis (1996), the founding father of wellness was inspired by Dunn's Ideas and his team of researchers developed a tool to assess one's levels of wellness known as Wellness Inventory, but more importantly the theoretical models explaining the links between human health, medical care and wellness was found application oriented. The concept of wellness aims to help people in achieving higher levels of health, more quality life, even physically ill person can live quality life. The Iceberg model of health and illness (Travis & Ryan, 2004) interprets wellness as an application of achieving positive definition of health. Applied health studies justified the relevance of illness cognition and wellness from socio-cultural perspective. Hence community specific understanding in achieving health for all should be the approach and anthropological methods should facilitate the process.

Anthropological Approaches on Health Studies

Health has been studied and perceived as an area of study for all disciplines. The resultant research has always been debated, summarised and hypothesised between these various disciplines. In spite of these differences health is the primary concern in the paradigm of development. Health from the social science perspective refers to the total fitness of an individual which would ensure performance of social roles to optimum efficiency. All societies equip their members through the process of socialisation and enculturation to play useful roles commensurate with their status. Society also provides institutional mechanism to look after the sick with a view to minimise the period and extent of disability and maximise the quantum of recovery in shortest possible period. Health is an aspect of culture, that is, a way of life of a group or a community equivalent to economic, political, social and religious aspects of a society. As a result specific study disciplines emerged to have a better understanding of these complex phenomena.

Medical anthropology emerged as an important sub-field within cultural anthropology. It takes both biological and cultural components of the society as independent variables for better understanding of health and disease among humans. Generally the definitions of health are usually infused with moral, ethical, and political implications in contemporary cultures. The universal definition of 'health' proposed by the World Health Organization (WHO), is "*overall sense of well-being*" which means that human should perceive health not as part but as a whole. Here, Glazier and Hallin (2010:925) report that a small percentage of the world's population can be classified as healthy.

Enough studies have justified that disease and illness are separate concepts. **Disease** is a physical condition which can be objectively measured and scientifically validated. It varies by groups (e.g., ethnicity and socio-economic status), geography, incidence, and severity whereas *Illness* is more of a cognitive behaviour. Illness becomes a disease when psychological or spiritual factors are tied to an individual's worldview. Miller (2011) expostulates, *health systems* discern cultural perceptions and classification of health-related issues, healing practices, diagnosis, prevention, and healers.

Three theoretical approaches have been given by Barbara Miller that attempt to understand world health systems. *Ecological/Epidemiological Approach* tries utilising the rich information from public health sectors and combined with the factors of natural environment, culture causes illness and influence the spread the same through a population. *Interpretive Approach* initiated by Claude Lévi Strauss describes the cognitive pattern of community and individuals towards health and cure attained through healing systems. The assumption here is healing system provides meaning for suffering. *Critical Medical Anthropology Approach theorises* how health systems are impacted by structural elements, e.g. social inequality, political economy, global media etc. These approaches elucidate the importance of health and wellness theories from socio-cultural perspective.

The Socio-cultural and Political System of Health

The symbolic and magico-religious dimension of any cultural group plays a prominent role in the process of understanding health. It includes the knowledge, perceptions and cognitions of the disease perceived by cultural groups. All cultures constructed the concepts of illness, diseases depending on the environment and natural resources. They also have disease classifications, and these are organised according to criteria of symptoms, severity etc. Hence classification, as well as the concepts of health and illness, are not universal and are rarely reflected in the biomedical definitions. Indigenous knowledge diagnosed and treated illness and diseases transmitted and the efficacy has been validated through the system. Culture provides etiological theories based on the culture specific worldview, and these theories can frequently indicate multiple causes of illness. Similarly, the taxonomy of specialist and the therapeutic methods has also been well structured according to the cultural values of the community.

The concept of cultural relativism evaluated the interpretations and interventions in health and illness processes, whether for individuals/ patients or for bio-medically trained health professionals, avoiding ethnocentric attitudes and analysis through the subjects of culture, who experience it in several ways, during sickness and treatment. However, professionals and researchers in the area of health, when they encounter other cultural systems, cannot process information without applying relativism to medical knowledge. While, West tries to *naturalizse* the medical field, attributing to it universal and absolute truth, distancing it from *culturalised* forms of knowledge, where truth is particular, relative and conditional.

Health and Wellness in Development and Applied Studies

The Bio-psychosocial Approach, formulated by Engel in 1977, is a comprehensive and integrative framework for understanding development, human health and wellbeing. This approach is based on the perception that—humans are inherently bio-psychosocial organisms in which the biological, psychological and social dimensions are inextricably intertwined (Melchert, 2007). This approach uses a holistic perspective focusing on psychological, biological and socio-cultural influences on development and functions along with their interactions. The main focus of developmental studies is to understand the social and psychological contexts; from family systems, developmental science, psychological, sociological, public health, feminist, and other perspectives. There is a clear difference in applied research and biomedical research. Applied research is problem-oriented, directed towards the solution of an existing problem. Biomedical research deals primarily with basic research involving processes at the cellular level and deals with issues in the environment, which promote changes at the cellular level; and behavioural research deals with the interaction of human and the environment in a manner reflecting the beliefs, attitudes and practices of the individual in society.

The above theories consistently establish the socio-cultural component and its relevance in understanding health and wellness not just dialectic. Studies have tried to understand the relationship between food literacy and food consumption that brought out the importance of hygiene and nutrition awareness with regard to health and wellness (Cullen *et al.*, 2015; Vidgen and Gallegos, 2011). Studies on food security and food consumption also have established a similar association with health and wellness (Deaton and Drèze, 2009; FAO, 2011; Patel *et al.*, 2015). Anthropological studies have established a strong interrelationship between Indigenous knowledge systems and food security (Kamwendo and Kamwendo, 2014; Lunga and Musarurwa, 2016). *Ethnomedicine* became a popular approach in anthropological cross-cultural studies of health systems. Pioneer ethnomedicine research focused on the health systems of indigenous people whereas Western biomedical practices identified these outputs as 'other knowledge systems' related to curative practices with specific causal explanations for health-related problems and included it in the scope of *ethno-etiology*.

World-view of Curative Practices

The world-view of health care process prioritised curative care/practices that treat patients with the intent of curing them, not just reducing illness. Healing is perceived as holistic where culture and spirituality are intertwined. In Western biomedical approach, *private healing* is the norm where the patient and the professional health practitioner alone interact and others are hardly permitted. In *Community healing* the social context is an important factor and viewed as collective experience. Healing practices take place in front of the whole community and often involve their participation.

Humoral healing system is an approach to treat illness by maintaining the balance between the elements of the body. The ideology of hot and cold food plays a vital role in traditional five element theory. Food and drugs are administered to offset these imbalances. In this system, healing is commonly done through informal methods, e.g. self-diagnosis and treatment (*Naattu or Kai Maruindhu* or 'Grand Ma remedies'). There are healing specialists like Shamans Midwives, Bonesetters, Chiropractors, Herbalists, and Acupuncturists who were established through practice over generations.

The health care system in traditional communities constitutes knowledge about the origins, causes and treatment of the disease, types of therapy, practitioners and their roles, agents in interaction. Over and above the knowledge, the system equipped the power relationship with other social institutions which maintain and restore the state of health and wellbeing of the community which has always been reflected through a set of symbols that are expressed through the practices, interactions and institutions; consistent with the general culture of the group, and in turn, defines, classifies and explain the phenomena perceived and classified as health and wellness. The present chapter tries to relate the role of food as a major variable in the process of substantiating health and wellness.

The social values, resource availability and cultural interpretations of food consumption are vital with regard to health and wellness. Many health conditions are caused by food and lack of nutrition and the quality of food can influence the progress of health and wellness. Particularly traditional foods of Indigenous communities acknowledge the nutritional and medicinal values of foods prepared from traditional crops, but because of manufactured social taboos, people refrain from eating such foods that have perceived lesser social value (Gartaula *et al.*, 2012). Various aspects of food security, including production, processing and consumption are derived from these social values. There are both internal and external factors which influence the choices of food decisions and bring about a paradigm shift (Cullen *et al.*, 2015). The World Development Report 2015 identified three principles; thinking automatically, thinking socially, and thinking with mental models which highlighted the influence of emotion of the people in food decision making along with contextual indication, local social networks, social norms, and shared mental models' (World Bank, 2015: 5). The report does not explicitly specify the role of food providers, but the logic in human decision-making presupposes the concept of food literacy, as it indicates human cognition.

Food Literacy and Health & Wellness

The knowledge about the production, distribution, utilisation and consumption of every food product has been well established in every culture and evolved as food literacy. It classified the information on nutrition in a reliable manner to promote and achieve optimal nutritional goals and food well-being. Conceptual or declarative knowledge, procedural knowledge and the ability to apply knowledge (Block *et al.*, 2011) constitute the food literacy. In precise, food literacy is knowledge about access to nutritious food, understand the process, analyses its efficacy and apply this knowledge in achieving good health and wellness. It brought out the relevance of access to knowledge and applying in everyday life (Vidgen and Gallegos, 2011). Contemporary food system includes social, economic, cultural, environmental and technical factors as important parameters of food literacy in contrast to traditional knowledge about nutrition, health and wellness (Cullen *et al.*, 2015; Sumner, 2013). Hence, *food literacy can also be viewed as 'cultural literacy'* (Snyder, 2009). In recent times, food literacy scholars have considered the term as learning (food skills, knowledge and behaviours) from everyday dietary practicalities which will lead to healthy living (Vidgen and Gallegos, 2014).

Everyday food practices meet the country's nutritional guidelines under the umbrella of agricultural education which can be explored and integrated with the contents of science, social studies, and health aspects of agricultural commodities. Research in food literacy has identified nine separate factors that influence food choices, namely fuel, health, culture heritage, memories celebrations, human connection, expression of love, emotions, creative outlet, and personal struggles. Aligning dietary advice with these factors in mind can improve options for health and wellness.

The Culture of Food in India

Food as a feast is an important and universal phenomena of everyday human life justified in the process of social evolution. In India, eating food is not just an activity; it is an important social tradition. Eating meals as a family is an important social occasion where all generations of the family gather, cook and eat traditional meals together. Most family social gatherings happen with little effort in India because it is common for generations of a family to live under one roof, or at least, very nearby one-another and food is an important component in festivals, rituals or celebrations.

Anthropology debates on health and wellness is relatively new and their critical engagement has been well considered (Fischer, 2014; Mathews and Izquierdo, 2008; Sarmiento Barletti, 2011). Anthropological research scholarship evidence has established the multiplicity of 'health and wellbeing' and justified the ethnographic profile of the studied communities (Mathews and Izquierdo, 2009). Studies have re-affirmed the role of food as markers of identities at different levels, ethnic to national. Linda Keller Brown and Kay Mussell (1987) studied the ethnic and regional food ways in the United States of America, Tanaka, (1995) and Ohnuki-Tierny (1993) assessed the role of rice in Japanese identity, while Harbottle (2000) examined both ethnic and gender identity issues among the British Iranian Communities. Quite a number of studies examined different dimensions of gender issues related to food.

Politics of food, which incorporates issues related to colonialism, has inspired several significant studies. Sokolov (1991) discussed the universal impact of colonialism, both in the old and new worlds, on the choice of food. Archetti and Napolitano's study on Ecuador exposes the conflict at the level of knowledge (1997), while Ochoa examines the use of food as a political tool in Mexico (2000). Several other authors like Nabhan (2001), Watson and Caldwell (2005) described the political roles of food in different parts of the world. Food security has been identified as a crucial political issue in the post-colonial world by the anthropologists as well. Pottier (1999) discussed the social dynamics of food security as part of his anthropological study.

All cultures have their own body of knowledge on food and on human behaviour. When the folklore, riddles and anecdotes found among the people are studied, those might reveal important insights into culture contacts of the distant and near past, changes in the collective value system and various culture dynamics of more recent times. Till date much of the knowledge has had been transmitted orally, only a fraction of it has been written down or documented. The existing literature can be classified into several distinct genres. Starting from economic discourses on procurement, production, distribution, availability, affluence, wastage and scarcity of food, there are innumerable studies on nutritional and other physiological impact of food on human groups. The anthropological writings on food have examined various dimensions of human behaviour; those studies have critically examined the traditional knowledge as well as the political and historical perspectives to the recent perceptions and popular discourses on the subject.

The theoretical and conceptual analysis has brought out the relevance of culture of food, indigenous knowledge system, identity and the power of politics and its interrelation with health and wellness. In this chapter we try to bring about the conceptual understanding and substantiate it with empirical evidence. The case study analysis of a community re-affirmed the role of food, food providers, knowledge system, habitat, and social status, as markers of identities at comparative levels.

Methodology Applied

The philosophical approach to research is basically of two types: empirical and theoretical. Health research in general follows the empirical approach, i.e. it is based upon observation and experience with theory and abstraction. Epidemiological research, for example, depends upon the systematic collection of observations on the health-related phenomena of interest in defined populations. Empirical and theoretical research complement each other in developing an understanding of the phenomena, in predicting future events, and in the prevention of events harmful to the general welfare of the population of interest. Empirical research in the health sciences can be qualitative or quantitative in nature. Generally, health science research deals with information quantitative nature. Observational types of studies generally employ the method of sample surveys, where a sample of the population is observed for various characteristics. This may be by actual interviews of the subjects, by obtaining information from existing sources. The key *anthropological perspectives* are holism, relativism, comparison, and fieldwork. There are also both scientific and humanistic tendencies within the discipline that, at times, conflict with one another.

The present empirical study followed 'Case study' method, as a part of 'situational analysis,' in anthropological research of the post-colonial world. The narrations of individuals and groups within these situations to exhibit the morphology of a social structure, which is most often held together by conflict itself. Each case is taken as evidence of the stages in the unfolding process of social relations between specific persons and groups. When seen as such, we can dispense with the study of sentiment as accidental eruptions of emotions, or as differences of individual temperament, and bring depth to the study of society by penetrating surface tensions to understand how conflict constructs human experiences and gives shape to these as 'social dramas', which are the expressions of cultural life. "Narrative anthropology suggests that to capture and convey passion, to "accurately convey the lives of strangers, their systems of significant symbols, and the plots and counterplots of life" (Langness and Frank, 1978:21) requires not only difficult research to understand the plot in others' lives, but also a rich and flexible prose style. The content and discourse analysis facilitated the interpretation drawn. Besides, the secondary sources data were substantiated through archeological and literary evidences.

The above mentioned theories and methods have been used for our empirical understanding of the studied agricultural community of south India called as *Devendra Kula Vellalar*. Their role as the *food providers* for the society, their indigenous knowledge in *ensuring food for the health and wellness* of the communities, and the use of indigenous irrigation techniques in particular to integration of ecology and environment in their space and time. Lastly, to establish their unique identity for shading of their derogative and humiliating social stigma imposed by the oppressive dominant community has been empirically substantiated. The revivalist movement for three centuries fought by the community has been validated by the policy makers following the norms adopted by the government. The narrative analysis of the case and its interpretations are as follows.

Case Study

The government of Tamil Nadu had requested for an ethnographic study, categorised into the nomenclature of Scheduled Caste (SC), to the Department of Anthropology, University of Madras, to understand community who were claiming their collective identity as *Devendrakula Velalar* for about three centuries. The other dominant agricultural communities who own the lands used the term *Vellalar as* suffice were strongly objecting the community claim and socio-politically limiting the same. The "community" who claim for the collective identity were inhabitants demographically placed across the thirty-eight districts of Tamil Nadu. Intensive fieldwork was for a year started and initially started with key informant Interviews, studying Government G.Os issued from the time of Colonial rule, decrypting the archeological evidences from the copper plates. Collecting and understanding the land documents which were at times more than a 200 years old. The next stage was focus group discussions, one on one interviews and participant observation among the three hundred odd villages which were researched by the team of anthropologists.

The thick description data collected, consolidated around their agricultural knowledge system, unique irrigation technique, their pride as a food providers and as determinants of health and wellness of the society. This study has followed the ethnographic approach and process documentation. For the purpose of this chapter, the repetitive occurring narrations, the dominating discourse and iterative content were identified and interpretation drawn as follows:

Historical Precedence and Archival Evidence

Their population distribution is across Tamil Nadu in the districts of *Madurai, Virudhunagar, Ramanthapuram, Thoothukudi, Tirunelveli, Tiruchirappalli,* and *Thanjavur*. They have significant number within the SC communities as seen from the given table below. The community claim that they are descendent from *Lord Devendra* who is the rain god (*Mazhai Kadavul*). The major concentrations of community was in the Pandya, Chola and Kongu regions. The Palani Cheppedu (1528) is an archival evidence available in the Madurai Museum proclaiming them as indigenous agriculturalists. The same has been further reaffirmed in the year 1749 through another copper-plate. The community claim they had a strong relationship with the local ecology which is validated through Classical Tamil literature poems (*thinais*) or modes which classified the emotions of humans depending on the nature, location, mood and type of relationship represented.

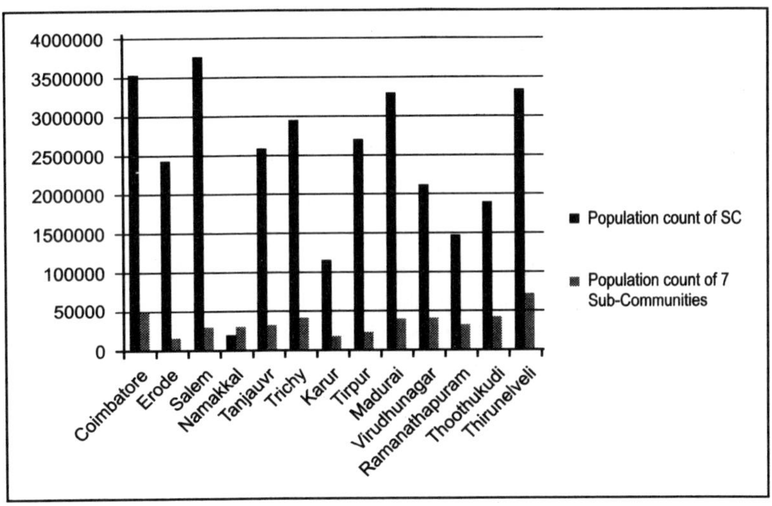

Interpretation

The community overwhelmingly believed that they are descendants of lord *Devendra* and proclaimed their pristine position in the social structure by identifying themselves with the creator and providers. The narration was always connected with them being the custodians of wellness of the society. The archival and literature evidences give validated interpretation to how each of these five *thinai are* closely associated with a particular landscape, and imagery associated with that landscape — its flowers, trees, wildlife, people, climate and geography.

Livelihood and Economic System

Agriculture and its associated work was the mainstay of the community and the major crop cultivated was Paddy. Both men and women work in the land. Traditionally, they shared their grains with all the other service communities like Aasaari, (goldsmith, Ironsmith and carpenter), Kuyavan (Potter), Pandaram (ritual service provider), Vannaan (*dobhi*), Ambattan (barber), Chakilis (cobbler), and Pusaari (Temple priests) through barter system.

Interpretation

As Food growers they ensured the all-round wellbeing of the members of the society by distributing the grown crops to each and every family that resided in their geography. It was their responsibility to provide nutritious diet to all while ensuring a healthy environment that had an abundance supply of resources. Traditionally, the hierarchical society saw them as food providers for the service communities which placed them in the top of the pyramid in the power structure. The modernisation and industrialisation process pushed them to the lowest position by the dominant communities and neglected their knowledge system, their role as food providers, ensuring the wellness of the entire community and ultimately referred them with derogative names.

Power and Politics

They have a strong traditional political system, the leaders within the community are elected by heredity and voice vote. The *Oor Kudumban* is the leader. To assist him the community has *Oor Kaaladi* and *Variyan*

(Messenger) and this is a heredity post. Both of them look after the village deity's temple and organise festivals. All disputes, including divorce, are settled by the traditional political system, cash fines are imposed for the grievance. Usually this political system does not permit divorce. To conduct village *thiruvizha* (festivals) the community head fixes the *Vari* (tax) which is compulsory for all households. There is a reduction only for widows and, who can pay half of the *Vari* (tax). The system was well organised and socially sensitive enough.

Interpretation

They had a mature political system which saw '*the welfare state*' being practiced, in their system of taxing the under privileged were given certain exemptions. The ables were given appropriate roles this saw an emergence of rigorous power structure within the community. Considering the evolved political structure as an indicator of development, the community justified those they never in a subjugated position.

Knowledge System and Mastery

As an agricultural community they were conservators of the social welfare of the community and environment. Their ability and vision to manage the food requirement of the then existing communities was based on the oral tradition of knowledge in which each generation passed on the information to their children. This is mentioned in the book 'Dying Wisdom' from the Centre for Science and Environment which exalts the water management in Tamil Nadu through the cascade tanks.

The *Devendrakula Velalars* had mastered Agriculture, Man and Ecology (AME) integration. Their skill in agriculture starts from their ability to identify the taxonomy of land in the traditional division of *Kurunji,* (Hill Agriculture), *Mullai* (Forest land), *Maruda* (Plains and fertile pasture land along the water source), *Neidal* (Seashore—Livelihood along the sea coast) and *Palai* (Desert or infertile Land). They were highly skilled in *Neer Pasanam* (Water management), for example the *Aaru pasanam* (River water management), *Kulathu Pasanam* (Pond water management) and *Kamma Pasanam* (Lake water management). These were three main sources of water for the livelihood of the society. River water was used for household and irrigation, pond water was used for the animals and plant life forms and lake water was again used for irrigation purposes. They still predicate the weather for the next day in the traditional observation method, this traditional wisdom was drawn from an intimate knowledge of plant and animal life. Just by observing Butterflies, ants and snakes which usually show up and move around just ahead of rainfall. Goats flapping their ears indicate imminent rain. A few repetitive proverbs which justify their ability as food provider for health and wellbeing are given here,

For example,

'*Nila Vattamitta mazhai oondu*' (meaning if there is a circle around the moon to would rain the next day).

'*Saamai soru Aamai Aayul*' (Little millet rice gives you the longevity of a turtle).

'*Kolundri nadapavarum Kambangkuzhaal Kaalundri Nadapaar*' (A old person walking with a stick will start walking without a stick if he had pearl millet porridge).

'*Thinai oondaal thekkupol oodal valuvaagum*' (If one has foxtail millet their body will be as strong as teak).

Interpretation

They were great strategists in water resource management for both the people and ecology, this ensured health and wellbeing of not only humans but for other life forms, like animals, plants and trees. They exhibited oneness with nature; air pollution and contamination of soil and food were unknown during the times when these communities were the guardians of land and water. The *Madai Kudumbans* were the water managers and it was a hereditary occupation where the father mentored and coached his son on how to manage the water resources for all the villages which depended them. Their expertise was to ensure water for irrigation as well as for potable drinking water.

As food providers for the society the proverbs mentioned above were strictly adhered and these communities ensured that health and wellness were more important that wealth. They lament that the health and wellness system fell apart when the British took over the administration and water resource management. The ecological rationality was overlooked by the colonial bureaucracy who could never understand the relationship built between nature and agriculture.

Today in the Western world Health and Wellness have become buzzwords and have gone corporate, Profit and loss studies on wellness programmes show return on investments is about $3.00 for every $1.00 spent (Baicker, Cutler, and Song, 2010). Wellness is a word which captures the sense that the period of fighting diseases has given way to a more complex situation of modernity: 'living well', as many of us live long lives, without the diseases that affected our ancestors. an idea that medical sociologist David Armstrong (2009) expounds. Today we speak of *health behaviours* or *risk factors*, but these are simply current terms for individualised explanations for health outcomes, however, these ideas have been with us a longtime as the roots of the concept extend far back into the history of ideas about health, morality, and responsibility. Longtime wellness researcher Dee Edington (2009, 2012) argues about taking a broader cultural and environmental approach in implementing a wellness programme, *wellness* is indeed a defining buzzword that captures so much about our relationships to health and personal responsibility. In "Wellness as a Worldwide Phenomenon", awareness of the importance of wellbeing can be discerned across the human and social sciences, with over 3000 studies on the topic published since 1960 (Nettle, 2005). The core dilemma of modernity is that in Western societies, although we have seen an unprecedented growth in wealth and comfort over recent decades but average levels of wellbeing have not increased.

In conclusion as Cohen and Strohecker said traditional culture of communities aimed for balanced human body, mind and spirit and perceived human health from its holistic perspective. Capitalist system of production and consumption has dominated the contemporary society, resulting in widespread social change which involved the abandonment of traditional sources of meaning, such as religion or a fixed place in the social hierarchy. A sense of self and purpose in life are no longer assigned or, so their development becomes a key task (Featherstone, 1991). The case study of *Devendrakula Velalar* community showed their cognitive ability was far superior in agriculture, ecology, climate change which led to health and wellness of the society. The community's claim as food providers for health and wellness was affirmed through continuous revivalist ethos. These identity claims of health determinants received universal approval as development criteria prioritising holistic wellness was the prime factor. The chapter tries to substantiate that indigenous knowledge of parochial communities was sagacious when the advancement of technology was at its prudent best. Health and wellness for all was the motto that was the unwritten law. Healthy relation with climate, environment and land is the way for the future generation of the community.

REFERENCES

Ardell, D.B. (1979). *High level wellness, an alternative to doctors, drugs, and disease*. Bantam Books.

Atkinson, S., S. Fuller and J. Painter (2012b), "Introduction", In *Wellbeing and Place*, (ed.) S. Atkinson, S. Fuller and J. Painter (Farnham: Ashgate), pp. 1–14.

Atkinson, S., S. Fuller and J. Painter (eds.) (2012a), *Wellbeing and Place* (Farnham: Ashgate).

Bina, O., and Vaz, S.G. (2011). "Humans, environment and economies: From vicious relationships to virtuous responsibility". *Ecological Economics*, Vol. *72*, pp. 170-178.

Block, L.G., Grier, S.A., Childers, T.L., Davis, B., Ebert, J.E., Kumanyika, S., ... and Bieshaar, M.N.G. (2011). "From nutrients to nurturance: A conceptual introduction to food well-being", *Journal of Public Policy and Marketing*, Vol. *30* (1), pp. 5-13.

Brown, L.K., and Mussell, K. (1984). *Ethnic and regional foodways in the United States: The performance of group identity*. University of Tennessee Press.

Christopher, J.C. (1999). "Situating psychological well-being: Exploring the cultural roots of its theory and research", *Journal of Counseling and Development*, Vol. *77* (2), pp. 141-152.

Conradson, D. (2012), "Wellbeing: Reflections on Geographical Engagements", In *Wellbeing and Place*, (ed.) S. Atkinson, S. Fuller and J. Painter (Farnham: Ashgate), pp. 15–34.

Corbin, C.B. and Pangrazi, R.P. (2001). "Toward a uniform definition of wellness: A commentary", *President's council on physical fitness and sports research digest*.

Corsín Jiménez, A. (ed.) (2007), *Culture and Well-being: Anthropological Approaches to Freedom and Political Ethics* (London: Pluto Press).

Cullen, K.W., Chen, T.A., and Dave, J.M. (2015). "Changes in foods selected and consumed after implementation of the new National School Lunch Programme meal patterns in southeast Texas". *Preventive medicine reports*, *2*, pp. 440-443.

Cullen, T., Hatch, J., Martin, W., Higgins, J.W., and Sheppard, R. (2015). "Food literacy: Definition and framework for action", *Canadian Journal of Dietetic Practice and Research*, Vol. *76* (3), pp. 140-145.

Deaton, A., and Drèze, J. (2009). "Food and nutrition in India: facts and interpretations", *Economic and Political Weekly*, pp. 42-65.

Dunn, H.L. (1959). "High-level wellness for man and society", *American journal of public health and the nations health*, Vol. *49*(6), pp. 786-792.

Fisheries, F.A.O. (2011). "Aquaculture department, 2013". *Global aquaculture production statistics for the year*.

Gartaula, H., Niehof, A., and Visser, L. (2012). "Shifting perceptions of food security and land in the context of labour out-migration in rural Nepal", *Food Security*, Vol. *4*(2), pp. 181-194.

Gilbert, J.L. (1962). "Hormones and the Metabolic Processes of the Body", *Humors, Hormones, and Neurosecretions*, p. 40.

Glazier, Stephen D. and Mary J. Hallin. (2010). "Health and Illness," In 21st Century Anthropology: A Reference Handbook, Vol. 2, edited by H. James Birx, pp. 925-935. Thousand Oaks, CA: SAGE Reference.

Harbottle, L. (2000). *Food for health, food for wealth: Ethnic and gender identities in British Iranian communities*, Vol. 3. Berghahn Books.

Jiménez, A.C., and Willerslev, R. (2007). "An anthropological concept of the concept: Reversibility among the Siberian Yukaghirs", *Journal of the Royal Anthropological Institute*, Vol. *13*(3), pp. 527-544.

Kamwendo, G., and Kamwendo, J. (2014). "Indigenous knowledge-systems and food security: Some examples from Malawi", *Journal of Human Ecology*, Vol. *48*(1), pp. 97-101.

Langnes, L.L., and Frank, G. (1978). "Fact, fiction and the ethnographic novel", *Anthropology and Humanism Quarterly*, Vol. *3*(1-2), pp. 18-22.

Lewith, G.T. (1982). *Acupuncture: its place in western medical science*. Harper Thorsons.

Lunga, W., and Musarurwa, C. (2016). "Indigenous food security revival strategies at the village level: The gender factor implications", *Jàmbá: Journal of Disaster Risk Studies*, Vol. *8*(2).

Marcus, G.E., and Fischer, M.M. (2014). *Anthropology as cultural critique: An experimental moment in the human sciences*. University of Chicago Press.

Mathews, G., and Izquierdo, C. (2009). "Anthropology, happiness and well-being", *Pursuits of happiness: Well-being in anthropological perspective*, pp. 1-19.

Mathews, G., and Izquierdo, C. (Eds.). (2008). *Pursuits of happiness: Well-being in anthropological perspective*. Berghahn Books.

Maxwell, S., and Smith, M. (1992). "Household food security: A conceptual review", *Household food security: Concepts, indicators, measurements*, Vol. *1*, pp. 1-72.

Miller, Barbara. (2011). "Cultural Anthropology", 6th edition. Boston: Prentice Hall.

Miller, G., and Foster, L.T. (2010). "Critical synthesis of wellness literature".

Nabhan, H. (2001). *Soil fertility management in support of food security in sub-Saharan Africa*. Food and Agriculture Organisation.

Oniang'o, R., Allotey, J., and Malaba, S.J. (2004). "Contribution of indigenous knowledge and practices in food technology to the attainment of food security in Africa", *Journal of food science*, Vol. *69*(3), CRH87-CRH91.

Patel, A., Sindhu, D.K., Arora, N., Singh, R.P., Pruthi, V., and Pruthi, P.A. (2015). "Biodiesel production from non-edible lignocellulosic biomass of Cassia fistula L. fruit pulp using oleaginous yeast Rhodosporidium kratochvilovae HIMPA1", *Bioresource Technology*, Vol. *197*, pp. 91-98.

Patel, R. (2009). "Food sovereignty", *The journal of peasant studies*, Vol. *36*(3), pp. 663-706.

Pottier, J. (1999). *Anthropology of food: the social dynamics of food security*. Polity Press.

Prior, I.A. (1971). "The price of civilization". *Nutrition Today*, Vol. *6*(4), pp. 2-11.

Sarmiento Barletti, J.P. (2011). *Kametsa asaiki: The pursuit of the 'good life' in an Ashaninka village* (*Peruvian Amazonia*) (Doctoral dissertation, University of St Andrews).

Shlygin, G.K., Lindenbraten, L.D., Gapparov, M.M., Vasilevskaia, L.S., Ginzburg, L.I., and Sokolov, A.I. (1991). "Radiothermometric research of tissues during the initial reflex period of the specific dynamic action of food", *Meditsinskaia radiologiia*, Vol. *36*(5), pp. 10-12.

Snyder, S. (2009). "Ethnographies of taste: cooking, cuisine, and cultural literacy", *Journal of agricultural and environmental ethics*, Vol. *22*(3), pp. 273-283.

Spielmaker, D.M., and Leising, J.G. (2013). "National agricultural literacy outcomes", *Logan, UT: Utah State University, School of Applied Sciences and Technology. Retrieved September*, *12*, 2015.

Steven Connor. (2001). "Deadly malaria may have risen with the spread of agriculture," *National Geographic*. http://news.nationalgeographic.com/news/2001/06/0625_wiresmalaria.html.

Strohecker, J., Barter, M., and Cohen, K. (2010). "Bilateral Adrenal Hemorrhage from Prophylactic Subcutaneous Low-Molecular-Weight Heparin Injections: 361", *Journal of Hospital Medicine*, Vol. *5*, pp. 185-186.

Sumner, J. (2013). "Food literacy and adult education: Learning to read the world by eating", *Canadian Journal for the Study of Adult Education*, Vol. *25*(2), pp. 79-92.

Tanaka, S. (1995). "Emiko Ohnuki-Tierney. Rice as Self: Japanese Identities through Time", Princeton: Princeton University Press. 1993. pp. xi, 184. $19.95.

Thin, N. (2008). "Realising the substance of their happiness: How anthropology forgot about Homo gauisus", *Culture and well-being*, pp. 134-155.

Travis, J.W., and Ryan, R.S. (2004). *Wellness workbook: How to achieve enduring health and vitality*. Random House Digital, Inc.

Travis, S.S., Duncan, H.H., and McAuley, W.J. (1996). *Mall walking: An effective mental health intervention for older adults*.

Vidgen, H.A., and Gallegos, D. (2011). "What is food literacy and does it influence what we eat: A study of Australian food experts".

Vidgen, H.A., and Gallegos, D. (2014). "Defining food literacy and its components", *Appetite*, Vol. *76*, pp. 50-59.

Watson, J.L., and Caldwell, M.L. (2005). *The cultural politics of food and eating: a reader*. Blackwell Publishing.

Armstrong, David. (2009). "Origins of the Problem of Health-Related Behaviours," *Social Studies of Science* 39, No. 6: 909–26.

World Bank. (2015). Millennium Development Goals.

World Health Organization. (2013). World Health Organization Health Impact Assessment. www.who.int/hia/evidence/doh/en/

7
PVTGs Health Status and Health Access Livelihood Framework

Sonia Kaushal

Introduction

We are living in a world of inequalities. Inequality is evident in all aspects of life, including social, economic, political, educational, and health. The concept of equality is utopian and no known state in history ever completely provided equal rights to its citizens. Although most of the governments take necessary steps to minimise the disparity, yet the inequality prevails (Kaushal, 2019). One of the important areas where inequality is evident and requires appropriate measures to minimise it, is health. Health is a fundamental right of every individual and the health facilities and resources should be within the reach of every person so that he/she could economically and socially lead a productive life.

The healthcare system in every country strives to provide better care and the primary health services are designed in such a manner that they are available to everyone. Access to healthcare is determined by the community's use and supply of health services (Travassos & Martins, 2004). According to studies, certain communities, such as refugees, settlers, and indigenous peoples, are still vulnerable (Oliveira, & Pereira, 2013). Ensuring better healthcare access is the goal of every countries healthcare system. Regardless of massive efforts to improve the healthcare access especially among vulnerable population remains a serious issue. For instance, the study conducted on Mexican immigrants in USA indicates that undocumented immigrants were excluded from the patient protection and affordable care act and they were not entitled to access health care services (Vargas *et al.*, 2012). Another study focused on the rural settlement in the north-west region of the State of Rio Grande do

Sul states that the families are not able to access the health services due to poor living conditions (Wunsch *et al.*, 2014). The quilombola communities in the state of Goias also stressed on the difficult healthcare access issue and quality care (Santos & Silva, 2014). Therefore, healthcare access is a critical problem that needs immediate attention. Despite the fact that various countries are taking measures to reduce health disparities, there is no globally recognised concept of "equitable access" (Oliver & Mossialos, 2004). Hence, provision of comprehensive health care to the vulnerable people is a complicated issue. The governments across the world are coming up with various strategies to meet the health needs of vulnerable tribal people.

The inequality among vulnerable tribal people is more pronounced in India because the concept of tribe in Indian context is debatable and complex. The concept carries not only the colonial burden and stereotypes but it has also created a division between tribal and non-tribal communities. The gap is also widened the way the concept of tribe has been perceived in the popular discourse. This popular discourse is value loaded with assumptions and glorifies the certain image of tribe. On the contrary, the 'tribal reality' is far more away from what has been perceived and written (Srivastava, 2008). The tribal communities are not any more isolated living groups in the hilly terrains or forested areas. Tribal communities are interacting with the mainstream societies. Moreover, the rapid deforestation, conflict, loss of land, depletion of natural, economic and social resources compelled the tribals to migrate to cities in search of livelihood. The migration has no doubt ensured the survival but has also resulted into the distress, anxiety and low health care access.

The expert committee on the tribal health in India, in their report, voiced that the comparison of 9 indicators to assess the social and health outcomes reflect poor outcomes for the tribal population in most of the countries (MoHFW, 2018). The study claims that tribes' health has improved dramatically as a result of the Government of India's efforts after Independence, but that their condition is still worse than that of other social classes. Apart from a lack of numbers, efficiency, and funding, tribal health care suffers from a significant design issue of appropriateness and lack of involvement.

The health system represents contrasting health care access in India. It is evident from the health research that the huge disparities are present in the rural-urban healthcare services (Nagaraja & Veeradhrappa, 2018; Barik & Thorat, 2015). Even the extent of health care services disparity in vulnerable or marginal tribal population is aggravated due to livelihood instability. In healthcare access, livelihood insecurity is a major factor. Studies based on the Health access livelihood framework reveals that the relationship between access to household and community assets fall under the umbrella of livelihood resources and economic, political, and technical powers influence these assets, and people have little control over them. Access to health care must be enhanced, as well as the alignment of health care assets with livelihood assets needed (Obrist *et al.*, 2007). Therefore, the present chapter tries to explore the relationship between healthcare status of PVTGs and their livelihood insecurity through Health Access Livelihood Framework.

Health Status of Particularly Vulnerable Tribal Groups (PVTGs)

Tribal groups have traditionally lived in or near forests, relying on forest resources for survival. For centuries, their needs were fulfilled but their association with the forests changed with the colonisation. The Indian Forests Act (1865) established by British was first attempt to control the forest resources and imposed restrictions on the tribes to access the forest resources. However, after Independence, legislatures have been made to rectify the afflictions. The tribes have been reclassified as Scheduled Tribes (ST) and they were granted some administrative and political privileges. However, the criteria to identify any community as ST were not specific. Therefore, the Lokur Committee was formed in1965 to resolve the issue but unfortunately the criterion identified by the committee has no relevance in today's context (Srivastava, 2008). The criteria to identify the tribe as ST are: (i) primitive traits, (ii) distinctive culture, (iii) geographical isolation, (iv) shyness of contact with the outside world, and (v) backwardness. According to the Dhebar Commission study, 52 groups of underdeveloped, low-populated people are recognised as a Scheduled Tribe's subcategory known as "Primitive tribal community" in 1979 and then 23 more tribal groups were added, bringing the total number of tribal groups in PTGs to 75. These tribal communities renamed as Primitive Tribal Groups (PTGs) in 1979 and renamed again as Particularly Vulnerable Tribal Groups (PVTGs) 2006 (Kumar & G.K., 2019).

The PVTGs are considered vulnerable as they have declining or stagnant population, low level of literacy, inaccessible habitation, pre-agricultural level of technology. These PVTGs are experiencing socio-economic and political, educational and health marginalisation. The UNDP (2013) report on Livelihood Promotion Strategies for PVTGs highlights that in 2002, Ministry of Tribal Affairs, Government of India has decided to minimize the disparity among tribal groups and to achieve this goal the state governments are directed to conduct a survey to understand the socio-economic condition and other factors which hamper the upliftment of these PVTGs. The state governments even charted out various development schemes for these PVTGs. The efforts by state governments could not bring any kind of change in the socio-economic status of these tribal and none of the tribal group was removed from the PVTGs list. Unfortunately after so many efforts no state government has proposed the removal of any group from the list. Therefore, the Government of India (GoI) has made significant efforts to improve the socio-economic and health indicators, despite this, there are tribes which are at the verge of annihilation.

The health is determined by complex interplay of social-economic and other related factors. It does not exist in vacuum. The health status of vulnerable tribal population is shaped by the geographical isolation, lack of education, forest destruction, land-alienation, poverty, displacement and migration as all these factors together act as barriers to access the health care services. The other hindrances to the healthcare access of the tribes are the discrimination and lack of cultural understanding and sensitivity by the health staff. Even the health-care system ignores the marginalised tribal groups socio-cultural values and traditions related to health (UN, 2015).

Rural areas have a stronger primary healthcare system that is more structured and organised in comparison to tribal areas. The tribal areas are provided with the primary health care infrastructure for the first level contact with the community members and the health provider. These health care providers play important role in implementing the family welfare and health schemes. The specialised health services are given either in secondary or tertiary health centres. The PVTGs has to cover a long distance to reach the nearest health centre. The unfriendly behaviour of the health personnel, shortage of medicines and diagnostics, their own belief regarding certain illnesses etc. deter the PVTGs to utilise the health care services. The PVTGs tend to underutilise the healthcare services because the system is alien to them and it does not fit into their world view. Regardless of the fact that rural areas are provided with better health services and infrastructure, the attitude of staff, inaccessible area, language, specific belief system of the tribal groups and livelihood insecurity plays important role in the underutilisation of the health services by the PVTGs (SCSTRTI & AIPH, 2015).

The habitats and socio-cultural matrix of the PVTGs have been threatened by displacement and by ignoring their historical rights in lieu of conservation of wildlife and natural resources (Chakma, 2014).

The main subsistence economies of PVGTs are pre-agricultural based but developmental projects force them to uproot from their homeland. The Protected Area policies (National parks, Sanctuaries, Conservation reserves etc.) have displaced many such indigenous communities from their original abode and led to their impoverishment (Kothari, 2008). The food gathering and NTFP is affected by new conservation policies and forest regulations. Some of these PVTGs are even forced to evict the core areas of forest under Project Tiger (Rao, 2015). In Achanakmar Tiger Reserve, 2009, Baiga families had to leave their traditional source of livelihood. The Baiga families were removed from the tiger reserve and rehabilitated to another place without receiving *pattas* for farming and compensation under the Project Tiger Relocation Scheme (Bera, 2012). Likewise, the Dongriya tribe of Odisha's Niyamgiri Hills has been displaced and evicted from the forests, and their inability to access forest resources has had a significant effect on their socio-economic situation (Dash, 2016). The deprivation of traditional habitat has also resulted in the forced migration of these groups to the mainstream land and reduced their status to the unskilled labour workers.

The health inequities among tribal communities in selected districts of Chhattisgarh, Jharkhand, and Odisha are examined in a study published recently by SAMA Resource Group for Women and Health (2018) titled "From the Margins to the Middle." The report emphasised the connection between tribal communities' poor health and their social, economic, and political marginalisation. The SAMA (2019) report, shows that PVTGs from Chhattisgarh (Pahari Korwa and Baiga), Odisha (Bhunjia and Dongriya Kondh), and Jharkhand (Asur and Korwa) migrate to larger cities on a seasonal basis. They work as daily wage labour, which is a low-paid and insecure. The health status of the PVTGs is severely affected by the alien environment, poor sanitation and water facility as well as demanding workload. Furthermore, the unawareness of the health facility or unfamiliar health facility, language, loss of wage due to visit to the health facility have adverse impact on their overall well-being. The report also highlights the Health inequalities among tribal communities, tribal patients' tuberculosis and sickle cell disease care is halted due to migration. The migration has a particularly negative impact on pregnant women. Pregnant women are the ones who suffer the most because they do not have access to routine ANC and PNC facilities at work. The immunisation and nutrition of children are also affected. The tribes who migrate to the cities struggle to integrate into the host society. They have their own reservations regarding treatment process, perception regarding certain cultural specific illnesses and their traditional healing. The tribal identity and migration to the urban space has shaped new vulnerabilities. Thus double folded vulnerabilities of the migrant tribal people increases low health care access. However, the health care in the native place is easily accessible due to familiarity and location of the health services (Mishra, Kusuma & Babu, 2015).

The worsening of health status of PVTGs is aggravated by the developmental projects and forced migration. The developmental projects have displaced these PVTGs from their homeland and forced them to migrate and look for a new livelihood. The PVTGs heavily rely on the forest resources by selling them for livelihood. But with the commencement of new forest policy, these vulnerable tribal groups are unable to collect and sell the non-timber forest produce as they are forced to evict the area in the name of conservation. In addition to this, their displacement from the traditional homeland has resulted in the loss of subsistence and forced them to migrate to the urban areas. The loss of livelihood, displacement from the homeland and consequent constraint to mobilise the resources during ill health make PVTGs more vulnerable to disease and malnutrition. Besides, the search for new employment opportunities put these vulnerable groups to new kind of health challenges in the new setting. Additionally, the livelihood insecurity hugely impacts access to healthcare services. The PVTGs are not able to mobilise the available livelihood resources in critical health situations due to above cited reasons. Therefore, it becomes necessary to assess the health care access in the context of livelihood insecurity of PVTGs.

Furthermore, the low literacy rates among these PVTGs are the main hindrance for providing facilities and schemes related to health care. Their awareness level regarding the health schemes also affects their healthcare access. The low literacy rate naturally has negative impact on the health status of these PVTGs and the situation is more aggravated by the declining of their original natural habitats. These groups are forced to live in new ecological settings which have a negative impact on their health and nutritional status (Sahani, 2003). One study published by ICMR Jabalpur indicates high TB disease prevalence (3294 per 100,000) among Saharias of Sheopur (Rao, 2015). Even high rate of malnutrition is also documented among PVTGs (Damayanti & Chakma, 2003, 2004). The situations of the Baigas are also very bad. The incidence of high mortality and highest infant mortality rate, high level of infectious diseases, under nutrition, delayed menarche are very common among Baigas (Sahani, 2013).

In another study, it has been shown that the Baiga women have low level of awareness and utilisation of maternal child health services.

The study stresses that women are willing to opt for government health services but the accessibility and expenditure related to health, the unfriendly behaviour of the staff are some of the factors which hinders them to seek health care (Kumar *et al.,* 2016). The National Institute of Research in Tribal Health has been conducting research to assess the tribal health problem and come up with measures to improve the overall health status and maternal and child health MCH of the tribal groups of Madhya Pradesh (Balarajan *et al.*, 2011). To reduce the burden of health care expenditure and to improve the healthcare access, the government has launched the state government funded health insurance scheme called Rashtriya Swasthya Bima Yojana (RSBY). The scheme intends to reduce the IMR and MMR among the vulnerable section of the society. The study done by Kumar *et al.* (2016) indicates that tribal women are welcoming towards the scheme but face difficulty while using the RSBY as they lack necessary documents to open the bank account.

Thus, the tribes are compelled to approach traditional healers due to interior habitation, far-flung health centres, limited public transportation, local beliefs and traditions, and lack of access to health facilities. Furthermore, inadequate public health systems, poor behaviour by health personnel, and language barriers force them to rely on private practitioners, further depleting their financial resources. Another factor affecting tribal health is the lack of proper documents required to apply for health and nutrition programmes.

Besides, since PVTGs live in conflict areas, they are constantly afraid of violence and struggle for survival. This conflict is exacerbated by development projects that force them to relocate, resulting in the loss of traditional livelihood and migration in search of work. In terms of health, education, and other issues, the new setting presents new challenges to them.

Health Access Livelihood Framework and PVTGs Health Status

The Health Access Livelihood Framework was created in the context of malaria care in rural Tanzania as part of the ACCESS Programme. The Framework stresses on providing high-quality health care in resource-poor settings, especially in Africa. The framework primarily addresses health-care access and livelihood assets, which are essential for treatment. It is emphasised that once the illness is recognised and treatment decision is made, the access becomes critical issue. The treatment process is influenced by five dimensions of access, i.e. availability, accessibility, affordability, adequacy and acceptability. The interaction of health care services, and policies, as well as available livelihood resources that could be mobilised in critical circumstances, determines the accessibility of health services. Therefore, the framework basically integrates health care interventions as well as health seeking behaviour and situates access health care within the broader context of livelihood insecurity (Obrist *et al.*, 2007).

The 'health-seeking behaviour' approach focus on the people, while 'health service' approach focus on factors affecting access to health care, and 'livelihood approaches' emphasise assets and activities needed to achieve and maintain during livelihood insecurity.

In health seeking behaviour approach the social actors are considered as the main motivating factor towards health care access. But it has been observed that such social actors are controlled by the social-economic and political dynamics of the society at the macro and micro level (Montgomery *et al.*, 2006; Singer & Baer, 1995). Livelihood insecurity plays a very important role in healthcare access. Therefore, studies related to the livelihood approach demonstrate that the relationship between access to household and community resources affect the strategies to cope with the illness (Obrist *et al.*, 2007). The livelihood resources are encompassed human capital, social capital, natural capital, physical capital and financial capital. These assets are controlled by the economic, political and technological forces over which people have little control. It is necessary to improve health care access as well as align it with the livelihood assets.

The framework could be applied to understand the healthcare access of PVTGs in relation to livelihood insecurity. There is an evident paucity of studies on PVTGs concerning the health care access in relation to livelihood insecurity produced by displacement from the traditional land, migration and minimal access to the forest resources as well as in their natural habitat.

According to the above cited literature, PVTG studies are primarily focused on particular diseases such as sickle cell anaemia, G6PD deficiency, malaria, tuberculosis, and others, as well as studies relating to health seeking behaviour. However, there are few studies on health care access and livelihood insecurity as a result of relocation, land alienation, migration, poverty, conflict, and other factors. The tribal population, especially PVTGs, has undergone significant changes and is increasingly vulnerable to the resources on which they have relied for generations. The tribal population's livelihood opportunities have been severely impacted by land alienation. The loss of traditional land and limited access to forest resources has a direct effect on livelihood and health.

Therefore, the health services in the tribal areas require a comprehensive understanding of the health care access. It is important to explore the issue of health care access from the perspective of tribal peoples' livelihoods, especially PVTG. There is a need to understand the health care utilisation in association with the livelihood insecurity of the tribal population and PVTGs. Such knowledge production may help in identifying current gaps in health policy and implementing appropriate initiatives to increase tribal community access to health care. Thus, in tribal communities where livelihoods are in jeopardy, providing quality health care is a challenge. There is a need to improve the health care access as well as livelihood resources for care. Therefore, the studies conducted by considering the Health Access Livelihood Framework will be able to assist the health system in addressing the health needs of the tribal community.

Conclusion

Health is a fundamental right of every human being to lead a life with dignity, and necessary to participate in social, economic and political life without any discrimination. The vulnerable tribal population constantly subjected to inequality, oppression and social exclusion and have been deprived of basic amenities like education, livelihood, and health services which affect the quality of life. The PVTGs are vulnerable to many ill-health due to illiteracy, unawareness, malnutrition and loss of livelihood resources. The Government of India has come up with number of developmental and health-related schemes aimed at bringing PVTGs up to par with the mainstream population. Despite all these efforts, the health status of PVTGs continues to deteriorate. The migration, displacement, conflict and livelihood loss have exposed the PVTGs to new kind of health vulnerabilities. Therefore, there is a need to understand the PVTGs health status and livelihood insecurity posed due to developmental programmes, displacement, and poverty. The livelihood insecurity has major health repercussions in terms of health care access and services. The Health Access Livelihood Framework can be employed to understand the healthcare access in broader context of livelihood insecurity. The framework could help in capturing the health care issues during economic hardships. The framework could also highlight the efficiency and gaps of the health system and how tribal people mobilise the resources in relation to livelihood insecurity.

REFERENCES

Balarajan, Y., Selvaraj, S., and Subramanian, SV. (2011). "Health care and Equity in India", *Lancet, 3*(77):505-515.

Barik, D. and Thorat, A. (2015). "Issues of Unequal Access to Public Health in India", *Front Public Health.* 2015; *3*: 245.

Bera, Sayantan (2012). "Baigas in exile: Down to Earth", Centre for Science and Environment, India.

Chakma, S.B. (2014). "Conservation Refugees: A Methodology of Tribal Marginalisation", *Journal of Tribal Intellectual Collective India*, *2*(1), 25-38.

Damayanti, K. and Chakma, T. (2003, 2004). "Nutritional Status of Adolescents in Tribal Areas of Madhya Pradesh", Chapter-2: Nutrition. *Annual Report.* 2003-04. Regional Medical Research Centre for Tribals (ICMR), Jabalpur.

Dash, J. (2016). Supreme Court quashes Odisha's plea on Niyamgiri. Business Standard. https://www.business-standard.com/article/current-affairs/supreme-court-quashes-odishasplea-on-niyamgiri-116050601256_1.html

Kaushal, Sonia (2019): "Critical Medical Anthropology and Bio-power: A Review", In Rashmi Sinha (Ed.), Anthropology and Health (pp. 53-66). Rawat Publications, New Delhi.

Kothari, A. (2008). "The 4-C Factor: Community Conservation and Climate Change", *Biodiversity, 9*(3 and 4):19-23.

Kudimetha, G.K., and G.K., Dinesh. (2019). "Particularly vulnerable tribal groups (PVTG): An Ecological and Environmental perspective", In book *The Agraria,* (pp. 23-26), Issue 22, Publisher: IMoT Forum.

Kumar, D., Goel, A.K., Ghanghoria, V. and Ghangoria, P. (2016). "A Qualitative Study on Maternal and Child Health Practices among Baiga Tribe of Madhya Pradesh State in Central India", *The Journal of Community Health Management*, *3*(1): 23-27.

Ministry of Health and Family Welfare, (2018). Report of the Expert Committee on Tribal Health—Bridging the Gap and Road Map for the Future. Publisher MoHFW. https://drive.google.com/open?id=1Jpf7CXQ-mXVrLaJDv9PEG_4Z-lgIFBU5

Montgomery, C.M., Mwangee, W., Kong'ong'o, M., and Pool, R. (2006). "To help them is to educate them: Power and pedagogy in the prevention and treatment of malaria in Tanzania". *Trop Med Int Health, 11*: 1661–1669.

Nagaraja, K., and Veerabhadrappa, B.P. (2018). "Rural-Urban Health Disparities in India", *Indian Journal of Applied Research*, *8*(8).

Obrist, B., Iteba, N., Lengeler, C., Makemba, A., Mshana, C., Nathan, R., *et al.* (2007). "Access to Health care in Contexts of Livelihood Insecurity: A Framework for Analysis and Action", *PLoS, 4*(10): 1584–88.

Oliveira, M.A.C. and Pereira, I.C. (2013). Primary Health Care Essential Attributes and the Family Health Strategy. *Rev Bras Enferm, 66*(Esp):158-64.

Oliver, A., and Mossialos, E. (2004). Equity of Access to Health Care. Outlining the Foundations for Action. *J Epidemiol Community Health, 58*: 655–658.

Rao, P.V. (2015). "People of India—Particularly Tribal Groups". In P.C. Joshi (Ed), *Symposium of India,* Department of Anthropology, University of Delhi, pp. 50-53.

Report Health Status of Particularly Vulnerable Tribal Groups (PVTGs) of Odisha, India. SCSTRTI and AIPH, 2015.

Report of the High Level Committee on Socio-Economic, Health and Educational Status of Tribal Communities of India. (May 2014) Ministry of Tribal Affairs. Government of India.

Report on 'From Margins to the Centre: A Study on the Health Inequalities among the Tribal Communities in selected Districts of Chhatisgarh, Jharkhand and Odisha, Research Report (2019) by Sama — Resource Group for Women and Health; *SAMA Final Report.pdf (nhrc.nic.in)

Sahani, R. (2003). Nutritional and Health Status of the Jarawas: A Preliminary Report. *J. Anthropol. Surv. India*, *52*: 47–6 5.

Sahani, R and Nandy, S.K. (2013): Particularly Vulnerable Tribal Groups in India: An Overview. *Journal of Anthropological Survey of India*, *62*(2):851-865.

Santos, R.C., and Silva, M.S. (2014). Living Conditions and Therapeutic Paths in a Quilombola Community in Goiás, Brazil. *SaudeSoc, 23*(3):1049-63.

Singer, M., and Baer, H. (1995). Critical medical anthropology. Amityville (NY): Baywood. 28. Penchansky, R., and Thomas, J.W. (1981). The concept of access. Definition and relationship to consumer satisfaction. *Med Care, 19*:127–140.

Srivastava, V.K. (2008). Concept of 'Tribe' in the Draft National Tribal Policy. *Economic and Political Weekly (EPW)*.

Suchismita, Mishra; Yadlapalli S., Kusuma; and Bontha V., Babu (2015): Migration and health-care access: Barriers to access government health services by migrant tribal community living in an eastern Indian city. *International Journal of Medical Science and Public Health, 4*(11), 101-108.

Travassos, C., and Martins, M. (2004). A Review of Concepts in Health Services Access and Utilization. *Cad SaúdePública*, 20:190-98.

UN. (2015). *State of the World's Indigenous Peoples: Indigenous Peoples' Access to Health Services*. 2 vols.

UNDP (2012). Identifying Livelihood Promotion Strategies for Particularly Vulnerable Tribal Groups under NRLM. Delhi: UNDP India.

Vargas, B.A., Fang, H., Garza, J., Carter-Pokras, O., Wallace, S.P., Rizzo, J.A., and *et al.* (2012). Variations in Healthcare Access and Utilization among Mexican Immigrants: The Role of Documentation Status. *J Immigr Minor Health, 14*(1):146-55.

Wunsch, S., Budó, MLD., Girardon-Perlini, N.M.O., Garcia, R.P., and Oliveira, S.G. (2014). Care as a Commitment of All: A Study in a Rural Settlement. *Rev Gaucha Enferm*, *35*(4):65-71.

PART II

Health, Disease and Health Seeking Behaviour

8
Building a Bio-Social Understanding of Diseases
An Overlooked *Sine Qua Non*

M.P. Sachdeva, Naveen Kumar, Architha Tandon, and *Vipin Gupta*

Introduction

When a disease insinuates itself so potently into the imagination of an era, it is often because it impinges on an anxiety latent within that imagination. AIDS loomed so large on the 1980s in part because this was a generation inherently haunted by its sexuality and freedom; SARS set off a panic about global spread and contagion at a time when globalism and social contagion were issues simmering nervously in the West. Every era casts illness in its own image. Society, like the ultimate psychosomatic patient, matches its medical afflictions to its psychological crises; when a disease touches such a visceral chord, it is often because that chord is already resonating (Mukherjee, 2010).

The historical triage of the anthropologists dealing with the issues of disease and illness, not as therapists or rapporteurs but as the societal gatekeepers and significant stakeholders in the ethnology of the aspects of treatment in various societies, in itself reflects the unspoken need of inciting a societal perspective into the mediated solo biological attenuation of the human medical problems. As a species, achieving a stance of not merely curing ourselves but rendering service to affliction of the other species, incorporates not merely a habitat but a niche, that accustomed our gargantuan thought of *Homo sapiens*, the literal wise! Undoubtedly with the marvels of science and technology, physiology has gone a long way from facelifts to transplants and with a thought of answer to all biological problems, yet the enigma remains faded and an intertwining importance of the socio-cultural aspect looms this enigma.

Homo sapiens is a relatively younger species that emerged around 195,000 years ago, though it seems like a very long time but in comparison to these other species, humans are very young. Lifestyles of humans have been changing drastically in quest of the time period lapsed in exposure to adaptations and natural selection. Humans have indeed come a long way, from the naive bipedal settlers of the savannah to the world of agriculture and further to the extent of the urban marvels. The pace of the world sets the change, reflected by the transition of the lifestyle primarily through a dialectic interaction between biology and society. The lithic culture, and the existence of the subsistence-based collecting and foraging, marvels the ecology which yet supports the simplest amidst the advanced. With a rapid turn of events, the change in the human's perception of problems in terms of diseases, was not merely a physical affliction any more.

The concepts of health, disease and illness are interrelated yet different. Health is a universal notion but every culture holds different aspects of 'health' and what they mean by 'healthy'.

According to the World Health Organization, 'health' is a state of physical, mental and social wellbeing in the absence of disease and infirmity. Health is a fundamental right of every individual to enjoy the highest attainable standard of health irrespective of race, religion, political belief, economic or social condition (WHO, 1995).

So, a bigger question that arises is 'What does it mean to be healthy?' WHO's definition of health tries to cover all dimensions of health and at times is a little bit too idealistic *per se*. Indeed, it is depicted as a universal concept but the looming lacuna of the socio-cultural interface that facilitates the adaptation to diseases in all societies, needs an anthropological revelation, an impact on particularism rather than generalizations. As Ackerknecht stated, 'disease and its treatment are only in the abstract purely biological processes. Actually, such facts as whether a person gets sick at all, what kind of disease he acquires and what kind of treatment he receives depends largely upon social factors' (Ackerknecht, 1947).

Certain behavioural and/or physical traits are adaptive, which increase an individual's ability of survival and reproduction. These traits are passed on to next generations. And as the lifestyles become more modern and technologically advanced, certain changes lead to new lifestyle characteristics and become maladaptive. Glaring prevalence of obesity in most parts of the world, in this regard can significantly ascribe to the lacuna of biology meeting society, as a part of disease and illness. With the globalized world and the onset age of the franchise eateries, the local and the ongoing environmentally suited lineage of diet has taken a back seat. The indigenous routines of workouts have been shoved off by the art of the gyms.

Every individual will go through different diseases throughout their life. It is universal to every society, but how we accept, act and treat it, varies across societies as well as individuals. For example, in the current times of a postmodernist world, if someone catches a cold, people react to it and treat it, differently. For instance, one might go to a physician and take the prescribed medicine or one may wait for three to four days or someone might have turmeric milk and go with the traditional method of treatment.

Humans are developing rapidly and with the development of technology, lifestyles and health care, we have succeeded in finding cures and treatments of many deadly diseases, thereby improving the life expectancy. With the increasing development and advancement, diseases and illnesses are also increasing in tandem. Millions and billions of dollars are being spent on the health industry to seek treatments, medications, vaccines and cures for diseases that are recent and also for the ones which have been with us since decades and centuries. If this touted general way would have worked marvellously or even the tailored pharmacogenetics-based medicines would have, then where would have the human made technology failed?

The answer is, it's not enough, what lacks here is the social aspects of disease and illness which have been ignored by the foremost scientists, researchers and doctors. Researchers have started focusing on the social aspect as well, but the traverse is a long labour.

The 18th and 19th century medical work could be seen emphasizing on the role of social components in the disease genesis. Occupational disease studied by Bernadino Ramazzini (Ramazzini, 1940) in 1700, and Benjamin McCready in 1837 (McCready, 1972) in the United States are prime examples. In 1848 Rudolph Virchow started a new journal *Die Medizinische Reform* in which he fought for the concern of social situation as etiological factors in disease and famously declared 'Medicine is a social science'.

Most of all, the socio-cultural lacuna is somehow tried to be filled by the mental health workers, although garnering not much of the attention. Psychiatry is a discipline in biomedicine which explains the mental illness and its framework. But in medical anthropology, mental illness or mental health conditions are much more complicated than the biological model illness suggests (Brown *et al.*, 2020). These illnesses are not just biological or chemical, but are a conglomeration of responses to social and cultural relationships of individuals.

Lee argued that each culture understands and responds to mental health concerns differently. In China patient's suffering from depression did not describe feelings of sadness, instead complained of boredom, discomfort, feeling of inner pressure, and symptoms of pain, dizziness and fatigue (Lee *et al.*, 2007).

Social Aspect of Diseases: Anthropologists, the Human Mirrors

Intervention is a crucial and most sought venture by all therapists, doctors and practitioners. Yet with all people being biologically and socially varied, it is a difficult task. The need of the hour is to stabilize the virtue of anthropological networking into the latent of the society and come up with reflections on the ethnological aspects of those interventions which even existed way before the hijacking by the technology. An anthropologist is the only stakeholder not affecting the people's natural and socially mediated ways of resilience towards the diseases (Castro, 2004). When we compare the work, a social scientist does in comparison to a surgeon or a physician, it is always looked down upon and neglected. Working in a clinical setting is not so easy and social scientists cannot work as a doctor does; also doctors regard themselves as superior to these social scientists, thereby expecting them to work quickly and hasten to the conclusions. But gradually with time things are changing and doctors are also understanding the importance of the social aspect of disease and illness.

Social aspects of a disease can be understood in terms of the environmental, religious, cultural, familial, emotional, behavioural, psychological, or economical, effects on an individual or patient, because of a specific disease/s before, during and post treatment. Also, when we cannot find a cure or treatment of a disease then it is often the social aspects that come into play in order to mediate an understanding that helps in curing, avoiding, managing or living with the disease (Singer *et al.*, 2019).

Anthropologists while working in clinical settings or in public health related fields must understand that they are in the situation as a social scientist and not as the physician, nutritionist or psychologists. So, they must maintain their role as an anthropologist or a social scientist; if they notice anything serious which needs to be treated, corrected or modified they should recommend the person or patient to the appropriate personnel in the field. This may sound easy and simple but that is not the case in the field setting and one often has to make decisions according to the situation which is often very stressful (Kleinman *et al.*, 1978).

To understand the social aspects of disease and illness, the following three examples of different diseases tend to elucidate how the prioritizing attribute functions with rendering society as one of an overriding importance as AIDS and COVID-19 are the two outbreaks (Schell, 2021) that shook the entire globe, while transplantation stays as the most advanced in the medical field (Bezinover & Saner, 2019).

1. Acquired immunodeficiency syndrome (AIDS) which is caused by human immunodeficiency virus (HIV), that attacks the immune system is a life-threatening disease. Currently there is no cure for this disease as it interferes with the body's function to fight against infections and diseases. Strict antiretroviral regimens (ARVs) drastically slow the development of disease and prevent secondary complications too. This is a global pandemic. It is believed to have been transmitted from a non-human primate to humans (Sharp and Hahn, 2010). It is transmitted through sex, blood transfusion and intravenous drug use (Chu and Judith, 2005). This disease has a lot of social stigma attached to it.

The fear ascribed to AIDS was at its peak for a long time after the 1980s and the affected individuals were discriminated against and looked down on, which made their lives harder. As the societies were not accepting the infected persons, it almost came down on, whether being infected was a worry or being excommunicated because of it. Biology was failing in finding a cure or treatment. When we were not able to find a cure of disease biologically, we started looking for other factors to reduce the effect of HIV/AIDS in order to cope up with the disease, to provide a better quality of life to patients, and significantly focused on how to normalize the panic around the patients in a society, so that one does not feel abandoned by the society as it could affect the mental health of the patient severely. In the beginning people were afraid of even touching the infected person and thought they might catch HIV too. Then a lot of awareness programmes were organized worldwide to spread awareness about HIV/AIDS, its spread and prevention (Marshall & Bennett, 1990). The overriding social aspect associated with this pandemic comes up in various forms of advertisements that guide the society to act carefully towards the contraction of this disease or even suggesting them to normalize their behaviour towards the patients. Even the rise in the sub-branch, queer anthropology, tends to elucidate the debates on how the biology of a disease can affect drastically if it is not handled carefully by the society. The racket of prostitution along with the issues of homosexuality, associated with HIV/AIDS, questionably target a sect of subaltern communities amidst the perplexed social perceptions of the biological explanations of the etiology of the disease (Bolton *et al.*, 1994; Ramin, 2007; Susser, 2009).

Another dimension of the social aspect of AIDS is classically entailed in the study by Mahajan *et al.* on the stigma of HIV/AIDS patients. He pointed out the subjective experience of the illness which can also be influenced by social attitudes. Research in many countries showed that people including the health workers, categorized between patients into "innocent" as the ones who are innocent victims of AIDS and "guilty" ones who contracted HIV through sex or intravenous drug use. HIV transmitted from blood transfusion, or inherited are viewed as innocent and are subjected to superior treatment as compared to the 'guilty' patients, who are treated with disrespect, indifference in medical settings and have difficulty in accessing the medical facilities and care. 'Guilty' patients suffer from social marginalization and exclusion while 'innocent' patients receive greater social acceptance, practical assistance to their need of support and care (Mahajan *et al.,* 2008).

2. COVID-19 and locally known as CORONAVIRUS. COVID-19 is the disease caused by SARS-CoV-2, a virus from the family *coronaviridae*. The whole world is affected by this and it has become a global pandemic. There was no cure found for the virus and millions of people were being infected by it causing lakhs of death worldwide. Hospitals were flooded with patients; doctors, nurses and medical staff were exhausted by working overtime. Almost all the countries were locked down. Flights were cancelled. Transportation being shut down and everyone advised to stay home. It is crucial here to build after this narration the role of social aspects and that came and still come into play when there were no available cures in the form of the vaccine, which is yet not a confirmed cure. Social distancing, hygienic habits, the importance and use of culture like for instance in form of greeting people with a '*Namaskar*' instead of a 'handshake' includes some of the examples of how the culture came to the rescue in avoiding the disease. Although we all looked forward to a biological tool to indefinitely put this to an end, but till then the indigenous *ashwagandha, nimbu* (lemon), *haldi* (turmeric) were coming into use, and the panorama widens with respective cultures and societies dealing with the pandemic (Srivastava, 2020). The beautification of masks, for them being an easy add on in the human lives, has already been started by the capitalist fashion enthusiasts. Thus, societal interface is a huge key player in even manifestation of the war models of India responding to the pandemic, and other countries dealing in their own ascribed ways (Manderson & Levine, 2020).

Another social dimension of the disease is the effect of lockdown on population. For months people were locked in their homes, protecting themselves from the virus. This had led to people getting vulnerable to the sudden change in the situation and thus leading to psychological harm. People were facing problems that never existed such as cancellation of clinical appointments, difficulties in accessing medications, women were facing difficulties in accessing abortion facilities, reduced exercise, increased frustration and stress level. Men often faced boredom, anxiety and frustrations for staying in for such a long time and it often resulted in domestic violence (Singer & Rylko-Bauer, 2021). The fear of catching viruses, the workload of work at/from home, for students the online lectures and classes, financial crisis, ruined business, companies firing employees, were some of the impending effects of the pandemic, which were best dealt socially and culturally. If someone got infected then it was very hard to get a bed in hospital, neighbours or friends were reluctant to come and help the patient, and even the financial burden in admitting at private healthcare facilities was prohibitive. People were losing their loved ones and in many countries the relatives were not even allowed to even bid a final goodbye to them as the authorities undertook the death rites, in fear of the spread of the virus. COVID-19 has not only created biological issues, but also the social, economic, familial, psychological, emotional hue and cry, seem a bigger crisis, that can also be more crippling and life-long. The virus was the same, yet garnered different reactions from people in the form of their resilience to it, which were socio-culturally mediated (Hahn & Schoch-Spana, 2021).

3. Transplantation is an end stage treatment for organ failures when conventional treatment methods are unable to offer survival (Rios *et al.*, 2006). Kidneys, liver, lungs, heart are the most common human organs that are likely to fall prey to the failure. There are options like dialysis, medications, ventricular assist devices, assisted respiration through mechanical devices but these are not permanent solutions assuring the quality of life. Organ transplant challenges nature and gives an individual another chance to live and have more years added to one's life. Organ transplant is a procedure of procurement of an organ from one individual, living or dead and transplanting it to another individual (Sharp,1995). Even though dialysis is an alternate option for end stage renal failure patients but still kidney is the most transplanted organ globally, according to the World Health Organization (WHO, 2013). Dialysis of an individual accounts for an average of 3 sessions each Week, with all of the sessions lasting for 3-4 hours which is a highly cumbersome process, which brings the so-called normal life of people to halt. This is the major reason that end stage renal failure patients choose transplantation over the dialysis (Fotheringham *et al.,* 2021). Whereas in case of failure of liver, lungs or heart, the patient does not have such an option and has to have a transplant.

Even after achieving the advancement in medications, surgical techniques, compatibility tests, the field of transplantation is lacking behind. There is a huge gap between the need and supply of organs. Organs can be recovered from either a living donor or a brain-dead donor. Hearts and lungs can be procured only after brain death. Besides this a living individual can donate one kidney, a segment of liver or a portion of pancreas (THOA, 2014). The decision to donate is huge and has social, psychological, emotional, physiological realms that pertain to the fear, belief and an idea of self-attachment to one's body. Living donors agreeing to donate, have to live with a missing part for the rest of their lives. This is a big decision to take which does not stem up primarily from the arena of a biological understanding of organ failure (Joralemon, 1995). Yet it is the care and attachment that people have for the person in this end stage treatment that leads to this altruistic behaviour of humans. Money is a peripheral attachment to procurement of organs, as many times organs of the poor and underprivileged are trafficked to meet the needs of the other. Similarly, in case of a deceased or a brain-dead donor, the family has to consent for donation (Shih *et al.,* 2001). The consent to donate comes along with the religious and cultural beliefs, traditions, death rites and rituals, family's reaction, personal attachment, the right over the body of loved one, and the fact that the organ of loved one is still functioning in someone else's body, are deeply integrated in the social fabrics, which, of course, if looked at from this perspective would lead to break this divide between need and supply of organs. The field (Ebner *et al.,* 2019; Kerstis & Widarsson, 2020; Siminoff *et al.,* 2007) of transplantation cannot be developed without considering these aspects.

After an organ transplant, recipients are prescribed a strict and a high regimen, they have to take immunosuppressants regularly, to suppress their immune system in order to prevent it from attacking the transplanted organ. These medications increase the risks of secondary diseases like infections and cancers (Vial & Descotes, 2003). The recipients always have the fear of organ rejection and other health problems. The patient-healthcare interface and the role of social environment too comes to the advent of patient recovery in cases like this (Raia, 2020). Anthropologists study the quality of life of living donors and recipients post-transplant; the experience, feelings and emotions of recipients as well as the living donor; the non-reciprocal gift and its pressure; how to adjust with the fact of living with someone else's part; the fear of rejection; fear of catching diseases; fear of cancer; fear of life; the social, behavioural, and mental effect pre- and post-transplant; economic burden; familial relationships; family's care; and organ trafficking and medical tourism. This significantly upholds the social aspect of disease, as mirrored by the anthropologists (Lock, 2003).

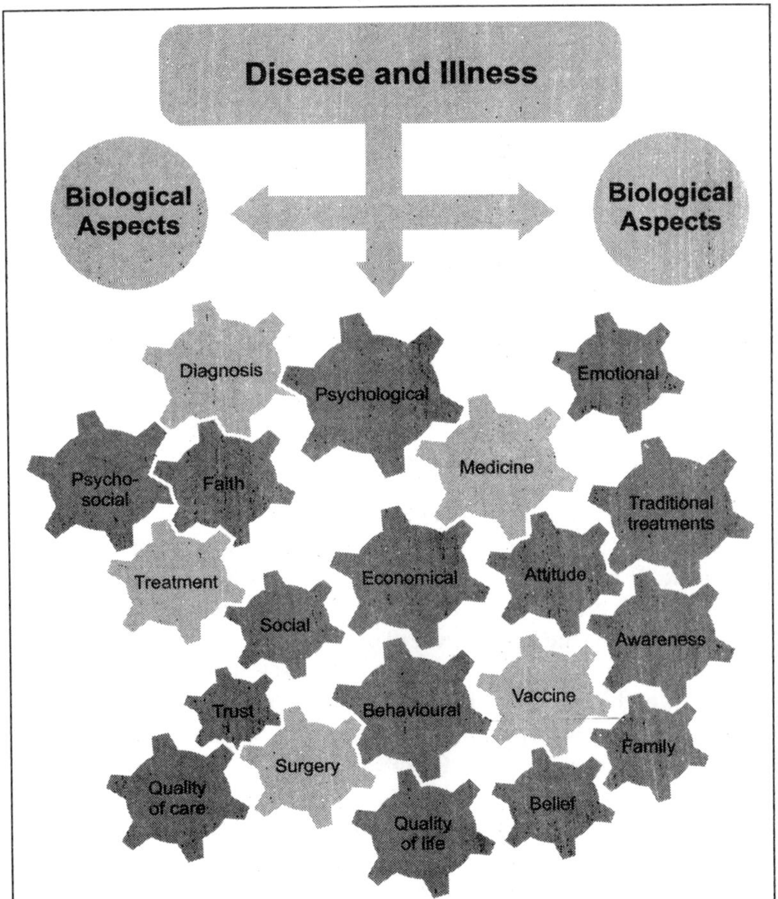

Fig. 8.1: Interdependence of social and biological aspects of disease and illness.

Illness is a social manifestation of a disease and Figure 8.1 is representative of the dialectic, criss-crossed and interdependent nature of determinism and possibilism of biological and societal factors.

Thus, it is clear that social scientists or more specifically anthropologists are *sine qua non* in clinical settings and/or public health. Mahoney pointed out some of the key roles and contributions that anthropologists can make to public health as listed below (Mahony, 1960):

- To study the concept of health and illness held by the people to be served, suggestions of particular approaches which may be helpful with such groups.
- Helping public health personnel to understand their own attitudes and how these attitudes affect their work.
- Promotion of understanding of public health programmes among communities.
- Contributing directly to the knowledge of therapy, disease and disease patterns.

In addition to these, presently the anthropologists also focus on the emotional factors attached with a disease, social suffrage and pressure, psychosocial, quality of life, changes in lifestyle and many other aspects which affect the individual's life. A disease is not just a disease, it has its own kinship, family, economy, politics, and other perspectives, requiring an anthropological crucial examination. Thus, an affliction is not merely of an individual but it does affect an entire family (Singer *et al.*, 2019).

These listings render us to believe that no matter what, society has all the curbs of prevention under its jurisdiction, in cases where cure is not possible. It is hence not merely an 'anthropology of health' but an 'anthropology in health' approach, which classically entails the power of society in the delineation of the sick, ill or diseased. Diseases come handy in this fast-moving world, and the human niche acts as a guardian against the fatalities of these. Indeed, the social aspect kills the anxiety of biology, by generating an intercorporeal as Merleau-Ponty suggests, that makes it easier for people to cope with it (Landes, 2013).

Faith: A Peripheral Attachment of Cure

Another prime dimension of social aspect is 'faith' that is evidently illustrated in most public health-based research. William Osler, founder of Johns Hopkins Hospital and a Canadian physician believed that the success and ability of physicians healing is based on the ability of doctors to inspire patients with a faith that they could be cured and will be able to have a better life (Bliss, 1999). Osler wrote, Faith in the Gods or in the Saints cures one, faith in little pills another, suggestion a third, faith in a plain common doctor a fourth… if a poor lass, paralyzed apparently helpless, bed-ridden for years, comes to me having a worn out in mind, body, and estate a devoted family; if she in a few weeks or less by faith in me, and faith alone, takes up her bed and walks, the Saints of old could not have done more (Osler, 1910).

There are several researches indicating the role of placebo effects in healing and treatment. A placebo effect is a response of an individual in treating oneself because s/he believes that they are getting better with the said treatment, as due to their faith in the treatment and not evidently because of the placebo itself. Here the faith and will to recover, process and programme the body to respond in a way the drug will. A simple act of writing prescription by a trained professional on which an individual has faith, leads to successful recovery of individuals (Bud, 2007).

Benson *et al.* (2006) study on therapeutic effects of intercessory prayers on cardiac bypass patients reveals very interesting results. In this study patients who underwent heart surgery were divided into two groups. In the first group patients were aware that they are receiving prayers from others and in the second group patients were not aware of the prayers they were getting. This study portrays very beautifully the relation of mind-body and how it works. The groups which knew they are receiving prayers had more complications and problems as compared to the group which was unaware of the fact that they are receiving prayers. What happened here is that the group which knew of the prayers became more stressed and perceived that they are at a greater risk, which is why their doctors have asked others to pray for them (Benson *et al.*, 2006).

Curiously enough the anxiety of biology meets society, in the heart of the diseases, a mere rendition of family, support, care and faith can turn the physical ailments into a psychological offset which gets cured with the social conditions of the humans.

Conclusion

'Anthropology of Care', 'Ethnography of Hospital', 'Domestic violence to hospitals', ethno-medicine, belief in shamanistic practices are some of the crucial advents into the societal understanding of the disease, which have significantly gained momentum in the recent era (Pool &

Geissler, 2005; Baer, 2017). While some of them, regaining their place in anthropology, aside from the studies of religion or as a mere structural perseverance of the society, but finally as the community health interface mechanism to fight against the diseases. The genetics of the human body is indeed enigmatic for the mutations to change the entire perception of the viscera in a lapse of time, but the society no matter under the dynamic spectra of change, will, however, take time to adapt fully to the biological changes. Had it been so easy! Why would the world have WHO, campaigning for people to maintain distance, wash hands or wear masks to save their own lives! The complacency comes from the lived social experiences, in the form of socialisation and perceptions. The socially accepted becomes viable and survives. The anxiety of biology truly represents the visage of the unfulfilled human capacities, even after generating an entire Human Genome, to whose rescue comes the society. Indeed, this anxiety brings up the very notion of interaffectivity amongst the entire species of *Homo sapiens* which is guarded by the society.

Medications, vaccinations and operations cannot treat everything is a social fact, in a Durkheimian approach (Durkheim,1894; 2014). One cannot neglect the emotions, feelings, experiences and faith of an individual that are attached pre and post the diseased phase. The aspects of healing also come with the underpinning of the experiences of the people or of oneself. Thus, a bio-culturally mediated anthropological examination of the patterns of people during diseases, aspects of complacency and the latent community resiliency will definitely render an end to the anxiety of biology, as it meets the society. Making people believe in the change is not easy, especially when it comes to medicines and treatments. People have their societal ways to combat the diseases. If the medical anthropologists need to lead the bandwagon of universal answering of the disease patterns and experiences, one must lead through the *Aristotelean,* Persuasion Triad of the *logos* (rational mind), *ethos* (sense of credibility) and *pathos* (emotion), wherein the road to logos is often paved through *pathos* that tends to the horizon of the anxiety of biology meeting society, in context of diseases (Allen, 2007).

REFERENCES

Ackerknecht, E.H. (1947). "Primitive Surgery", *American Anthropologist, 49*(1), 25-45.

Allen, J. (2007). "Aristotle on the disciplines of argument: Rhetoric, dialectic, analytic", *Rhetorica, 25*(1), 87-108.

Baer, H.A. (2017). *Democratic eco-socialism as a real utopia: Transitioning to an alternative world system*. Berghahn Books.

Benson, H., Dusek, J.A., Sherwood, J.B., Lam, P., Bethea, C.F., Carpenter, W.,... and Drumel, D. (2006). "Study of the Therapeutic Effects of Intercessory Prayer (STEP) in cardiac bypass patients: a multicenter randomized trial of uncertainty and certainty of receiving Intercessory prayer", *American heart journal*, *151*(4), 934-942.

Bezinover, D., and Saner, F. (2019). *Organ transplantation in the modern era.*

Bliss, M. (1999). *William Osler: A life in medicine.* Oxford University Press.

Bolton, R., Orozco, G., and Lindenbaum, S. (1994). "The AIDS Bibliography: Studies in Anthropology and Related Fields", *American Anthropological Association.*

Brown, N., McIlwraith, T., and de González, L.T. (2020). *Perspectives: An Open Introduction to Cultural Anthropology.*

Bud, R. (2007). "Antibiotics. From germophobia to the carefree life and back again: the lifecycle of the antibiotic brand". *Medicating modern America: Prescription drugs in history,* 17- 41.

Castro, A. (2004). "COMMENTARY: Anthropologists as Advocates: Power, Suffering and AIDS". *Anthropology News*, *45*(7), 9-11.

Chu, T.X., and Judith, A.L. (2005). "Injection drug use and HIV/AIDS transmission in China", *Cell research*, *15*(11), 865-869.

Durkheim, E. (1894). "Les règles de la méthode sociologique". *Revue Philosophique de la France et de l'Étranger*, *37*, 465-498.

Durkheim, E. (2014). *The rules of sociological method and selected texts on sociology and its method.* Simon and Schuster.

Ebner, K., Ostheimer, J., and Sautermeister, J. (2020). The role of religious beliefs for the acceptance of xenotransplantation Exploring dimensions of xenotransplantation in the field of hospital chaplaincy. *Xenotransplantation*, *27*(4), e12579.

Fotheringham, J., Latimer, N., Froissart, M., Kronenberg, F., Stenvinkel, P., Floege, J.,... and Wheeler, D.C. (2021). Survival on four compared with three times per week haemodialysis in high ultrafiltration patients: an observational study. *Clinical kidney journal*, *14*(2), 665-672.

Hahn, R.A., and Schoch-Spana, M. (2021). "Anthropological foundations of public health; the case of COVID-19". *Preventive Medicine Reports*, 101331.

Joralemon, D. (1995). "Organ wars: The battle for body parts". *Medical anthropology quarterly*, *9*(3), 335-356.

Kerstis, B., and Widarsson, M. (2020). "When Life Ceases—Relatives' Experiences When a Family Member is Confirmed Brain Dead and Becomes a Potential Organ Donor—A Literature Review". *SAGE Open Nursing*, *6*, 2377960820922031.

Kleinman, A., Eisenberg, L., and Good, B. (1978). "Culture, illness, and care: clinical lessons from anthropologic and cross-cultural research". *Annals of internal medicine*, *88*(2), 251-258.

Landes, D.A. (2013). *Merleau-Ponty and the paradoxes of expression.* A&C Black.

Lee, D.T., Kleinman, J., and Kleinman, A. (2007). "Rethinking depression: an ethnographic study of the experiences of depression among Chinese". *Harvard Review of Psychiatry, 15*(1), 1-8.

Lock, M. (2003). *Twice Dead: Organ Transplants and the Reinvention of Death.*

Mahajan, A.P., Sayles, J.N., Patel, V.A., Remien, R.H., Ortiz, D., Szekeres, G., and Coates, T.J. (2008). "Stigma in the HIV/AIDS epidemic: a review of the literature and recommendations for the way forward". *AIDS* (London, England), 22(Suppl 2), S67.

Mahony, F. (1960). "Anthropology and Public Health". *Community Development Bulletin,* 71- 77.

Manderson, L., and Levine, S. (2020). "COVID-19, risk, fear, and fall-out". *Medical Anthroppology, 39*(5), 367-370.

Marshall, P.A. and Bennett, L.A. "(1990). "Anthropological contributions to AIDS research". *Medical Anthropology Quarterly, 4*(1), 3-5.

McCready, B.W. (1972). *On the influence of trades, professions, and occupations in the United States, in the production of disease.* Arno Press.

Mukherjee, S. (2010). *The emperor of all maladies: a biography of cancer.* Simon and Schuster.

Osler, W. (1910). "The faith that heals". *British Medical Journal*, 1(2581), 1470.

Pool, R. and Geissler, W. (2005). *Medical anthropology*. McGraw-Hill Education (UK).

Raia, F. (2020). "The temporality of becoming: care as an activity to support the being and becoming of the other". *Mind, Culture, and Activity, 27*(3), 292-312.

Ramazzini, B. *De Morbis Artificum* Translated by WC Wright (1940). *Diseases of Workers*.

Ramin, B. (2007). "Anthropology speaks to medicine: the case HIV/AIDS in Africa", *McGill Journal of Medicine: MJM, 10*(2), 127.

Ríos, A., Ramírez, P., Martínez, L., Montoya, M.J., Lucas, D., Alcaraz, J.,... and Parrilla, P. (2006). "Are personnel in transplant hospitals in favour of cadaveric organ donation? Multivariate attitudinal study in a hospital with a solid organ transplant programme", *Clinical transplantation, 20*(6), 743-754.

Schell, N.L.P.A.E.N.R.G.D. (2021, May 11). "Visualizing the History of Pandemics". *Visual Capitalist.* https://www.visualcapitalist.com/history-of-pandemics-deadliest/.

Sharp, L.A. (1995). "Organ transplantation as a transformative experience: anthropological insights into the restructuring of the self", *Medical Anthropology Quarterly, 9*(3), 357-389.

Sharp, P.M. and Hahn, B.H. (2010). "The evolution of HIV-1 and the origin of AIDS", *Philosophical Transactions of the Royal Society B: Biological Sciences, 365*(1552), 2487-2494.

Shih, F.J., Lai, M.K., Lin, M.H., Lin, H.Y., Tsao, C.I., Duh, B.R., and Chu, S.H. (2001). "The dilemma of 'to-be or not-to-be': needs and expectations of the Taiwanese cadaveric organ donor families during the pre-donation transition". *Social Science and Medicine*, *53*(6), 693-706.

Siminoff, L., Mercer, M.B., Graham, G., and Burant, C. (2007). "The reasons families donate organs for transplantation: implications for policy and practice", *Journal of Trauma and Acute Care Surgery*, *62*(4), 969-978.

Singer, M., and Rylko-Bauer, B. (2021). "The syndemics and structural violence of the COVID pandemic: Anthropological insights on a crisis", *Open Anthropological Research*, *1*(1), 7-32.

Singer, M., Baer, H., Long, D., and Pavlotski, A. (2019). *Introducing medical anthropology: A discipline in action*. Rowman & Littlefield.

Srivastava, A.K., Chaurasia, J.P., Khan, R., Dhand, C., and Verma, S. (2020). "Role of Medicinal plants of Traditional Use in Recuperating Devastating COVID-19 Situation", *Med Aromat Plants* (*Los Angeles*), *9*(359), 2167-0412.

Susser, I. (2011). *AIDS, sex, and culture: global politics and survival in southern Africa*. John Wiley & Sons.

TRANSPLANTATION OF HUMAN ORGANS ACT (THOA), 2014 (Rep.). (2014, March 27). Accessed: January 28, 2021, from *The Gazette of India*. website: https://notto.gov.in/WriteReadData/Portal/images/THOA-Rules-2014.pdf

Vial, T., and Descotes, J. (2003). "Immunosuppressive drugs and cancer", *Toxicology*, *185*(3), 229-240.

World Health Organization. (1995). *Constitution*. Retrieved June 3, 2020, Constitution of the World Health Organization. Retrieved from https://www.who.int/about/who-we- are/constitution

World Health Organization. (2013, December 11). Retrieved June 3, 2020. WHO | Human organ transplantation. Retrieved from https://www.who.int/transplantation/organ/en/

9

Myths and Misconceptions about Diabetes (T2DM) in Chandigarh Tricity

Anil Kishore Sinha, Rajnish Kumar Singh, Nutan Kumari Jha, Rita Kumari, Ramandeep Kaur, Kiran Jyoti Kaur, Jagriti Mehta, Shalu, and *Sanjay Bhadada*

Introduction

The knowledge, awareness, belief and attitude towards the self-health care with a sense of self-efficacy of an individual or group of individuals determine their behaviour towards the health and disease. Diabetes Mellitus (DM) is a hereditary and lifestyle related acute major health hazard with long term complications and increased risk of myriad of associated disorders, which entails complex behaviour of an individual 'living with the disease'.

In recent decades diabetes has become one of the most prevalent diseases of the world, the International Diabetes Federation (IDF), which produces estimates of diabetes prevalence from time to time since year 2000, had estimated in 2017 that worldwide about 451 million people were diabetic and by 2045, it is expected to increase to 693 million (Cho *et al.*, 2018). According to NCD Risk Factor Collaboration (2016) diabetes is highly prevalent in five countries: China, India, USA, Brazil, and Indonesia. Earlier India was considered as 'diabetes capital of the world', but now China claimed this crown and has superseded India with around 110 million diabetics as opposed to 72 million diabetics in India in 2017 (Anjana *et al.*, 2017; Bhansali and Bhansali, 2018).

The Union Territory of Chandigarh also known as 'The City Beautiful', which also has non-aberrant diabetes prevalence as reported in recent studies; Chandigarh Urban Diabetes Study (CUDS), 2009, reported the prevalence of diabetes and pre-diabetes as 11.1 per cent and 13.2 per cent, respectively among the adults of age group ≥20 years (Ravikumar *et al.*, 2011); with 13 per cent of diabetes prevalence which is in contradiction to the 7.3 per cent of prevalence of the disease at the national level, Chandigarh is sometimes also called as "Diabetes Capital of India" by scholars (Anjana *et al.*, 2017; Bhansali and Bhansali, 2018).

The diagnosis of diabetes in India is mostly done through opportunistic screening, like while antenatal and pre-anesthetic check-up or due to repeated infections etc. In T2DM patients there are bunch of asymptomatic health complaints such as chronic fatigue, malaise etc., however, the detection of the disease in most of the patients are circumstantial. Sometimes, patients introduce to the health exigency with noted symptoms and metabolic decompensation such as hyperglycaemia, lack of insulin, ophthalmic complications, deterioration of tissues or organ etc., thus it needs to be followed up lifetime once diagnosed, even if all the set health parameters returned to normal (Pearson and McCrimmon, 2014). The carelessness or aggressive management of the disease may increase the risk of critical low blood sugar which may lead to serious brain injury or high blood pressure etc. There is lack of proper counselling and health education including lifestyle modifications, due to which people construe their own opinion and ideas as per their understanding, which may not have any scientific explanation and that leads to myths and misconceptions about the disease.

The word myth comes from the Greek mythos which means fiction or story or narrative. Myths are defined as stories shared by group of people as a part of their cultural identity, which may have strong influence in the life and way of living of individuals including their health seeking behaviour and practices 'during as well as in the absence' of any illness (Adler and Paauw, 2003). The prevalence of myths in a population may be due to poor education, cultural beliefs, and social misconceptions. Myths with respect to any disease among any community or society or at individual level reflect their basic health awareness, outlook and health care seeking behaviour. These false collective beliefs become part of cultural identity and are used to justify a social behaviour (Rehman *et al.*, 2013).

There are several myths related to T2DM which are very common in practices and people have strong beliefs over them as these have not been correctly evaluated. The myths often lead people to shuffle between treatment options and therefore, they are not able to effectively cure themselves. This is important as better patient self-management ability is related to improved diabetes control. Perceived quality of life is also lower in patients being managed aggressively, due to lack of dramatic disease-related symptoms and side-effects of interventions. This can affect patient's compliance with medical advice (Venkataraman *et al.*, 2009). The transmission of myths and misconceptions in any society are also passed over to generations, therefore, there is dire need of understanding to provide excellent care and health education to patients, their caregivers as well as to healthy individuals.

The present study aims to understand and identify the prevailing myths and misconceptions about T2DM in Chandigarh tri-city, among diabetes patients, their attendants or caregivers and non-diabetic individuals, comparatively.

Methodology

The present study was a cross-sectional study conducted in the tertiary care hospital, i.e. Postgraduate Institute of Medical Education and Research (PGIMER), Chandigarh (Union Territory) and also in the Chandigarh tri-city, as a part of UGC-Major research project during 2015-2019. Ethical clearance was taken from Institute Ethics Committee, PGIMER, Chandigarh, as well as Ethical clearance from the Panjab University Institutional Ethics Committee, prior to the data collection.

Sample Size and Universe of the Study

The present study was conducted among 180 adult diabetic patients (males—94, females—86) attending the treatment at the Post Graduate Institute of Medical Science and Research (PGIMER), Chandigarh, their 80 attendants, i.e. their friends/relatives who accompanied these patients to the diabetic clinic (males—46, females—34) and age-sex-ethnicity matched 180 non-diabetic healthy individuals (males—95, females—85) from Chandigarh tri-city. The study population consisted of total 440 respondents, i.e. 235 males and 205 females.

An attempt was made by the research team to explore the myths and misconceptions prevalent in the study population. A pretested semi-structured interview schedule was administered by the researchers among the respondents seeking information about their myths and misconception related to diabetes, to understand the perception of the respondents pertaining to myths in relation to diabetes. The schedule was translated and interpreted in the language, i.e. Hindi and Punjabi, as per the convenience of the respondents. All respondents were well informed about the purpose and objectives of the present study, and the interview was taken with their prior informed consent.

Statistical Analysis

The qualitative data collected were subjected to the thematic analysis and then transformed to quantitative data. The present study used mixed-method for the statistical analysis. All quantitative data were analysed for group-wise percentages, and z-test (for comparison of proportions between groups) etc. by using Ms Excel and SPSS 20.0 software.

Results and Discussion

The distribution and comparison of prevalent myths among the diabetics (N = 180), non-diabetics (N = 180) and the attendants (N = 80) has been well represented in Table 9.1 (gender-wise distribution) and Table 9.2 (all respondents of each group). Detailed analysis for the prevalence of myths are as follows:

Myth 1: Consumption of Sugar Causes Diabetes

Among the diabetic patients, 20.21 per cent male and 31.39 per cent of the female respondents believed that consumption of sugar causes diabetes, while 79.79 per cent male and 68.61 per cent female respondents did not have such myth. Thus, overall only 25.55 per cent of the diabetic patients believed myth-1 to be the causal factor for diabetes, while remaining 74.45 per cent patients considered this as a myth propagated over generations and has no scientific explanation.

Similarly, among non-diabetics, 53.68 per cent male and 91.76 per cent of the female respondents believed that myth-1 causes diabetes while 46.32 per cent male and 8.24 per cent female respondents had not such myth. Thus, in total 71.66 per cent of the non-diabetic patients had believed in myth-1.

Furthermore, among the attendants, i.e. relatives/friends accompanying the patients, 43.47 per cent male and 94.11 per cent of the female respondents believed in myth-1 as casual factor of diabetes while remaining others denied this myth as cause. Thus, overall 65.0 per cent of the attendants believed in myth-1 as the cause for diabetes while remaining others considered this as a myth.

Myth 2: Diabetics should Never Consume Sweets

Among the diabetic patients, 65.95 per cent male respondents and 93.02 per cent of the female respondents believed in myth-2 while 34.05 per cent male and 6.98 per cent female respondents denied belief in such myths. Total 78.88 per cent of the diabetic patients believed sweets ought not to be consumed by diabetic patients while remaining others opined that diabetic patients can consume sweets in moderation while monitoring their carbohydrate intake, and keeping in mind its impact on the blood sugar levels.

Furthermore, 67.36 per cent male and 88.2 per cent female non-diabetics believed in myth-2 while rest of others do not have such myth and opined that sometimes diabetics can consume sweets while taking precautionary measures regarding their diet and making certain lifestyle changes (i.e. exercising regularly). Hence, majority, i.e. 77.22 per cent of the non-diabetics have myth-2.

Among the attendants, 63.04 per cent male and 88.23 per cent female respondents had myth-2. Thus, 73.75 per cent of the attendants believed in myth-2. Among those who did not have full belief in myth-2, some have perception that diabetics can consume certain sweets keeping in mind the carbohydrate intake and monitoring their sugar levels, whereas some were in favour of moderate consumption of sweets by diabetics being acceptable with suitable precautionary measures.

Myth 3: Diabetics can Eat Anything Once the Treatment Begins

The majority (81.12%) of diabetic patients were not agreed with myth-3, and believed that dietary restrictions need to be observed even after treatment to control blood glucose levels. However, only 14.89 per cent male and 23.25 per cent female respondents had myth-3.

Among the non-diabetics, 44.21 per cent male and 62.35 per cent female respondents had myth-3 and they believed that no dietary restrictions need to be observed while rest of the respondents believed that diabetics need to observe certain dietary restrictions and have to avoid certain foods that raise blood sugar levels despite the ongoing treatment. Therefore, only 47.23 per cent non-diabetics considered myth-3 as a myth with no scientific explanation.

Similarly, among the attendants, only 42.50 per cent believed in myth-3. Further with respect to gender, 26.08 per cent male and 64.70 per cent female respondents had myth-3, while remaining respondents believed that diabetics still need to take care of their eating habits to maintain healthy blood glucose levels.

Myth 4: Diabetes (T2DM) is an Inherited Disease

Among the diabetic patients, 25.53 per cent male and 34.88 per cent female respondents believed that diabetes is an inherited disease while 74.47 per cent male and 65.12 per cent female respondents believed that heredity is not a factor for diabetes. Thus, 70 per cent of the diabetic patients believed this to be a myth. Furthermore, 53.88 per cent of the non-diabetics believed in myth-4. With reference to gender, 36.84 per cent male and 72.94 per cent of the female respondents believed that diabetes is an inherited disease. About more than half (55%) attendants had myth-4, where 41.30 per cent male and 73.52 per cent of the female respondents believed that diabetes is inherited (*see* Table 9.1 & 9.2).

Myth 5: Diabetes is an Infectious Disease

Majority (88.89%) of the diabetic patients were aware that diabetes is not infectious. However, only 7.44 per cent male and 15.11 per cent female diabetics think it is infectious. Moreover, among the non-diabetic patients, 34.73 per cent male and 68.24 per cent female respondents believed that diabetes can be transmitted to other persons coming in contact with a diabetic person while remaining others believed that diabetes is non-infectious. Thus, overall 50.55 per cent of the non-diabetic patients were agreed with myth-5. Similarly, among the attendants, 63.75 per cent respondents considered this as a myth. However, with reference to 23.91 per cent male respondents and 52.94 per cent female respondents believed in myth-5.

Myth 6: Insulin Treatment is used in Final Stage of Diabetes

Majority, i.e. 63.88 per cent of diabetic patients believed that insulin is used for patients in final stage of the disease, while rest of patients explained that insulin treatment is used depending on the nature of the diabetes and various factors decide the use of insulin in treatment of diabetes. With reference to gender, 47.87 per cent male and 81.39 per cent of the female respondents had myth-6, while others were not agreed with this statement.

Among the non-diabetics, 71.58 per cent male and 84.70 per cent of the female respondents believed that insulin is an end term treatment for diabetes, while rest of the respondents did not believe in myth-6 instead they think that insulin is not used throughout the treatment process of diabetes. Thus, overall 77.77 per cent non-diabetics had myth-6.

Table 9.1: Gender-wise distribution of prevalent myths in diabetics, non-diabetics and attendants

Sl. No.	Myths	Diabetics (N = 180)				Non-diabetics (N=180)				Attendants (N=80)				Comparison of groups					
		Male N=94		Female N=86		Male N=95		Female N=85		Male N=46		Female N=34		Diabetics Male vs. Female N=180		Non-Diabetics Male vs. Female N=180		Attendants Male vs. Female N=80	
		n	%	N	%	n	%	N	%	n	%	N	%	z-test value	p-value	z-test value	p-value	z-test value	p-value
1.	Consumption of sugar causes diabetes	19	20.21	27	31.39	51	53.68	78	91.76	20	43.47	32	94.11	1.7	0.09	5.7**	<0.0001	4.7**	<0.0001
2.	Diabetics should never consume sweets	62	65.95	80	93.02	64	67.36	75	88.2	29	63.04	30	88.23	4.4**	<0.0001	3.3*	0.0008	2.5*	0.012
3.	Diabetics can eat anything once the treatment begins	14	14.89	20	23.25	42	44.21	53	62.35	12	26.08	22	64.70	1.4	0.15	2.4*	0.016	3.5*	0.0006
4.	Diabetes is an inherited disease	24	25.53	30	34.88	35	36.84	62	72.94	19	41.30	25	73.52	1.4	0.17	4.8**	<0.0001	2.9*	0.004
5.	Diabetes is an infectious disease	7	7.44	13	15.11	33	34.73	58	68.24	11	23.91	18	52.94	1.6	0.10	4.4**	<0.0001	2.7*	0.0076
6.	Insulin treatment is used in final stage of diabetes	45	47.87	70	81.39	68	71.58	72	84.70	28	60.86	31	91.17	4.7**	<0.0001	2.1*	0.035	3.0*	0.0023
7.	Insulin completely cures diabetes	14	14.89	20	23.25	49	51.57	75	88.23	18	39.14	21	61.76	1.4	0.15	5.2**	<0.0001	2.0*	0.046
8.	Insulin treatment is a lifelong treatment process	67	71.27	72	83.72	74	77.89	80	94.11	24	52.17	31	91.17	1.9*	0.05	3.0*	0.002	3.7*	0.0002
9.	Insulin treatment can be stopped once blood sugar level is under control	8	8.51	13	15.11	34	35.78	50	58.82	14	30.43	19	55.88	1.4	0.17	3.1*	0.002	2.3*	0.022
10.	Insulin treatment causes impotence in diabetic patients	19	20.21	12	13.95	36	37.89	20	23.52	17	36.95	12	35.29	1.1	0.27	2.0*	0.043	0.1	0.883
11.	Alternative medicine can treat diabetes	55	58.51	75	87.20	41	43.15	58	68.23	28	60.86	33	97.05	4.2**	<0.0001	3.4*	0.0008	3.8*	0.0002

12.	Diabetes can affect sexual life	27	28.72	21	24.41	33	34.73	30	35.29	17	36.95	15	44.11	0.7	0.52	0.1	0.944	0.6	0.53
13.	Diabetes affects vision over the long term	60	63.82	80	93.20	59	62.10	72	84.70	17	36.95	24	70.58	4.7**	<0.0001	3.4*	0.0007	3.0*	0.003
14.	Diabetics cannot participate in rigorous physical activities	33	35.10	41	47.67	36	37.89	60	70.58	30	65.21	33	97.05	1.7	0.086	4.4**	<0.0001	3.6*	0.003
15.	Artificial sweeteners are safe	68	72.34	63	73.25	75	78.94	73	85.88	30	65.21	21	61.76	0.2	0.88	1.2	0.227	0.3	0.75

Note: * indicates significant p-value <0.05 and ** indicates highly significant p-value <0.001.

Table 9.2: Comparison of myths between the respondents (diabetics, non-diabetics and attendants)

Sl. No.	*Myths prevalent among the study population*	*Diabetics (N=180)*		*Non-diabetics (N=180)*		*Attendants (N=80)*		*Comparison of groups*					
								Diabetics vs. Non-diabetics		*Non-diabetics vs. Attendants*		*Diabetics vs. Attendants*	
		N	*%*	*n*	*%*	*n*	*%*	*z-test valve*	*p-value*	*z-test value*	*p-value*	*z- test value*	*p-value*
1.	Consumption of sugar causes diabetes	46	25.56	129	71.67	52	65	9.6**	<0.0001	6.1**	<0.0001	1.9	0.0635
2.	Diabetics should never consume sweets	142	78.89	139	77.22	59	73.75	0.4	0.7036	0.9	0.3621	0.5	0.5445
3.	Diabetics can eat anything once the treatment begins	34	18.89	95	52.78	34	42.5	6.7**	<0.0001	4.0**	<0.0001	1.5	0.1264
4.	Diabetes is an inherited disease	54	30.00	97	53.89	44	55	4.6**	<0.0001	3.8**	<0.0001	0.2	0.867
5.	Diabetes is an infectious disease	20	11.11	91	50.56	29	36.25	8.1**	<0.0001	4.8**	<0.0001	2.1*	0.033
6.	Insulin treatment is used in final stage of diabetes	115	63.89	140	77.78	59	73.75	2.9*	0.0037	1.6	0.1185	0.7	0.48
7.	Insulin completely cures diabetes	34	18.89	124	68.89	39	48.75	9.6**	<0.0001	4.9**	<0.0001	3.1*	0.002
8.	Insulin treatment is a lifelong treatment process	139	77.22	154	85.56	55	68.75	2.0*	0.0423	1.4	0.1475	3.1*	0.0016
9.	Insulin treatment can be stopped once blood sugar level is under control	21	11.67	84	46.67	33	41.25	7.3**	<0.0001	5.4**	<0.0001	0.8	0.418
10.	Insulin treatment causes impotence in diabetic patients	31	17.22	56	31.11	29	36.25	3.1*	0.0021	3.4*	0.0008	0.8	0.418
11.	Alternative medicine can treat diabetes	130	72.22	99	55.00	61	76.25	3.4*	0.0007	0.7	0.497	3.3*	0.0012
12.	Diabetes can affect sexual life	48	26.67	63	35.00	32	40	1.7	0.0867	2.2*	0.0315	0.8	0.4397
13.	Diabetes affects vision over the long term	140	77.78	131	72.78	41	51.25	1.1	0.2716	4.3**	<0.0001	3.4*	0.0007
14.	Diabetics cannot participate in rigorous physical activities	74	41.11	96	53.33	63	78.75	2.3*	0.0202	5.6*	<0.0002	3.9*	<0.0002
15.	Artificial sweeteners are safe	131	72.78	148	82.22	51	63.75	2.1*	0.032	1.5	0.143	3.2*	0.0012

Note: * indicates significant p-value <0.05 and ** indicates highly significant p-value <0.001.

Similarly, among the attendants, 60.86 per cent male and 91.17 per cent female respondents agreed to myth-6 statement, while other respondents opined that insulin use is independent of the stage of the disease. Therefore, 73.75 per cent attendants believe this myth as a fact while other attendants considered this as only a myth.

Myth 7: Insulin Completely Cures Diabetes

Among the diabetic patients, 14.89 per cent male respondents and 23.25 per cent female respondents believed that insulin therapy completely cures diabetes or in myth-7, while 85.11 per cent male respondents and 76.75 per cent female respondents believed otherwise. Thus, 18.88 per cent of the diabetic patients believed in myth-7, while 81.12 per cent of the diabetic patients believed it to be a myth propagated over generations, only helps in controlling the blood sugar levels, and, dietary and lifestyle changes go hand in hand in controlling diabetes.

Similarly, among the non-diabetics, 51.57 per cent male respondents and 88.23 per cent female respondents believed in myth-7, while 48.43 per cent male respondents and 11.77 per cent female respondents believed that diabetes was incurable and could only be controlled by insulin therapy. Thus, 68.88 per cent non-diabetics believed in myth-7, while 31.12 per cent non-diabetics considered myth-7 was propagated over generations and with no scientific explanation.

Further, among the attendants, 39.14 per cent male respondents and 61.76 per cent female respondents believed in myth-7, while 60.86 per cent male respondents and 38.24 per cent female respondents believed that diabetes could only be controlled and not cured. Thus, 48.75 per cent of the attendants believed in myth-7, while 51.25 per cent of the attendants disregarded myth-7 and believed that diabetes could be controlled by insulin, proper diet and by leading a healthy lifestyle.

Myth 8: Insulin Treatment is a Lifelong Treatment Process

Among the diabetic patients, 71.27 per cent male respondents and 83.72 per cent female respondents believed that insulin treatment is a lifelong process or as in myth-8, while 28.73 per cent male respondents and 16.28 per cent female respondents believed that insulin need not be used for the entire life. Thus, 77.22 per cent diabetic patients believed in myth-8, while 22.78 per cent diabetic patients believed in myth-8 was propagated over generations, and believed that insulin treatment could be stopped once diabetes was under control. Also, some respondents believed the use of insulin as a treatment option and the duration of use of insulin therapy depended on the type of diabetes. They believed dependency on insulin to be harmful and suggested opting for alternative treatment for diabetes.

Among the non-diabetics, 77.89 per cent male respondents and 94.11 per cent female respondents believed in myth-8, while 22.11 per cent male respondents and 5.89 per cent female respondents believed that insulin treatment is used only if diabetes is very severe or in the final stages of the disease. A few respondents also believed that insulin treatment is used during pregnancy and it could be stopped later. Thus, 85.55 per cent non-diabetics believed in myth-8, while 14.45 per cent non-diabetics considered myth-8 was propagated over generations which had no scientific explanation.

Among the attendants, 52.17 per cent male respondents and 91.17 per cent female respondents believed in myth-8, while 47.83 per cent male respondents and 8.83 per cent female respondents believed that insulin only needed to be used as long as the disease was severe and alternative treatment options could be used to stop insulin use. Thus, 68.75 per cent of the attendants believed in myth-8, while 31.25 per cent of the attendants considered it as a myth and believed insulin use can be stopped once blood glucose levels were under control.

Myth 9: Insulin Treatment can be Stopped Once Blood Sugar Level is Under Control

Among the diabetic patients, 8.51 per cent male respondents and 15.11 per cent female respondents believed that insulin treatment can be discontinued once blood sugar level is under control or in myth-9, while 91.49 per cent male respondents and 84.89 per cent female respondents believed that insulin treatment once started could not be stopped. Thus, 11.66 per cent of the diabetic patients believed in myth-9, while 88.34 per cent of the diabetic patients believed in myth-9 to be false, as they believed insulin therapy to be a life-term treatment option.

Among the non-diabetics, 35.78 per cent male respondents and 58.82 per cent female respondents believed in myth-9, while 64.22 per cent male respondents and 41.18 per cent female respondents believed that insulin treatment needs to be continued throughout the life of a diabetic patient. Thus, 46.66 per cent non-diabetics believed in myth-9, while 53.34 per cent non-diabetics considered it as a myth.

Similarly, among the attendants, 30.43 per cent male respondents and 55.88 per cent female respondents believed in myth-9, while 69.57 per cent male respondents and 44.12 per cent female respondents believed that insulin cannot be stopped once it was recommended to the patient. Thus, 41.25 per cent of the attendants believed in myth-9, while 58.75 per cent of the attendants considered it as a myth.

Myth 10: Insulin Treatment causes Impotence in Diabetic Patients

Among the diabetic patients, 20.21 per cent male respondents and 13.95 per cent female respondents believed that insulin treatment causes impotence in diabetic patients or in myth-10, while 79.79 per cent male respondents and 86.05 per cent female respondents believed otherwise. Thus, 17.22 per cent diabetic patients believed in myth-10, while 82.78 per cent diabetic patients believed that it is a myth propagated over generations and believed it existed because of the disease itself.

Among the non-diabetic, 37.89 per cent male respondents and 23.52 per cent female respondents believed in myth-10, while 62.11 per cent male respondents and 76.48 per cent female respondents did not believe in myth-10. Thus, 31.11 per cent non-diabetics believed in myth-10, while 68.89 per cent of the non-diabetics considered it as a myth with no scientific explanation.

Among the attendants, 36.95 per cent male respondents and 35.29 per cent female respondents believed in myth-10, while 63.05 per cent male respondents and 64.71 per cent female respondents believed it to be a myth as impotence in diabetics was not caused by insulin treatment. Thus, 36.25 per cent attendants believed in myth-10, while 63.75 per cent attendants were of the opinion that diabetes led to impotence and not insulin treatment.

Myth 11: Alternative Medicine can Treat Diabetes

Among the diabetic patients, 58.51 per cent male respondents and 87.20 per cent female respondents believed that alternative medicine (i.e. Ayurveda, Homoeopathy, Naturopathy, Yoga etc.) can treat diabetes or in myth-11, while 41.49 per cent male respondents and 12.80 per cent female respondents believed that alternative medicine cannot treat diabetes. Thus, 72.22 per cent diabetic patients believed in myth-11, while 27.78 per cent diabetic patients believed it to be a myth propagated over generations, and believed that only alternative treatment was not sufficient to cure diabetes.

Among the non-diabetics, 43.15 per cent male respondents and 68.23 per cent female respondents believed in myth-11, while 56.85 per cent male respondents and 31.77 per cent female respondents believed that alternative medicine can help in controlling diabetes to some extent but alternative systems of treatment were also needed. Thus, 55 per cent non-diabetic believed in myth-11, while 45 per cent non-diabetics considered it a myth propagated over generations and had no scientific explanation.

Among the attendants, 60.86 per cent male respondents and 97.05 per cent female respondents believed in myth-11, while 39.14 per cent male respondents and 2.95 per cent female respondents believed that alternative medicine helped in controlling blood glucose levels but could not cure diabetes. Thus, 76.25 per cent attendants believed in myth-11, while 23.75 per cent attendants considered it as a myth.

Myth 12: Diabetes can Affect Sexual Life

Among the diabetic patients, 28.72 per cent male respondents and 24.41 per cent female respondents believed that diabetes affects the sexual life of the patient or myth-12, while 71.28 per cent male respondents and 75.59 per cent female respondents did not believe in myth-12. Thus, 26.66 per cent diabetic patients believed in myth-12, while 73.34 per cent (n = 132) of the diabetic patients believed it to be a myth propagated over generations.

Among the non-diabetics, 34.73 per cent male respondents and 35.29 per cent female respondents believed in myth-12, while 65.27 per cent male respondents and 64.71 per cent female respondents believed that the disease has no impact on the sexual health of a diabetic person. Thus, 35 per cent non-diabetics believed in myth-12, while 65 per cent non-diabetics considered myth-12 was propagated over generations and had no scientific explanation.

Among the attendants, 36.95 per cent male respondents and 44.11 per cent female respondents believed in myth-12, while 63.05 per cent male respondents and 55.89 per cent female respondents believed in myth-12 was untrue. Thus, 40 per cent of the attendants believed in myth-12, while 60 per cent of the attendants considered it as a myth.

Myth 13: Diabetes affects Vision Over the Long Term

Among the diabetic patients, 63.82 per cent male respondents and 93.20 per cent female respondents believed that diabetes causes ocular problems and affects vision over the long term or myth-13, while 36.18 per cent male respondents and 6.80 per cent female respondents believed in myth-13 to be untrue. Thus, 77.77 per cent diabetic patients believed in myth-13, while 22.23 per cent diabetic patients believed it to be a myth propagated over generations.

Further, among the non-diabetics, 62.10 per cent male respondents and 84.70 per cent female respondents believed in myth-13, while 37.90 per cent male respondents and 15.30 per cent female respondents did not believe in myth-13. Thus, 72.77 per cent non-diabetic patients believed in myth-13, while 27.23 per cent non-diabetics dismissed myth-13.

Similarly, among the attendants, 36.95 per cent male respondents and 70.58 per cent female respondents believed in myth-13, while 63.05 per cent male respondents and 29.42 per cent female respondents disbelieved in myth-13. Thus, 51.25 per cent attendants believed that diabetes causes vision problems in later stage of the disease while 48.75 per cent of the attendants considered it a myth.

Myth 14: Diabetics cannot Participate in Rigorous Physical Activities

Among the diabetic patients, 35.10 per cent male respondents and 47.67 per cent female respondents believed that diabetics could not participate in rigorous physical activities or myth-14, while 64.90 per cent male respondents and 52.33 per cent female respondents believed the opposite. Thus, 41.11 per cent believed in myth-14, while 58.89 per cent diabetic patients believed it to be a myth adding that the dietary pattern and lifestyle changes like monitoring sugar levels, maintaining a healthy blood glucose level, could help them endure rigorous physical activities.

Further, among the non-diabetics, 37.89 per cent male respondents and 70.58 per cent female respondents believed in myth-14 as they had less stamina and their blood glucose levels dropped drastically, while 62.11 per cent male respondents and 29.42 per cent female respondents believed that by taking necessary precautions a diabetic patient could even participate in rigorous physical activities. Thus, 53.33 per cent non-diabetics believed in myth-14, while 45.67 per cent non-diabetics considered it a myth for the patient with no health complications could pursue rigorous physical activities too.

Similarly, among the attendants, 65.21 per cent (n = 30) male respondents and 97.05 per cent female respondents believed in myth-14, while 34.79 per cent male respondents and 2.95 per cent female respondents believed otherwise. Thus, 78.75 per cent attendants believed in myth-14, while 21.25 per cent attendants considered it a myth propagated over generations and did not consider it impossible for a diabetic patient to participate in rigorous physical activities.

Myth 15: Artificial Sweeteners are Safe

Among the diabetic patients, 72.34 per cent male respondents and 73.25 per cent female respondents believed that artificial sweeteners are safe for consumption by diabetic patients or myth-15, while 27.66 per cent male respondents and 26.75 per cent female respondents believed that artificial sweeteners have adverse effects over prolonged use and should be avoided. Thus, 72.77 per cent diabetic patients believed in myth-15, while 27.23 per cent of the diabetic patients believed that myth-15 to be untrue.

Further, among the non-diabetics, 78.94 per cent male respondents and 85.88 per cent female respondents believed in myth-15, while 21.06 per cent male respondents and 14.12 per cent female respondents believed that artificial sweeteners are not safe and may have adverse health effects on prolonged use. Thus, 82.22 per cent non-diabetics believed in myth-15, while 17.78 per cent non-diabetics discarded myth-15.

Similarly, among the attendants, 65.21 per cent male respondents and 61.76 per cent female respondents believed myth-15 until taken in moderation, while 34.79 per cent male respondents and 38.24 per cent female respondents believed that artificial sweeteners are unsafe and should be avoided. Thus, 63.75 per cent attendants believed in myth-15, while 36.25 per cent attendants considered it as a myth.

On comparison of proportion (by using z-test) for myths among the above groups, it was found that non-diabetic patients had significantly higher prevalence (p-value <0.05) for myth-1, myth-4, myth-5, myth-7, myth-12, myth-13 than diabetic patients and the attendants. For myth-3 among significant difference was seen between diabetics and non-diabetics and the non-diabetic and attendants. It was also found that the diabetic patients had significantly higher prevalence (p-value <0.05) for myth-6, myth-8, myth-11 than non-diabetic patients and the attendants. However, the diabetics and non-diabetics had significantly higher prevalence (p-value <0.01) for myth-9, myth-10 than the attendants of patients. Furthermore, the non-diabetics and attendants had significantly higher prevalence (p-values <0.05) of myth-14 than diabetic patients. Similarly, it was found that diabetic patients and attendants had significantly higher prevalence (p-value <0.05) of myth-15 than the non-diabetic patients (Table 9.2). There are significant differences in prevalence of myths among the population for all variables with the exception of myth-2, and for myth-3 in the case of comparison between diabetic and attendants was non-significant.

The females reported more myths in comparison to the males. Among the diabetics, the variables showed significant association ($p < 0.05$) for myth-2, myth-6, myth-8, myth-11 and myth-13. Among the non-diabetics, the variables showed significant association ($p < 0.05$) for all myths except myth-12 and myth-15. Among the attendants, the variables showed significant association for all myths except myth-10, myth-12 and myth-15. The prevalence of myth about diabetes is high among both diabetic and non-diabetic population which could be associated with poor health seeking behaviour and poor compliance with treatment.

Graph 9.1 depicts the comparison of myths among the respondents: diabetic, non-diabetic and the attendants. Among the diabetic patients, the most prevalent myth is that the diabetic patients should never consume sweets (myth-2, 78.89%) and the least prevalent myth among the diabetic patients is that diabetes is an infectious disease (myth-5, 11.11%).

Among the non-diabetic patients, the most prevalent myth is that insulin treatment is a lifelong process (myth-8, 85.56%) and the least prevalent myth is that insulin treatment causes impotence in diabetic patients (myth-10, 31.11%).

Among the attendants, the most prevalent myth is that diabetic patients cannot participate in rigorous physical activities (myth-14, 78.75%) and the least prevalent myths are that diabetes is an infectious disease (myth-5, 36.25%) insulin treatment causes impotence in diabetic patients (myth-10, 36.25%).

The commonest myth among diabetic and non-diabetic respondents was that insulin treatment is a lifelong process (Myth-8, 81.38%) and non-diabetic patients and attendants was that insulin treatment is used in the final stage of diabetes (myth-6, 76.53%) and artificial sweeteners are safe (myth-15, 76.53%) while the most common myth among the diabetic and attendants was that diabetic patients should never consume sweets (myth-2, 77.30%) (*see* Graph 9.1).

Anthropological Perspective of Myths

Myths often are passed down the generations by word of mouth. It is often difficult to determine the origin of some myths. Understanding the myths and misconceptions about the care of patients with diabetes is important in providing excellent care to the patient with diabetes. Myths are defined as stories shared by a group of people which are a part of their cultural identity and history (Adler and Paauw, 2003).

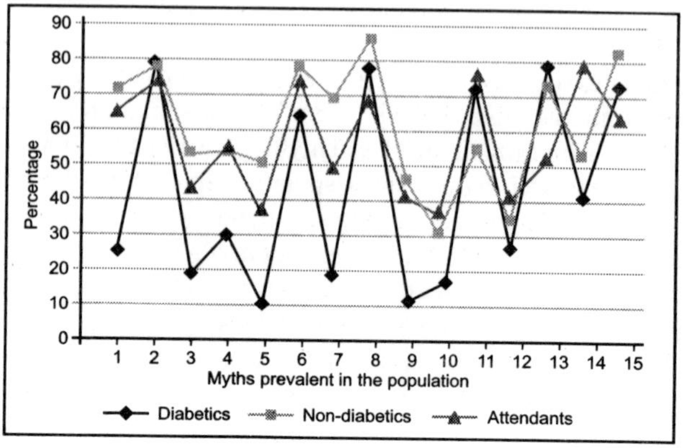

Graph 9.1: Myths prevalent among the population (diabetics, non-diabetics and attendants)

People often do not question many existing assumptions in order to not cause disturbance to the regularity and predictability of social life and order. In Indian society, myths are sometimes taken too literally and are believed to be self-evident truths and in cases of extreme behaviour it could be termed as orthodox. Myths are powerful to those who believe in them. They are persuasive because they offer explanations on human nature, society and their history. Anthropologists in the past have attempted to explain the meaning and the reason for its existence in our society. Levi-Strauss (1967) has a different way of looking at myth, as according to him a myth has meaningful structure that is worth studying in its own right which is apart from the use to which a myth is put. For him, myths are a tool to overcome logical contradictions. In conclusion it would be right to say that the meanings of myth may vary among societies but myths are meaningful because they reflect the capacity of humans to play with possibilities as they attempt to deal with many contradictions that exist (Schultz and Lavenda, 2005).

Myths are an integral part of society and are often not questioned because that always depends on the willingness of the members of the society. It is difficult to break this chain as it is deep seated in the society. We need to change the mindset and the behaviour of the population to eliminate the myths and educate the people about diabetes.

Myths surrounding diabetes are common and are usually attributable to practices that have not been evaluated rigorously. The present study was the exploratory research with the aim to identify the prevailing myths among diabetes patients, their attendants and non-diabetic healthy controls from Chandigarh tricity. To know the myths prevalent among the respondents and to understand the rationale behind them, a few facts related to the prevailing myths from the study have been listed as follows:

Myth: Eating sugar in excess raises blood glucose levels and can result in diabetes.

Fact: It is high calorie intake resulting in obesity or excess weight that increases the risk of diabetes. People are not aware about the normal blood sugar levels, role of lifestyle changes in control and treatment of diabetes and that if not treated diabetes can lead to complications. People with diabetes can eat sweets or chocolates with healthy meal plans and exercise, but people usually misconceive that eating sugar is completely prohibited in diabetes (Nisar *et at.*, 2007). Similar findings have been reported in a study conducted in China that low educational status was found to be an independent risk factor for diabetics.

Myth: Once insulin use starts, it continues for life.

Fact: Insulin is administered to patients before a major surgery or a baby's delivery. It can be stopped thereafter if strict diet regulations and medications pattern is adhered to.

Myth: There is a cure for diabetes.

Fact: It can only be treated not cured.

Myth: Blood sugar tests and reviews at the hospital should be done once there is fatigue, loss of appetite and sudden loss of weight — which are symptoms of diabetes.

Fact: As diabetes is a silent killer, it shows no symptoms at the beginning.

Myth: Diabetics should not continue with medicines once cholesterol level normalize.

Fact: Doctor's advice continuing with cholesterol medicines all through life. Diabetes increases the risk of cardiovascular diseases.

Myth: Diabetes is not a big deal.

Fact: If left unchecked, diabetes can cause serious complications and premature death.

Myth: People with diabetes should follow special diet and cannot eat sweets.

Fact: People with diabetes benefit from the same healthy food that is good for everyone else. They have to follow a balanced diet. So, total per day calorie intake is important.

Myth: Bitter foods can help lower blood sugar.

Fact: Just because some food is not sweet, does not mean it will help curb blood sugar. Bitter foods like *neem* and *karela* do not help.

Myth: Diabetics cannot have fruits.

Fact: Fibre in fruits helps slowly release fructose into blood. Apple, orange, mausambi, papaya, and guava can be taken.

Myth: Artificial sweeteners are safe.

Fact: Artificial sweeteners are 600 times sweeter than sugar, precipitating diabetes.

Myth: Diabetics are required to lose weight fast.

Fact: Obesity and diabetes are two sides of the same coin. Obese people are advised to lose weight but sudden weight loss through crash diet is not advisable.

Myth: Diabetes is caused by eating too much sugar.

Fact: T2DM results when the body does not produce enough insulin and/or is unable to use insulin properly.

Myth: Taking insulin means you have "failed".

Fact: People with T2DM may initially be able to manage with lifestyle modification and oral medication, but eventually, most people will need to go on insulin. Starting insulin helps better manage the diabetes.

Myth: Injecting insulin is painful.

Fact: Insulin injections shouldn't hurt if good injection techniques are practiced, and the experience will be virtually painless.

During the course of the study the researchers also came across a few myths that were prevailing in the study population. The respondents also believed that Type-1 diabetes leads to T2DM, skipping breakfast increases the risk for diabetes, soaking feet in water helps decrease blood sugar levels, normal blood sugar level should be < 200, diabetes occurs because of past sins and can be cured by spiritual treatment, diabetics should consume alcohol to lower blood glucose levels, there is no role of diet/lifestyle measures in cure of diabetes, diabetes occurs only in old age and no complications can occur even if diabetes is uncontrolled.

Preventive programmes targeted towards general population show greater benefits in this situation rather than targeting only high risk and diseased population. There has been little research to understand these myths. Not many studies have been done and we do not have much data related to this subject. Therefore, we have tried to find out the prevalence of common myths about diabetes and its treatment.

Conclusion

Myths and misconceptions in population prevail due to different reasons, for example, having inadequate knowledge. However, it has been known that knowledge alone is not sufficient to bring about behavioural change in population.

Due to rapid increase in the incidence of diabetes in India, preventive strategies are needed to be targeted towards the healthy population. Apart from treatment of diabetes we need to pay attention to the prevention and health education of people about the diseases. Educational level is protective against myths. Therefore, understanding the myths and misconceptions about diabetes mellitus is important in providing better care and health education to both patients and healthy individuals.

We need to educate people about this disease and its preventive as well as treatment options. This will play a very important role in control and prevention of diabetes in the country. Advocacy of diabetes programme is highly encouraged to deal with the myths and misconceptions in the society. Education serves as protective factor; hence efforts should be made to promote education and health awareness regarding the disease, with more emphasis on addressing myths regarding diabetes mellitus.

REFERENCES

Adler, E. and Paauw, D. (2003). "Medical myths involving diabetes", *Primary Care*, *30*(3), 607-618.

American Diabetic Association (ADA). (2005). Medical experts dispel myths about diabetes. JET. Retrieved http://findarticles.com/p/articles/mi_m1355/is_1_108/ai_n15681366.

Anjana, R.M., Deepa, M., Pradeepa, R., Mahanta, J., Narain, K., Das, H.K., ... and Bhansali, A. (2017). "Prevalence of diabetes and prediabetes in 15 states of India: Results from the ICMR–INDIAB population-based cross-sectional study". *The Lancet Diabetes and Endocrinology*, *5*(8), 585-596.

Bhansali, A., and Bhansali, S. (2018). "Diabetes: Easier to prevent, but difficult to tame", *International Journal of Noncommunicable Diseases*, *3*(3), 75.

Cho, N.H., Shaw, J.E., Karuranga, S., Huang, Y., da Rocha Fernandes, J.D., Ohlrogge, A.W., and Malanda, B. (2018). "IDF Diabetes Atlas: Global estimates of diabetes prevalence for 2017 and projections for 2045", *Diabetes Research and Clinical Practice*, *138*, 271-281.

Levi-Strauss, Claude. (1967). *L'antropologie structural*. Paris: Plon. Trans. Under the title *Structural Anthropology*, by Claire Jacobson and Brooke Grundfest Schoepf. New York: Doubleday Anchor.

NCD Risk Factor Collaboration. (2016). "Worldwide trends in diabetes since 1980: A pooled analysis of 751 population-based studies with 4.4 million participants", *The Lancet, 387*(10027), 1513-1530.

Nisar, N., Khan, I.A., Qadri, M.H., and Sher, S.A. (2007). "Myths about diabetes mellitus among non-diabetic individuals attending primary health care centers of Karachi suburbs", *J Coll Physicians Surg Pak, 17*(7), 398-401.

Pearson, E.R., and McCrimmon, R.J. (2014). "Diabetes Mellitus". In B.R. Walker, N.R. Colledge, S.H. Ralston, I.D. Penman, Eds. *Davidson's Principals and Practice of Medicine.* 22nd ed. London. Elseiver:797-8820.

Rai, M., and Kishore, J. (2009). "Myths about diabetes and its treatment in North Indian population", *International Journal of Diabetes in Developing Countries, 29*(3), 129.

Ravikumar, P., Bhansali, A., Ravikiran, M., Bhansali, S., Walia, R., Shanmugasundar, G., ... and Dutta, P. (2011). "Prevalence and risk factors of diabetes in a community-based study in North India: The Chandigarh Urban Diabetes Study (CUDS)", *Diabetes and Metabolism, 37*(3), 216-221.14.

Rehman, A., Mirza, U., Jehan, M., and Pasha, S.A. (2013). "Myths and misconceptions regarding diabetes mellitus among diabetic and non-diabetic Indian population", *International Journal of Current Research and Review, 5*(6), 26.

Schultz, E.A., and Lavenda, R.H. (2005). *Cultural anthropology*. New York, NY: Oxford University Press.

Venkataraman, K., Kannan, A.T., and Mohan, V. (2009). "Challenges in diabetes management with particular reference to India", *International Journal of Diabetes in Developing Countries, 29*(3), 103.

10

Health Seeking Behaviour and the Wellbeing of the Slum Dwellers of Delhi in Regards to Acute Respiratory Tract Infections

B.S. Aribam

Introduction

Health seeking behaviour in developing countries is mostly characterized by the availability of multiple alternative treatment choices (Young, 1981; Ryan & Martinez, 1996; Ryan, 1998). The alternatives include the application of a home remedy, self-medication with pharmaceuticals bought over-the-counter on the open market, herbal therapies provided by traditional healers as well as care provided by health centres or hospitals. Effective health seeking behaviour depends a lot on the types of health care or health care providers operating in and around the community.

The availability of increased health facilities and accessibility to health personnel also contributed to the change in the people's attitude towards the disease and health seeking behaviour (Rajamma *et al.*, 1996). Availability of transport, physical distance of the facility and time taken to reach the facility undoubtedly influence the health seeking behaviour and health services utilization. Patient satisfaction with the type of treatment available also plays an important role in the health seeking behaviour of the people (Shaikh *et al.*, 2004). A study by Kunda, on the health seeking behaviour of human brucellosis in rural Tanzania reported that distance to hospital, among other factors, was significantly associated with patients' delay in reaching in reaching to present themselves in the hospital (Kunda *et al.*, 2007).

However, there is a serious shortage of human resources to provide healthcare services in South Asian region (Wahed, 2010). As a result, informal healthcare providers, predominantly unqualified allopathic practitioners, provide a majority of healthcare for poor households in India, Pakistan, and Bangladesh (Hardings, 2003; Patil *et al.*, 2002; Kumar, 2004; Ahmed, 2005 and 2009). These providers are popular because of low cost, easy access, convenient hours, willingness to make house calls, and their acceptance by the community (Darmstadt *et al.*, 2006; Radwan, 2005). Therefore, there is a close relationship between the health seeking behaviour of a community and the people who are providing medical service. Consequently, in order to develop a rational policy to provide successful, suitable, cost-effective, inexpensive and easily reached health services, it becomes important to understand the health care providers who are channelizing the care seeking behaviour of the people.

Thus, the present paper tries to explore the health seeking behaviour of the two slum colonies in relation with the role of informal prescribers functioning in and around the two communities.

Materials and Methods

The present study was conducted in two slum clusters of Delhi in Timarpur over a period of six months from mid-October to March. The two study sites, namely J.J. Colony Patrachar Vidyalaya and Sanjay Basti have approximately 600 and 1500 households, respectively (MCD, J.J. Colony List, 2001). There was no linguistic variation in the two study sites as they are neighbouring colonies residing just across the road to each other. Majority of the people are predominantly Hindus and Muslims and a very few Christians. Most houses in this area are temporary tenements consisting of only a single room.

For data collection, a medical anthropologist was given intensive training to identify cases of pneumonia by a medical doctor who had experience of managing and treating ARI for many years. Qualitative methods used in the study were standardized in consultation with a social science expert. The basic training included explanation of ARI in the class room followed by on-the-field practice. Training was given on the classification of ARI, causes and factors that contribute to these infections, signs and symptoms of pneumonia and examination. The selection of the cases was done following the WHO guidelines for the symptoms of pneumonia which were specified as rapid or difficult breathing, cough, fever, chills, headaches, loss of appetite, wheezing and chest in-drawing (UNICEF/WHO, 2006).

The study was approved by the Institutional Ethics Committee. Verbal consents were obtained from the study respondents before proceeding with any form of interview. Research methods such as in-depth interviews, focus group discussions and case study methods were used for data collection during the fieldwork. A total of 610 respondents (587 mothers and 23 grandmothers) were interviewed. Overall, 410 cases/children were selected from J.J. Colony Patrachar Vidyalaya and 200 cases/children were selected from Sanjay Basti. Those children who were under five years of age and were showing symptoms of ARI at the time of visit or during the last two weeks were selected for study. A pre-design and pre-tested interview schedule was used for collecting data. These scheduled interviews were conducted to get a clear idea about the maternal perceptions of the key symptoms, severity of illness and its causation and the treatment strategies.

Around 10 focus group discussions (6 in Patrachar Jhugi and 4 in Sanjay Basti) with ten to twelve respondents in each FGD were conducted. In all, around 104 respondents participated in the focus group discussions. The mean age of the respondents of both the study sites was 25 years. Over three-fourth of the respondents were illiterate and the rest have studied up to primary level. The data was analysed using Statistical Package for Social Science (SPSS) version 15.0.

Results

All caretakers who were interviewed had heard about ARI and had prior idea about what ARI was. Most caretakers were also familiar with the term *nazlajukham* which was used interchangeably to mean common cold at the same time ARI as a whole.

Table 10.1: Knowledge of the caretakers regarding the symptoms of *nazlajukham*

Variables	*Frequency*	*Per cent (%)*
Nasal or eye symptoms	330	54.1
Difficulty or noisy breathing	91	14.9
Others	14	2.3
All the above	38	6.2
Any nasal and eye symptoms and difficulty in breathing	137	22.5
Total	**610**	**100.0**

From Table 10.1, it was observed that, caretakers had good knowledge about the symptoms of ARI. More than half of the caretakers (54.1%) identified the symptoms of ARI as nasal and eye symptoms. Nasal and eye symptoms mean block or runny nose and teary or watery eyes due to common cold. Around 22.5 per cent caretakers pointed out that a combination of nasal and eye symptoms and difficulty in breathing were symptoms of common cold. However, 14.9 per cent of them said that difficulty or noisy breathing were important symptoms of common cold. Around 6.2 per cent caretakers said that all the symptoms mentioned in Table 10.1 were symptoms of common cold, while 2.3 per cent caretakers pointed out that other symptoms like headache, fever, coughing, excessive crying etc. were also symptoms of common cold.

Table 10.2: Knowledge of the caretakers regarding the symptoms of Pneumonia

Variables	Frequency	Percentage (%)
Difficulty in breathing	82	13.4
Fast breathing	55	9.0
Chest in-drawing	183	30.0
Fever	110	18.0
All the above	83	13.6
Others	55	9.0
Cannot Say	42	6.9
Total	**610**	**100.0**

Table 10.2 showed that majority of the caretakers (30%) could recognize chest in-drawing as a symptom of pneumonia. A good number of caretakers also pointed out that fever could be a symptom of pneumonia as well. Many caretakers during FGD highlighted that high grade fever was the triggering point for seeking outside care or formal medical care. Around 13.4 per cent caretakers said that difficulty in breathing was also another symptom of pneumonia. A few caretakers mentioned fast breathing or rapid breathing as a symptom of pneumonia without any prompting. Approximately, 9 per cent caretakers believed that symptoms like excessive crying, loss of appetite, constant fatigue or lethargy or inactiveness among children were also some of the symptoms of pneumonia. They also pointed out that, these symptoms were often associated with fever if the child has pneumonia.

Causes of ARI According to the Caretakers

Majority of the caretaker (33.1%) believed that ARI was caused by seasonal change or onset of cold season. This was followed by the perception that ARI was caused by the exposure of nursing mothers and children to cold. However, 7.9 per cent said that ARI was caused by physical contact, i.e.

after mingling with ARI sick children. However, 3.9 per cent believed that ARI was caused by taking cold drinks and foods, while, 1.8 per cent believed that ARI was caused by evil eye alone. Finally, 14.6 per cent caretakers were of the perception that all the causal mechanisms mentioned in Table 10.3 could cause ARI when all these factors were together, while 15.7 per cent thought ARI was caused by a combination of seasonal change and exposure to cold (Table 10.3).

Table 10.3: Knowledge of the caretakers about the causes of ARI

Variables	*Frequency*	*Percentage (%)*
Seasonal change (onset of cold season)	202	33.1
Cold food or drinks	24	3.9
Physical contact	48	7.9
Exposure of mother or child to cold	140	23.0
Evil eye	11	1.8
All the above	89	14.6
Combinations of seasonal change and exposure to cold	96	15.7
Total	**610**	**100.0**

Treatment of ARI

Most caretakers were in favour of giving home remedies and self-prescribed medicines together for treating ARI. Around 18 per cent caretakers had the attitude that self-prescription medicines alone will cure ARI while, 10.2 per cent of them felt that home remedies alone could cure ARI. On the other hand, 16.2 per cent of the caretakers were of the attitude that ARI could be cured by consulting informal prescriber, whereas, 12.8 per cent favoured formal doctors for ARI (Table 10.4). A few caretakers were of the opinion that children would be alright or get well soon even without any form of treatment.

Table 10.4: Attitude of the caretakers regarding steps that should be taken up for ARI

Variables	*Frequency*	*Percentage (%)*
Giving Home remedies	62	10.2
Giving Self-Prescription	110	18.0
Both home remedies and self-prescription	152	24.9
Informal prescribers	99	16.2
Formal doctors	78	12.8
Any combinations	93	15.2
None	16	2.6
Total	**610**	**100.0**

A good number of the caretakers (64%) gave home remedies to their children who were showing symptoms of ARI. However, 36 per cent of them did not give home remedies because they felt that home remedies were not effective and they took time to heal the sickness.

Different forms of home remedies were given for treatment of ARI by the caretakers. Majority of the caretakers gave a combination of ginger honey tea and other herbal teas, milk and turmeric mixed together, nutmeg in hot water, boiled egg yolk of local egg mixed in milk (Table 10.5). Apart from these 8.9 per cent caretakers made their children inhale hot steam, rubbed their chest, nose and nape with Vicks Vaporub (brand name). In few serious cases or if the child was suspected to have pneumonia, caretakers rubbed hot mustard oil all over the child's body or rubbed the child's chest and back with a mixture of kerosene and camphor. This was followed by wrapping the child's chest where chest in-drawing was visible, with a piece of cloth. This was generally done to relieve to congestion in the chest and to free the air passage or to enable the child to breathe normally. A very few caretakers (1%) mentioned about giving proper bed rest, cleaning up the nasal and eye discharge and washing hands after that when their children showed symptoms of ARI (Table 10.5).

Table 10.5: Types of home remedies used for treating ARI among under-five children by the caretakers

Variables	*Frequency*	*Percentage (%)*
Ginger honey tea and other herbal teas	0	13.9
Bed rest, cleaning up the nasal discharge and washing hands	7	1.0
Inhale steam and balm rubs, camphor kerosene rubs	54	8.9
Milk and turmeric, *jaiffal* (nutmeg) and others	114	18.7
Any combinations	131	21.5
None	219	36.0
Total	**610**	**100.0**

Out of the total 610 cases, only 34 per cent took their children to seek health care provider for ARI including common cold and pneumonia. However, 66 per cent, i.e. majority of the caretakers chose to seek other forms of treatment instead of resorting to health care providers, mostly formal doctors or hospital care. The main reasons for avoiding hospital care were because most of the government hospitals were far from the two slum communities and the nearby ones were not well equipped to admit serious sickness. Other reasons given by the caretakers included lost of wages due to the time-consumed in the hospital (standing in queues and waiting for their turn), constraint of money and unavailability of people in the household for taking the child to the hospital.

It was observed from Table 10.6 that majority of the caretakers (66%) did not prefer health care providers for their children suffering with ARI. Around 18.4 per cent of the caretakers felt that hospital care should be sought only when the child started showing serious symptoms of ARI. This was followed by few caretakers (7.2%) who thought medical care was essential for children with ARI so children should be taken to a

Table 10.6: Attitude of mother concerning the importance of health care provider for ARI among under-five children

Variables	*Frequency*	*Percentage (%)*
Home remedies better for sickness	34	5.5
Only when the child was serious	112	18.4
Medical care essential	44	7.2
When the child was serious and medical care essential	18	2.9
No need to take to health care providers	402	66.0
Total	**610**	**100.0**

formal doctors or hospital when they had ARI symptoms. However, some caretakers (5.5%) felt that home remedies were better for ARI and other sicknesses too, as home remedies do not have side effects.

Table 10.7: Decision making in family for seeking health care for ARI

Variables	*Frequency*	*Percentage (%)*
Father	224	36.7
Mother	239	39.2
Grandparents	23	3.8
Both mother and father	124	20.3
Total	**610**	**100.0**

From Table 10.7, it was observed that decision making for seeking health care was mainly done by the mothers (39.2%) while fathers (36.7%) were also observed to be as much part of the decision making for seeking any form of health care for their children. Around 3.8 per cent grandparents helped in decision making for seeking health care for ARI. In 20.3 per cent cases, both mother and father made decisions together for seeking care from a health care provider.

Table 10.8: Services rendered by the health care provider for treating ARI among under-five children

Variables	*Frequency*	*Percentage (%)*
Check symptoms and examine	6	1.0
Prescription with medicine	2	0.3
Referral	22	3.6
Advises without seeing	4	0.7
Dispense medicine	84	13.8
Dispense medicines and advised without seeing	90	14.7
Did not seek health care provider	402	66.0
Total	**610**	**100.0**

From Table 10.8, it was observed that majority of the caretakers (66%) did not seek any health care providers for ARI. Among those who sought health care providers, 14.7 per cent were given advice without seeing the children and dispensed medicines on the basis of the symptoms reported by the caretakers. Health care provider mostly dispensed medicines (13.8%) for any symptoms related with ARI or advises (0.7%) without actually seeing the children with ARI symptoms. Around 3 per cent of the ARI cases were referred to hospital care since the cases were observed to be serious. Only 1 per cent children were examined and checked for ARI symptoms and only 0.3 per cent was given prescription with medicines for treating ARI symptoms.

Table 10.9: Commonly used medicines for ARI among under-five children

Variables	*Frequency*	*Percentage (%)*
Antibiotics	56	9.2
Anti allergic	2	0.3
Anti-pyretic	5	0.8
Unlabelled syrup/medicine	150	24.6
Combinations of unlabelled syrup and anti-allergic	49	8.0
Not given any medicine	348	57.0
Total	**610**	**100.0**

Table 10.9 showed the types of commonly used medicines for ARI by the caretakers. Around 24.6 per cent of the caretakers were reserving unlabelled syrup or medicines for treating ARI symptoms. These unlabelled drugs were believed to be antibiotics. About 9.2 per cent of the caretakers were giving antibiotics to their children for treating ARI. These antibiotics included Mox, Amoxicillin, Ampicillin, Tetracycline,

Cotrimoxazole etc. Around 8 per cent caretakers showed a combination of unlabelled syrups and anti-allergic medicines. Those anti-allergic medicines included Citrizine, Chlorpheniramine Maleate, Decongestants, and Antihistamines. On the other hand, 0.8 per cent caretakers showed anti-pyretic medicines given for ARI such as Aspirin, Acetaminophen, Paracetamol, Indomethacin, Brufen and cold packs.

Majority of the caretakers did not seek treatment from HCP (Table 10.10). Among those who sought treatment from HCP, 29 per cent of them continued for about 1-4 days. Whereas, 11 per cent gave the treatment for 5-8 days and only 3 per cent were given treatment by the HCP for around 2 weeks (Table 10.10).

Table 10.10: Number of days of treatment given by the health care providers to the under-five children who had symptoms of ARI

Variables	*Frequency*	*Percentage (%)*
1-4 days	177	29.0
5-8 days	67	11.0
Round 2 weeks	18	3.0
Did not seek treatment from HCP	348	57.0
Total	**610**	**100.0**

Table 10.11: Whether caretakers had already stopped treatment or not?

Variables	*Frequency*	*Percentage (%)*
Yes	48	7.9
No	214	35.1
Did not seek HCP	348	57.0
Total	**610**	**100.0**

Majority of the caretakers (35.1%) were still continuing with the treatment given by the HCP (health care provider) while, 7.9 per cent of them had already stopped giving treatment to their children as directed by the HCP (Table 10.11).

Table 10.12: Reasons for stopping treatment by the Caretakers

Variables	*Frequency*	*Percentage (%)*
Recovered	30	4.9
Child's condition not improving	4	0.7
Unable to afford	9	1.4
Not Applicable/Not stopped	567	93.0
Total	**610**	**100.0**

The common reasons given by the caretakers for stopping treatment for ARI were recovery of their children (4.9%), children's conditions were not improving (0.7%) and inability to afford the treatment any more (1.4%) (Table 10.12). Many caretakers had the general perception that if the symptoms of ARI were not improved after the administration of medicines within 1 or 2 days then they would start thinking about changing the type of treatment they were giving or they would either change the health care provider.

Most caretakers (19.5%) expressed their desire to stop treatment after the recovery of their children while some other caretakers said that they would stop treatment after 3 or 4 days. About 3.6 per cent of the caretakers said that they would wait until the completion of the duration prescribed by the HCP while a few caretakers gave multiple opinions like after complete recovery of the sickness or after 3 or 4 days (Table 10.13).

Table 10.13: When do caretakers stopped the treatment given by the health care providers

Variables	*Frequency*	*Percentage (%)*
After recovery	119	19.5
After 3/4 days	102	16.7
Completion of prescribed duration	22	3.6
Any combination	8	1.3
Not Applicable or continued treatment	359	58.9
Total	**610**	**100.0**

Discussion

The knowledge of ARI was universal among the caretakers of the two communities. Caretakers had a fair idea about the symptoms of mild ARI or common cold. It was encouraging that majority of the caretakers could recognize nasal and eye for example running nose, nasal congestions, teary eyes etc., as common symptoms of common cold. However, it was a thing of concern that onset of difficulty in breathing and noisy breathing were recognized as symptoms of common cold as well instead of pneumonia. On the other hand, these symptoms could be the early manifestations of the serious sicknesses like pneumonia and could prove to be dangerous if not treated on time.

The term pneumonia was familiar with almost all the caretakers and it was recognized by most of the caretakers in general. However, there was a great variation concerning the recognition of many specific symptoms of pneumonia. It was encouraging that a large number of the caretakers could recognize chest in-drawing as a symptom of pneumonia as the local terminology of pneumonia was *paslichalna* which itself meant chest in-drawing. This was similar with the findings of Hussain *et al.* (1997), where recognition of pneumonia was universal among the caretakers of the urban squatter settlements of Karachi, Pakistan (Hussain *et al.*, 1997). However, it was disturbing to find that most caretakers could not recognize difficulty in breathing and fast breathing as symptoms of pneumonia. It also showed that most caretakers were not aware of the early symptoms of pneumonia as a form of ARI. Similar findings were reported in earlier studies where pneumonia signs such as rapid breathing, by and large were not picked up by the caretakers (Hussain *et al.*, 1997; de Tejada, 1990; Nichter *et al.*, 1994; Steward *et al.*, 1994 and Dyal *et al.*, 1994).

Moreover, the present study also showed that caretakers gave much emphasis on the onset of high grade fever as a triggering device for seeking formal medical help rather than any other symptoms of pneumonia. Similar findings were reported from the urban squatter settlements of Karachi, Pakistan (Hussain *et al.*, 1997). Besides, a few caretakers did not have any clear idea of pneumonia and its symptoms as they could not give any concrete response when enquired about symptoms observed on their children. Therefore, it is important that caretakers should be given health education messages around specific symptoms of pneumonia. It would also be fruitful if caretakers were given awareness programmes on the early symptoms of pneumonia and incorporate the caretakers' perception about fever as the triggering mechanism for seeking any kind of formal medical help. This would make the ARI awareness programme to be more community sensitive and credible for application.

The common perception that ARI was caused by seasonal change or onset of cold season or weather was very popular among the two slum communities. Similar findings were reported from a study on the knowledge, attitude and practices of the mothers on ARI in Myanmar. In this study, most mothers did not know the etiology of ARI but rather attributed it to rain or cold weather as the etiological agents (Aung *et al.*, 1994). Another general perception about the cause of ARI was exposure to cold. According to the caretakers, if the nursing mother or child were exposed to cold then they were sure to get ARI. Many times nursing mothers were advised not to take bath with cold water or not to expose in rain or cold weather or not to take cold foods or drinks. The universal belief behind this perception was deeply rooted in the ancient system of humoral medicine proposed by Hippocrates and Gelan, which was derived from the Oriental system of medicine (Shah, 1996). People in these communities believed that if there were any imbalance in the 'hot' and 'cold' elements of the body then, the person would ultimately fall sick. In other words, a child gets ARI when the 'cold' element in the body is more than the 'hot' element. Similar kinds of findings were reported by Hussain *et al.*, in his study among the caretakers of the Mohajjir community and the Sindhi respondents in the urban squatter settlements in Karachi, Pakistan (Hussain *et al.*, 1997). Therefore, this deeply ingrained perception of getting ARI due to humoral imbalance in the body needs to be incorporated in framing any National level or State level ARI programme.

Caretakers had the general curative attitude rather than preventive outlook. Therefore, people believed in treating a sickness instead of preventing the sickness beforehand. Great proportion of the caretakers had the attitude to treat their children at the home level with available home remedies and self-prescribed medicines which were mostly procured without prescription and through over-the-counter. This very outlook of the caretakers was transformed to practice. In other words, greater number of the caretakers relied strongly on home remedies and self-medication for ARI. A report on the focused ethnographic study on acute respiratory infection among children revealed that mothers normally believed in curing ARI with home remedies and by giving herbal drinks, oil massage and keeping the child warm (Solutions Consultant Private Limited, 2005). The strategy of attempting to treat childhood ailments at home as a first line of treatment was explained as a cost-saving mechanism to avoid potentially high costs of medical care. Such costs could place further strains on already limited household economic resources in the case of a hospitalization (Luque *et al.*, 2008).

Majority of the caretakers were not in favour of seeking health care providers or prescribers. Many reasons had been cited for not wanting to seek health care provider and many caretakers believed that health care providers were needed only when the sickness was very serious. Moreover, it was not uncommon for the caretakers to keep hospital care as the last option for seeking care. Ankita a 35-year old housewife in Sanjay Basti said "We only go to the hospital if it is something really serious. You have to wait for hours in the hospital, and the cost for going there is much higher than to see our local doctor here." This was the general pattern of seeking care people follow in these two colonies. The common pattern of health seeking behaviour also revealed that caretakers depended heavily on over-the-counter medicines which were very worrying. A study on ARI and concepts of mothers in a Punjabi village also found that mothers relied heavily on allopathic medicines (Rehman, 1994).

Inappropriate use of medicines is a significant source of ineffectiveness in the health systems and management of its finances. Desired treatment results are not attained when medicines are or used more or less than their required doses and when not applied suitably according to scientific guidelines. When medicines are over-used, it calls for greater expenditure than the normal charge, to achieve the desired treatment results (Abegunde, 2010).

Similarly, when medicines are generally consumed below the appropriate dose, desired treatment outcomes are not achieved. Failure in the treatment also leads to prolonged treatment strategies. Anti-microbial resistance, a likely sequel of rampant inappropriate use of antibiotics also drives up treatment cost (Abegunde, 2010). For many prevalent diseases like malaria, diarrhoea and acute respiratory infection, if the medicines are not appropriately used, the cost of treatment can go up sharply. Self-medication in the present study also consists of reuse of the prescribed medicines for the same person and the same problem, but without seeking any medical advice for reuse (Drug Utilization Research Group, 1997).

Mothers usually make decision for seeking care in and around the slum colony and also for giving care at home concerning ARI. However, fathers were the ones who usually make decisions in case of seeking outside care. In other words, maternal autonomy was restricted in giving care to their children at home only and administer medicines procured OTC (Over the Counter) from the nearby drug shops or informal prescribers. Mostly, fathers do not interfere in any form of treatment given by their mothers, at home to their children for ARI but they get involved in decision making when it comes to seeking specific formal medical help or hospitalization (D'Souza, 2003). It was encouraging to see mothers being involved in decision making in some cases of ARI. Mothers' autonomy in decision making was limited in seeking care where there would be a need for money. Seeking a private health care provider or seeking hospital care definitely called for consultation with the father since he was the one who would be financing it. One another explanation could be that when mothers go to the hospitals, their housework and other children have to be taken care of, and they have to make arrangements for them. Delayed decision making due to consultation with other family members will postpone life-saving treatment and a mild illness can progress to serious one leading to the death of the child (D'Souza, 2003). Moreover, among the caretakers, mothers are the ones who are always with the children and they do know every minute detail and every change in the body or behaviour of their children. Therefore, mothers' autonomy in making decisions about the treatment of their children will help a lot in seeking prompt care as soon as symptoms start manifesting itself on the child's body. Education could be one of the factors likely to influence maternal autonomy (D'Souza, 2003). Consequently, both mothers and fathers of the children need to be educated about the necessities of seeking prompt care and importance of the role of the mothers in doing that.

Behaviour of the Health Care Provider

In the present study many of the health care providers mostly informal health care providers indulged in dispensing medicines without seeing the patient or the ARI sick children. Reported cases of ARI where the health care providers checked and examined the symptoms on the under-five children were very few. Moreover, the medicines dispensed by these health care providers were mostly allopathic which was constituted by a large proportion of antibiotics in the form of unlabelled syrup and many other brands (Nair *et al.*, 2019). They dispensed these antibiotics to be given for 3 days at the most. Health care providers often advised the caretakers to throw away these unlabelled syrup after using those for 3 days but all the same, caretakers, anyways, saved them for future use. It is supported by a study by Fischer *et al.*, among the patients showing symptoms of respiratory tract infections where antibiotic prescriptions by the general practitioners were found to be very high (Fischer *et al.*, 2005). Similar findings were reported Shaver *et al.* (2019) and Spellberg *et al.* (2008).

Irrational dispensing of antibiotics by the health care providers was worrisome and to top this, prescriptions were given to administer the medicines (mostly antibiotics) for 3 days. This widespread practice among the two slum colonies was quite alarming and need immediate attention from the government side agencies or local NGOs to rectify the rampant use of antibiotics. This was alarming because a minimum of 5 days of antibiotic therapy is needed to get clinical efficacy in serious ARI as well as to avoid creating strains of drug resistance bacteria (Rehman *et al.*, 1994).

It was common practice that caretakers stopped giving treatment to their children after seeing the improvement in the ARI symptoms without completing the course of the medicine. Most caretakers, after stopping the treatment would either change the health care providers or the types of treatment they were giving. This was one of the major problems reported from the caretakers among the urban squatter settlements of Karachi, Pakistan where mothers had the unrealistic expectations of quick cure. This led them to change the physicians often, with the child receiving 2 or 3 incomplete regiments of very potent antibiotics (Hussian *et al.*, 1997).

In Delhi, only a few of government clinics or dispensaries operate in and around the slum areas, despite the fact that two-thirds of the city's 14 million people live in urban slums (Gardner, 2008). Health experts say that the city cannot keep up with the arrival of poor rural dwellers seeking a better life in urban areas. Many Indians are treated by a number of informal prescribers and more so in the slum areas. These informal prescribers are commonly known as quacks, or "Bengali doctors" (since many of them come from West Bengal). The government estimates it needs 600,000 doctors and 1 million nurses to reach an acceptable level of health care for the nation's 1.1 billion citizens, according to a recent government report (Gardner, 2008).

Most caretakers also preferred to consult these informal prescribers due to many social and cultural reasons. These prescribers were more community friendly and used the same disease terminology as the slum communities. Moreover they normally do not make the show of high standard and highly qualified attitude which were often seen among the qualified doctors or the hospital doctors. As one of the mothers said that she felt more comfortable with their local doctor than the outside doctors and when enquired about the reason for that she said "because he belongs to our locality and he knows us more". This was the reflection of a commonly accepted impression of the two slum communities. Moreover, informal prescribers served as the easily accessible and inexpensive means of getting medical care in and around the locality itself. People do not need to go far by spending money and time due to the informal prescribers. Therefore, the role of informal prescribers in the slum communities needs to be recognized by the policy maker since they not only served as the first line of medical help but also accepted by the whole community (Aung *et al.*, 1994). Consequently it would be well served if the training for standardized care management of ARI is also extended to the informal prescribers.

Conclusion

Caretakers had a fair idea about the symptoms of mild ARI or common cold. The term pneumonia was familiar with almost all the caretakers and it was recognized by most of the caretakers in general. Recognition of last signs of pneumonia like chest in-drawing was high; however, early symptoms like difficulty in breathing and chest in-drawing were low. Onset of high grade fever marked as the triggering mechanism for seeking formal medical help rather than any other symptoms of pneumonia. Therefore, it is important that caretakers should be given health education messages around specific symptoms of pneumonia. It would also be fruitful if caretakers were given awareness programmes on the early symptoms of pneumonia and incorporate the caretakers' perception about fever as the triggering mechanism for seeking any kind of formal medical help. Seasonal change or onset of cold weather was believed extensively as the cause of ARI other than any causal agent. This needs to be incorporated in framing any National level or State level ARI programme since the common attribution of cold as the cause of ARI was deeply ingrained to the perception of the mind of people.

Caretakers had the general curative attitude rather than preventive outlook towards ARI. Huge reliance of the caretakers on home remedies for treating ARI rather than seeking health care providers was profound among the two slums. Widespread preference of self-medication by the caretakers or strong reliance on over-the-counter medicines for treating ARI could be highlighted. Restricted autonomy of the mothers in terms of seeking formal medical care or hospital care appeared to be one of the reasons for delay in seeking prompt care for ARI. Consequently, both mothers and fathers of the children need to be educated about the necessities of seeking prompt care and importance of the role of the mothers in doing that. Moreover, the perceived efficacy of treatment was an important factor in determining the use of health care.

Careless dispensing of antibiotics by the health care providers was worrisome and to top this, prescriptions were given to administer these medicines for 3 days. This was alarming because a minimum of 5 days of antibiotic therapy is needed for to get clinical efficacy in serious ARI as well as to avoid creating strains of drug resistance bacteria Health care providers, mostly informal health care providers indulged in dispensing medicines without seeing the patient or the ARI sick children. Caretakers, more often than not, see the attitude of the service provider and their comfort level in seeking the health care provider rather than their qualification or knowledge about ARI. Informal prescribers served as the first line medical help as well as easily accessible and inexpensive means of medical care in and around the slum locality. Therefore, the role of informal prescribers in the slum communities needs to be recognized by the policy makers.

REFERENCES

Abegunde, D. (2010). "Inefficiencies due to poor access to and irrational use of medicines to treat acute respiratory tract infections in children", *Background Paper, No 52, World Health Report.* World Health Organization.

Ahmed, S.M. (2005). "Exploring health-seeking bahaviour of disadvantaged populations in rural Bangladesh", Stockholm, Sweden: Karolinska Institutet.

Ahmed, S.M., Hossain, M.A., Chowdhury, M.R. (2009). "Informal sector providers in Bangladesh: How equipped are they to provide rational health care?" *Health Policy and Planning*, 1-12.

Aung, T. Tun, K.M., Thinn, K., Thein, A.A. (1994). "Knowledge, attitude and practices of mothers on childhood acute respiratory infections (ARI)", *Southeast Asian J Trop Med Public Health. 25*(3): 590-592.

D'Souza, R.M. (2003). "Role of health-seeking behaviour in child mortality in the slums of Karachi, Pakistan", *Journal of Biosocial Science, 35*: 131-144.

Darmstadt, G.L., Syed, U., Patel, Z., Kabir, N. (2006). "Review of Domiciliary New born care Practices in Bangladesh", *Journal of Health, Population and Nutrition. 24*(4):380-393.

De Tejada, S.S. (1990). Popular notions of ARI in Guatemala and Ghana. Unpublished manuscript, Department of Anthropology, University of Arizona, Tuscon.

Drug Utilization Research Group, Latin America. (1997). "Multi-center study on self-medication and prescription in six Latin American countries", *Clin Pharmacol Ther. 6*1, 488-493.

Dyal, A.D. and Bahattacharyya, K. (1994). "The Marathi 'taskonomy' of respiratory illnesses in children", *Medical Anthropology. 15*, 395-408.

Gardner, H. (2008). "India's sick poor turn to unlicensed doctors, Facing long trips and full clinics, ailing poor turn to unlicensed doctors", *Chronicle Foreign Service.*
https://www.sfgate.com/news/article/India-s-sick-poor-turn-to-unlicensed-doctors-3203439.php (Accessed on 12/04/2021; 4:17pm)

Harding, A. (2003). "Introduction to Private Participation in Health Services", In Private Participation in Health Services. Edited by: Harding, A. Preker, A.S. Washington: *The International Bank for Reconstruction and Development/ The World Bank;* 2003:11:100.

Hussain, R., Melvyn, A.l., Bazmi I., Amanullah, K., Asma, F.Q., and David, M. (1997). "Pneumonia perceptions and management: An ethnographic study in urban squatter settlements of Karachi, Pakistan", *Social Science and Medicine. 45*:991-1004.

Kumar S. (2004). "Much health care in rural India comes from unqualified practitioners", *BMJ. 328*(7446):975.

Kunda, J., Fitzpatrick, J., Kazwala, R., French, N.P., Shirima, G., MacMillam, A., *et al.*, (2007). "Health seeking behaviour of human brucellosis cases in rural Tanzania", *BMC Public Health.* 7(315).

Luque, J.S., Whiteford, L.M., and Tobin, G.A. (2008). "Maternal recognition and health care-seeking behaviour for acute respiratory infection in children in a rural Ecuadorian county", *Maternal and Child Health Journal. 12*:287-297.

Nair, M., Tripathi, S., Mazumdar, S., Mahajan, R., Harshana, A., Pereira, A., *et al.* (2019). "Without antibiotics, I cannot treat": A qualitative study of antibiotic use in Paschim Bardhaman district of West Bengal, India. *PLoS ONE*. 14(6): e0219002. https://doi.org/10.1371/journal.pone.0219002

Nichter, M. and Nichter, M. (1994). "Acute respiratory illness: popular health culture and mother's knowledge in the Philippines", *Medicine and Anthropology. 15*, 353-375.

Radwan, I. (2005). India-Private Health Services for the Poor: A Policy, Note. Health, Nutrition and Population (HNP) Discussion Paper Health NaPfHotWBsDN. Washington, DC: *The International Bank for Reconstruction and Development/World Bank, 13*:58-60.

Rajamma, K.J., Rao, D.V.B., Narayana, A.S.L., Ramchandran, R., Prabhakar, R. (1996). "Health seeking behaviour, Acceptability of available health facilities and knowledge about Tuberculosis in Tribal area", *Indian Journal of Tuberculosis. 43*: 195-199.

Rehman, G.N., Qazi, S.A., Mull, D.S., and Khan, M.A. (1994). "ARI concepts of mothers in Punjabi villages: A community based study", *Journal of the Pakistan Medical Association.* 44.

Ryan, G.W., and Martinez, H. (1996). "Can we predict what mothers do? Modeling treatments for infantile diarrhea in rural Mexico", *Human Organization. 55*(1), 1-12.

Ryan, G.W. (1998). "What do sequential behaviour patterns suggest about the medical decision-making process? Modeling home case management of acute illnesses in a rural Cameroonian village", *Social Science and Medicine. 46*(2), 209-225.

Shaikh, B.T., David, H. and Hadener, J. (2004). *Health seeking behaviour and health service utilization in Pakistan: Challenging policy makers. Journal of Public Health.*

Shaver, A.L., Jacobs, D.M., LaMonte, M.J. *et al.* (2019). Antibiotic prescribing for acute respiratory tract infections in the United States outpatient setting. *BMC Fam Pract.* 20, 91. https://doi.org/10.1186/s12875-019-0980-1.

Spellberg, B., Guidos, R., Gilbert, D., Bradley, J., Boucher, H.W., Scheld, W.M. *et al.* (2008). The epidemic of antibiotic-resistant infections: a call to action for the medical community from the Infectious Diseases Society of America. *Clin Infect Dis. 46*(2):155-64.

Stewart, K.M., Parker, B., Chakraborty, J. and Begum, H. (1994) Acute respiratory infections (ARI) in rural Bangladesh: perceptions and practices. *Medical Anthropology. 15*, 377-394.

Patil, A.V., Somasundaram, K.V., Goyal, R.C. (2002). "Current health scenario in rural India", *Australian, 10*(2):129-135.

Young, J.C. (1981). "Non-use of physicians: Methodological approaches, policy implications, and the utility of decision models", *Social Science and Medicine. 15*(B), 499-507.

11
Sanitation Practices and Behavioural Discourses

A Case of Karang, an Island village in Loktak Lake, Manipur

Oinam Hemlata Devi

Introduction

Historically, sanitation was conceptualized with human excreta disposal by cesspools, manual carriers, open pits etc. For the first time in human history, the sanitary awakening of Europe in the 19th century taught us a scientific outlook on the causes of illness and disease. However, places like India could focus on it in the late twentieth century only. India adopted the National Water Supply and Sanitation Programme in 1954, followed by the Accelerated Rural Water Supply Programme (1972-73) and then the Central Rural Sanitation Programme (1986). Later, it was followed by the Total Sanitation Campaign (TSC, 1999) and the Nirmal Bharat Abhiyan (NBA, 2012), aiming to focus on its successful outcomes rather than simply looking at the construction of latrines. NBA was restructured as Swachh Bharat Abhiyan (Clean India Mission) in October 2014, and so far, it is the largest and the most successful scheme that claims a tremendous figure of successful reduction of Open Defecation (OD) in India.

Sanitation in rural India is always challenging in the context of religious taboos, lack of water, gender, and power relations. The surrounding environment and settlement patterns add up to the existing challenges and issues of sanitation. Sanitation and its implications on health are inevitable; the difference lies with the nature of its interconnectedness derived and constructed by different communities. It is translated into different meanings, behaviours, and identities. With the scientific and cultural notion of sanitation, the causative factors of diseases related to sanitation are multifactorial.

Some of the issues of sanitation are geospatial and political (Mcfarlane, C., Desai, R., & Graham, S., 2014), related to water scarcity, particularly the practice of OD (*Deccan Herald,* May 17, 2019), linked to religious beliefs and taboos or purity and pollution or caste and social stratification (George, 2008, Coffey *et al.,* 2017). However, the issue that has been described in this chapter about Karang Island village in Manipur is different. There is no scarcity of water, no hierarchical structure among the villagers. Instead, sanitation is considered as a reflection of the island ecosystem that shapes the socio-cultural and economic status of the villagers. Availability of space and individual level consciousness is an issue that is unfavourable to the construction of toilets and sanitation related behavioural outcomes. In the light of this context, the present study focuses on understanding the determinants of sanitation and its discourses experienced by the Karang Islanders over a period of time.

For this, I consider six significant sanitation components in which I would give special attention to the first criteria. The six components are: (i) Safe disposal of human excreta, (ii) Disposal of waste (liquid and solid), (iii) Collection, storage, and use of drinking water, (iv) Home sanitation and food hygiene, (v) Personal hygiene; and (vi) Environmental hygiene (Kurukhshetra, 2005).

Methodology

It is a product of an ethnographic method of data collection in an island village in Manipur. The basis of it traces back to the data collection process of my Ph.D. research work during 2004 and 2005. Fieldwork for more than a year in the village provided a deeper understanding of the island life through the methods of participant observation and in-depth interviews. After that, I visited Karang Island regularly at least once every three years. My experiences and intermittent visits from 2004 to 2019 allowed me to observe many significant changes on the island village's ecology, including socio-economic conditions and interpersonal relationships.

Methodologically, it is a village study equipped with ethnographic methods such as participant observation, informal group discussions, interviews, case studies, key informant interviews to identify and assess the everyday constituent of their community life and living. Participant observations were the core of getting into sanitation practices in the village, mainly during 2004-05 when I was staying in the village. This method is significant as people prefer to pretend and portray the availability of minimally acceptable sanitation practices though its reality is different.

Informal conversations and group discussions provided enough knowledge about various challenges and sanitation issues at individual and household levels. Interviews provided a detailed account of the villagers' perceptions and behavioural attitudes to the new entries, such as the Assam Rifles Camp and their presence on the island, the establishment of tourism facilities, the creation of a local market etc. The key informant interviews act as a buffer to highlight and engage on some of the selected sanitation issues. Personal interviews of the villagers already migrated to the mainland in the Moirang and Imphal areas of Manipur provided the village's changing aspects and views about the island life. Interviewing them gives an alternative way of cross-checking the information.

Karang Island: Not many are familiar with an island village in the Loktak Lake of Manipur. Manipur is known in India's north-eastern states for its various attributes such as Manipuri classical dance, Brow antlered deer, Keibul Lamjao National Park, Siroy lily, Women's market (Ema market), Sports personalities, Loktak Lake etc. Loktak Lake is the largest freshwater lake in northeast India and is considered the lifeline of the people of Manipur. It is mainly inhabited by the Meities, the primary community of Manipur.

Loktak Lake has been fed by 30 rivers showing variation in its size from approx. 500 to 250 sq. km. during the rainy season to dry winter months (Gajananda, Kh. & Chanu, T.S., 2009). This lake's unique characteristic feature is the presence of floating grassy masses that are enriched with rich vegetative flora enhancing a healthier site for fish breeding. It also acts as a good fishing platform and the best site for building huts for many fishing families. The huts constructed are called floating huts. However, the recent scheme of removing the floating *Phooms* and huts led to various ecological and socio-economic implications reducing the production level of catching fish in the lake.

Karang Island is situated 48 km. away from the capital city, Imphal. It is the only inhabited island in the Loktak Lake of Manipur, separated from the nearest mainland by 5 km. The closest mainland is Thanga which is divided into two Gram Panchayats, Thanga Part I and Thanga Part II under the Moirang CD Block in Bishnupur district. Karang comes under the Thanga Part I sharing beneficiary level schemes with the other three villages listed in Part I. However, the standard of living in Karang is comparatively low compared to the other villages of the same Panchayat due to its isolation as an island.

Settlement Pattern

The island is mainly constituted of a hillock in which a clustered form of settlement pattern is present on the slope and foothills nearby the shore of the lake called '*Patpan*' (*Pat*=Lake; *Pan*=border). The island village is divided into five localities (called *leikais*) as east, west, middle, north, and south. Within a locality, there are small lanes (*leirak*) for people's passage from one house to another. Karang has around 1.5 km. long serrated weathered main road on the western side of the hillock. In Karang, this single village road is the only means of thoroughfare for moving across the village. The eastern part of the hillock does not have a proper road due to its unsystematic road and scattered settlement pattern. The road on the east side at six points will have to pass the lanes, or side yards of specific houses settled there. So, the eastern side road is much narrow compared to the road on the western side. Above, it is less used by the passerby unless there is work-related to pass through. The lanes/*leirak* (intra-village roads) concept is very important to the villagers for their day-to-day transactions and interactions. The lanes/*leiraks* of Karang are made by connecting several side yards, backyards, and courtyards of their houses. It doesn't mean that they pass through all settlement areas/ households, but if we wish to go through the village domicile areas, we must pass by, the houses as intra-village road.

As a tradition, a house in Manipur is always constituted with an open courtyard (*sumang*), a granary (*kei*), a cowshed (*sankol*), toilet/ latrine (*amangsang*), a pond (*pukhri*) and a space for kitchen gardening (*ingkholkoiba*). However, in Karang, cowshed and granary are not desirable due to their occupation of fishing. Some families keep paddy that are produced from the fields of the mainland agricultural areas owned by them. However, they prefer taking rice grain instead of raw paddy as transportation of rice is easier and lighter.

The tradition of constructing a house with the front always facing the east direction has a cultural reason and facilitates sunlight inside the house right from the morning. However, houses in the island village are built and faced according to their convenience and thus located haphazardly. The majority of the houses are oriented towards the south. There are no social restriction in the settlement pattern, but it is usually the people of one surname (*Yumnak Sagei*) of the same clan who are neighbours.

Sanitation

In general, sanitation facilities and arrangements are challenging considering the lifestyle and surrounding environment; however, some recent developments directly or indirectly facilitate the village's behavioural pattern and consciousness of sanitation practices.

1. Safe Disposal of Human Excreta:

Villagers must construct latrines to dispose of excretal remains in a community. Any form of contamination may link to various communicable diseases, particularly a village located in the lake where water accessibility is not an issue. However, there is the highest chance of sewerage contamination if the latrines are not constructed properly.

Construction of latrines: In Karang Island, there were no latrine before 1999 except 18 *kutcha* latrines. The 18 households were considered as those who can afford latrines of *kutcha* category economically and spatially. All the houses in the village are of *kutcha* category with thatched and tin (CGI) roof. The nature of the settlement pattern was so much closely packed that it is not feasible to build *kutcha* latrines or open pits as it may lead to disturbances of foul smell circulating the congested settlement areas. However, the scheme provided under the Loktak Development Authority facilitated the low-cost pit latrines, and availability of it was increased starting from 1999 to 2001. Afterwards, most houses could access to latrines when some families used them on a shared basis. During the fieldwork of 2004-05, it was informed that five families do not use latrines; instead, they use surrounding areas, particularly the space available in the lake.

Outcomes I Latrines were preferably used by the people of the island on emergency, else menfolk in every household gets up before dawn and reach out to the lake to their respective fish traps or nets to pick up their day's catch and then arrange new traps and nets, some of them return at home, but the majority stay on the lake, and all their natural requirements are performed into the lake including defecation. The wife or female members or children of the family go to the lake to give the lunch packed and helped her husband/parents in the afternoon for a good catch. Thus, almost 70 per cent of the village population spends their time in the lake, and their consumption of the facilities of latrines becomes very limited. It is observed from their livelihood practices that they spend maximum hours of almost 14 hours in the lake from around 3 a.m. to 5 p.m. There were also years of fishing they spent on floating huts and returning to their houses once a month or occasionally. Such a prolonged stay was possible before implementing the scheme of removing floating huts in 2011 under the Manipur Loktak Lake Protection Act, 2006.

Regarding children and women, they will just paddle the oars and go out to a nearby distance of around 100-200 metres, and then any of the nearby floating *Phooms* will be used as bathing platforms and for open defecation. In this process, they will also pluck vegetables available on the *Phooms*. It serves many purposes at a time. As the *Phooms* keep moving following the direction of the winds, they usually try to get a nearby new *Phoom* for different purposes. They felt that excreta go down deep inside the lake or converted to manure with its own. Therefore, the rest of the activities, such as bathing and collection of vegetables, do not get affected by OD. Instead of using the foul smell latrines that is already used by someone, or sitting above the same place that is believed to be polluted already, they prefer using *Phooms* and canoe which is much cleaner and smell-free platforms than the latrines. Therefore, open defecation in the lake remains one of the common practices.

The most pertinent issue is the process of washing and cleaning at times of defecation where, they would use the oars of the canoes to remove the water that comes inside the canoe. There is no concept of using soaps or sanitizers after defecation though there are high chances of contamination.

Frequency of cleaning latrines: The concept of cleaning latrines is almost absent; cleanliness is always compromised against the priority of earning a livelihood. However, the idea of cleanliness improves with the improvement of their household income. It shows that they are aware of it while the focus was on feeding all the family members and other basic requirements such as daily meals, treatment costs of diseases and illnesses, social ceremonies, and religious festivals. The majority of the islanders never consider cleaning the latrine as a required chore in a dwelling. Instead, it may clean once in a while when visitors come or any specific rituals such as the beginning of a year (April) as per Manipuri calendar, *Emoinu Ahongbi puja* (worshipping of the Goddess of wealth) etc. However, there were instances where they will splash water for cleaning. The concept of washing hands after using the latrine simply remains to wash hands with plain water. In some rare instances, families of better economic conditions keep soap outside the latrine, but the same soap is used for bathing purposes. Members of the family do not have the habit of ablution and thus missed using soaps after using the latrines.

Recent Development: In 2007, under the AFSPA (Armed Forces Special Power Act), the government of Manipur installed a camp of a paramilitary force of Assam Rifles on the hilltop of Karang Island for political and security purposes. It was also the timing where there were major efforts made to reduce and check the conflict of insurgency groups and their activities in Manipur. The Assam rifles stayed there for ten (10) years until 2017. During their stay, there was regular patrolling and checking of all the entry of outsiders into the island village. As it is an island and there are possibilities of people reaching any house from different directions using different waterways, there were strict surveillances all over the island.

The repercussions of Assam Rifles' presence are mainly observed in the behavioural attitudes and changed practices of the villagers towards open defecation. The practice of open defecation by children in the vicinity of the village or village road has completely stopped. Girls and womenfolk who usually prefer taking baths or defecate in the open on the nearby *Phooms* have gradually reduced. Instead, they have started making small enclosures designated for bathing and washing. They had spent money buying motor pumps or cheaper technology to draw water from nearby areas that are clean for consumption. Suddenly, the latrines constructed and shared by 2-3 houses have become functional regularly. Some have also tried to build their own by taking the help of available government schemes. Currently, every house has its latrine. However, it is still difficult to claim that this area is entirely free from open defecation as their livelihood practice compels the fisher folk to spend maximum hours in the lake. Bringing any change on their open defecation behaviour is impossible when they are still spending maximum hours in the lake for a hand-to-mouth existence of fishing.

It is also important to note that after the Assam Rifles left in 2017, the last three years are mainly marked by a sudden spurt of tourists on the island. Earlier, people did not wish to come to this village unless there is a dire need for it as the place was considered unclean and not safe to visit. It was considered unclean in the '70s, and '80s as there were no latrines and told that the roadsides and empty spaces of the hillocks were filled with excretal remains. Children and the aged were compelled to use open spaces during that time and this made outsiders conclude that the village was not at all good and clean to visit. There were times where insurgency issues were so strong that it was considered unsafe to go there. However, after the stay of the Assam Rifles for ten (10) years and improvement of village lifestyle, particularly in the use of latrines, other development activities such as total electrification and progress in the health care facilities could gain and this, in turn, provided a better scope of tourism which has now increased successfully. The availability of motorboats adds to boost it further.

Outcomes II: The coming up of tourists is responsible for significant changes in the village lifestyle and sanitary practices; some of the village's prominent families have started maintaining proper use of latrines and facilities of hand wash. However, tourists who plan to visit and spend a whole day, including preparing lunch in the village, usually come prepared with all the essential cooking requirements such as oil, spices, potatoes, and other ingredients that are not readily available on the island. It reduces the burden to the host family for making the required arrangements for the meal. There are no homestay or dedicated hosting services available except a floating resort in the lake. The floating resort is available for night stays, and it can be occupied by some travellers or explorers of up to 2-3 individuals. With the help of the local contacts, visitors plan to spend their one-day holiday on the island. However, families from different parts of Manipur visiting the island for a day would prefer to reach in the morning and leave the island before dark. They usually prepare food on the spot after their arrival, where they also lend a helping hand by participating in the preparation and cooking of food. Sometimes, people visit the place without prior contact, and on the island, there are village guides and volunteers to support such visitors in which they get some token amount as a gesture of appreciation from the tourists.

Tourism has further favoured developing a thriving local market for selling fishes of various kinds, particularly the dried, roasted ones. Such local vendors are more active on weekends and holidays as the tourists, particularly families and groups of families, visit on such days.

Altogether, sanitary awareness and conscious practice arising out of various reasons have now provided an avenue for alternative livelihood opportunities within the village.

2. Disposal of Waste (Liquid and Solid)

One of the crucial aspects of sanitation includes waste of both liquid and solid forms generated from the village other than the human excreta or feces. The solid waste materials or refuse in the village include kitchen waste, dust and dirt generated in the homestead area, dry twigs from kitchen gardens, broken or discarded parts of nets and other fishing traps, unused sachets/packets of groceries and household items etc. The liquid waste or sullage includes all the liquid waste generated from the kitchen, mopping activities, washing areas.

Every household tries its best to maintain some cleanliness level in the kitchen space as it is also considered a sacred area. Everyday refuse and sullage generated from the kitchen is immediately thrown outside, where it is thrown directly on the shore of the lake by the majority, while some maintain a dedicated open space for it. As the settlement pattern is made on the slope of the hillock, the sullage gets absorbed naturally or drain down towards the lake in case of excess amount. During the rainy season, some of the houses located closer to the lake will throw the refuse and sullage by standing from the house's side yard or verandah. Regarding the dust and dirt generated in the homestead area, every house usually sweeps the verandah and courtyard regardless of its cleanliness, simply because of the aged old tradition of cleaning the verandah courtyard in the early morning for everyday ritual offerings. Every Meitei household will begin a day with a prayer to their respective deities, and before it, sweeping and cleaning are compulsory. It does not mean that they are very conscious of hygiene; instead, it is an act of rites to be performed and thus not necessarily connected with proper cleaning and mopping. For some families, they would simply clean the place dedicated to making ritual offerings. The refuse and sullage are dumped at their convenient sites rather than thinking of its negative implications about becoming a breeding ground for flies, mosquitoes, and other micro-organisms. The distance of throwing the waste by some are so close to houses that smells are expected anytime. There is no concept of converting waste into compost or fertilizers. Very few sometimes casually happen to use it as manure for kitchen gardening, but most prefer not to give any attention to it.

3. Collection, Storage, and Use of Drinking Water

Water in the village are collected and stored in various ways for their daily purpose starting from cooking, drinking to washing clothes. For kitchen use, water is stored in two forms, one for drinking and the other for cooking and washing vegetables. The drinking water is mainly collected from the treated water supply public stand post placed at different village road intervals and in between the lanes (*leikais*). This water is poured into a non-electric ceramic candle filter/chalk and stone filter or clothe strainer. Sometimes, they choose to boil water, mainly during the monsoonal days when there is a high rate of water-borne diseases. If no such requirement is felt to them, they do not follow it. They also use alum to purify water.

Every house does have a piece of alum which they use whenever required. Rainwater harvesting with the help of containers up to 1000 litres are commonly used.

Some families were hesitant to consume the treated water supply as the water tank at the hilltop is an open rectangular structure with no cleaning. The maintenance of the water tank was so poor that they prefer taking lake water only. They were not ready to share much about the dissatisfaction they had but simply maintained silence about drinking water quality. Altogether, the island had a treated water supply of its kind, though not appropriate for all purposes of their daily life. They thus use both types of water, and lake water is unavoidable in their life and living. The water nearby the shore area or closure to the settlement places of around 200 metres were not clean enough for washing clothes and bathing. They usually sail out the canoes beyond such distance to get clean water. It provides scope for anyone to guess the nature of contamination already happened in and around the village's vicinity. People were very much aware of its implications and possible connections with illnesses and diseases, particularly water-borne diseases. However, people consider it as part and parcel of their life; they did not feel that it should be brought into the authorities' notice or some forms of social service and awareness about hygiene should be made.

4. Home Sanitation and Food Hygiene

The level of living in the village is again very much related to the types of housing present. There were no concrete houses in the village. All are categorized into *kutcha* houses with CGI (Corrugated Galvanized Iron) rooftop. Three houses in the village do have cemented verandah, while the rest of their houses are *kutcha* type. There were around ten (10) houses whose verandah (the front part called '*Mangon*') were cemented partially towards the front end of around 2-3 feet in width. It is mainly helpful in improving its durability as this is the area of a house which is mainly exposed during the rainy season. Houses in the village are structurally more or less similar. There is no proper ventilation available in their houses' structural arrangement though a small window for each of the rooms is present. The presence of windows in each of the rooms somehow helped the entry of sunlight into the interiors. However, despite the presence of windows, some of the houses could not receive sunlight due to their clustered settlement form.

Kitchen space is an important area where two fireplaces are usually present: one for cooking and the other for informal conversations and gatherings. It is the place where every member gathers around the fireplace and interacts about a day's experience and their other familial matters. It is also used as a place for cooking non-vegetarian items such as chicken. Fish is allowed to cook in the main kitchen. Some of the families converted this place as a fireplace for drying and roasting the fishes. However, many families prefer separate rooms for roasting and drying as it is always found to be continuously used throughout the day depending on the amount of catch they could collect from the lake. Due to its continuity, the whole room turns black from the shoot released from the fireplace. Womenfolk also do have lots of health complaints such as coughing and other respiratory tract infection-related issues.

Food is cooked using firewood only. They use LPG facilities mainly during emergency cases or at the arrival of guests in the family to make tea and snacks in a short duration. The usual meals are prepared using firewood only. Children would prefer playing all over the places, including the kitchen spaces when their mother would be preparing food. They will throw things from here and there or eat foods that are scattered on the floor. Mothers will sometimes remind children not to eat food from the floor, but usually, it remains a verbal attitude; no responsive action is taken either by the children or the mother. Instead, it is advised that children should learn all of these to remain active and strengthen their immunity.

The concept of washing hands before taking food is there in principle; practically, it remains a simple dip of few fingers to moisten the hand, meaning that proper hand wash is not usually done before eating, especially when the person was not doing any activities or chores which needs to wash the hands before eating. After food, hand wash is done using simple water. No soap or detergents are used for this purpose.

Overall, there is ample scope for improving the sanitation aspects related to home and eating food. This might be expected more as the level of tourism increases.

5. Personal Hygiene

It is one of the significant attributes of a person to live a healthy life. Personal hygiene in the village is again not so appropriate to interpret that they are conscious of it. Some practices have become so habitual that they did not even consider it essential to maintain a disease-free lifestyle. Many people brush their teeth using ash or salt or slabs of bamboo twig instead of toothbrushes and paste. However, it is also not deniable that villagers use brush and paste. Ash and salt is mainly used by menfolk who spend their maximum time in the lake for fishing and old-aged ladies who are not ready to accept toothbrush and toothpaste. Growing up, girls and middle-aged women prefer toothbrushes and toothpaste. If any girl or woman in the village uses ash or salt or other traditional alternatives, they have been looked down by the others. Grooming is mainly vital for girls as they will get better husbands from well-to-do families and thus beauty, good mannerism and good household management skills particularly cooking and roasting or drying fishes are expected as the desired personality of a marriageable girl. Menstrual hygiene is treated as confidential, private and hardly shared in the open, no matter how many problems a girl would be facing. However, in rare cases, girls will share their concerns with the mothers or girl siblings. They use cloth as a napkin and usually hide them from others at times of drying for reuse. Women of middle age do not use any cloth or materials; instead used two loincloths; the one inside is worn to absorb the flow.

Bathing is a regular practice for everyone except children. Children sometimes do not take baths regularly. Children tend to go in groups and swim inside the lake at around 100-200 metres distance. Small children usually are found to be left under the care of older siblings and aged people. They will get a bath only when the caregivers provide the support, and they cannot get a regular bath due to the nature of livelihood that their parents have. People go to the lake for bathing with or without soap; a simple splash of water over the body making the clothes all over the body wet can be considered the complete bathing process. A woman should take a bath before making daily prayers and stepping into the kitchen to cook a day's meal. Children in the village will roam around all places without caring about bathing, cutting nails, wearing washed, clean clothes. They enjoy running behind the visitors or outsiders who come to the island, playing on the ground among the youth and aged who would be spending their leisure time with games such as football/volleyball, cards, informal group conversations etc.

Much improvement is required in personal hygiene. Competition and conflicts among the girls to maintain better physique, appearance, and behaviour are becoming more with the changing socio-economic condition and livelihood patterns.

6. Environmental Hygiene

There are lots of factors that contribute to contamination of the surrounding environment. They do not have proper disposal of waste; all end up throwing into the lake. The periphery or shore area (*Patpan*) becomes the most contaminated area and is frequently used daily. *Patan* is the area where all the respective canoes of groups of households are parked. Some will use the canoes as a platform for bathing and washing clothes; some will be piling up all the fishing traps, vegetables, and many more transportation items. Poultry and pigs are usually inhabited in this area. Domesticated animals such as dogs and cats will roam around. Children under five years generally defecate wherever they feel like. Altogether, the *patpan* area becomes the breeding ground for mosquitoes, flies, and microbes. At night, mosquitoes are very active, and one finds it difficult to stay in the rooms of a house except for the area where fireplaces are present. In all the fireplaces, there are lots of smokes as drying, and roasting fishes need smoking as well. Such availability of smokes keeps the mosquitoes away. Mosquito repellers available in the market are not sufficient to fight the volume of mosquitoes available, and their frequency increases closer to the shore area. In the daytime, flies are all over the place, especially over those baskets and trays where raw fishes are sundried. Nobody feels terrible eating uncovered food in practice though some showed that they would not eat uncovered food.

Discussion and Conclusion

From the above findings, rural sanitation is not an easy way out; it implies different facets of our behavioural attitudes and practices. The determining factors of sanitation are enormous. It could be tradition and culture, economy and livelihood practices, environmental factors, competition and conflicts, power relations present among the family members/neighbours/villagers etc. Post LDA Scheme of construction of latrines in 1999 show differential attitudes to the successful use of latrines. The denial narrative has been slowly replaced by the acceptance of latrines, including bathrooms that were spontaneously compelled by the Assam Rifles camp's coming up in the village in 2007. The personal safety and security of women and children played an important role in determining the changing behavioural attitudes and widespread acceptance of latrines in the village. The gender aspect of safe sanitation and power dynamics in rural India, as discussed by Khanna and Das (2015), shows that sensitization programmes and sanitation policy for the poor will strengthen toilets' use and adoption. Here, the factors influencing the use of latrines may differ when agreeing that it is gendered due to the known risk of various kinds, either safety or health issues. Therefore, awareness, sensitization and facilities are a must.

Open defecation in the lake is one of the discourses that remains an unsolved agenda till today. Because, most of the village population including women and sometimes children spend their maximum hours in the lake for fishing, and they do not have other alternatives. This discourse of open defecation in comparison to other rural villages is quite contradictory. Coffey *et al.* (2017) explain it in the lines of belief system, purity and pollution, caste and untouchability and Routray *et al.* (2015) mention incomplete structures of government-subsidized latrines. While Karang villagers' constraints were mainly connected with the nature and duration of occupation that they have. However, in the end, these arguments meet up together towards the question of affordability as Coffey *et al.* (2017), Routray *et al.* (2015), and Karang study highlight the importance of income to the practice of open defecation.

Likewise, other sanitation components have also been found to be improving slowly despite their level of inappropriateness compared to other places.

The science of sanitation to avoid many diseases, particularly communicable water-borne diseases in the village, is coupled with the people's changed behavioural attitudes. The medical facilities, particularly doctors' availability, have improved compared to no doctors in the late 90s and beginning of 2000. There is a need to sensitize people about the values and implications of better use of sanitation. Sanitation discourses already available to them, awareness and reflexivity will help each of the villagers decide the better practice and maintain a healthy lifestyle.

REFERENCES

Coffey, D. and Spears, D. (2018). "Open defecation in rural India, 2015–2016: levels and trends in the NFHS-4", *Economic and Political Weekly, 53:*10–13.

Coffey, D., Gupta, A., Hathi, P., Srivastava, N., and Vyas, S. (2017). "Understanding Open Defecation in Rural India: Untouchability, Pollution and Latrine Pits", *Economic and Political Weekly (EPW), LII*(1): 59-66.

Deccan Herald (May 17, 2019). Acute water shortage leading to open defecation. Retrieved from https://www.deccanherald.com/state/mangaluru/mangalore-university-postpones-ug-exams-till-april-10-amid-rising-covid-19-cases-971839.html Date of Access: 9/4/2021.

Gajananda, Kh. and Chanu, T.S. (n.d.). The Fate of Loktak Lake. Retrieved fromhttp://www.e-pao.net/epSubPageExtractor.asp?src=education.Scientific_Papers.fate_of_loktak_lakeDate of Access: 6/4/2021.

George, R. 2008. *The big Necessity: Adventures in the world of human waste* (pp. 90-100). London: Portobello Books.

Khanna, T. and Das, M. (2015). "Why gender matters in the solution towards safe sanitation? Reflections from rural India", *Global Public Health,* DOI: 10.1080/17441692.2015.1062905

Mcfarlane, C., Desai, R., and Graham, S. (2014). "Informal Urban Sanitation: Everyday Life, Poverty, and Comparison", *Annals of the Association of American Geographers*. DOI: *104*. 10.1080/00045608.2014.923718.

Routray, P., Schmidt, W.P., Boisson, S., Clasen, Th., and Jenkins, M.W. (2015). "Socio-cultural and behavioural factors constraining latrine adoption in rural coastal Odisha: An exploratory qualitative study". *BMC Public Health.* DOI 10.1186/s12889-015-2206-3.

12
Medicalization of Health Systems
Anthropology on Vigil

M.P. Sachdeva, Archita Tandon, Naveen Kumar and *Vipin Gupta*

From Anthropology in Health to Anthropology of Health: The Historical Breakthrough

The ontology of human life is a product of the authority of the interaction between biology, culture and environment. Yet, the gold standard of biomedicine's control over this life as a mere biological category that predominantly evaporated from its occidental genesis, was challenged by anthropology (Brotherton & Nguyen, 2013). Anthropology's conquest of breathing reality into the fact that humans are not the same everywhere, shook the pillars of biomedicine that rested upon the foundation that bodies were biologically the same everywhere (Andelson *et al.*, 2013; Brotherton & Nguyen, 2013).

The perceived objectivity of biomedicine that predominantly did not believe in the ideologies of the 'non-Western' world on health, disease or sickness, were knocked off by Pritchard's study of the Azande witchcraft (Pritchard, 1937), as one of the pioneering attempts of anthropologists, though classically from a modernist premise, led to empower a perspective, other than biological into studying the metaphysical origins of a thinking about disease or illness by the people who were then untouched by biomedicine (Pool, 1994). This reality of disease and cure, existed out of the mind alone, but, in the shared agency of culture, where prepositions that came as a part of Azande socialization, were the workforce behind their beliefs in witchcraft rendered an explanation to, why affliction struck a single individual and not the others. He contested that this ideology was not alone resting on the premise of moral accentuation, rather on empirical evidence that Azande derived from autopsy, to validate a witchcraft.

This bestowed the fact that though Azande knew that witches did not exist, yet their ascription of the evidence in form of what Pritchard calls undigested material from the intestine, was enough for them to believe in 'why me'(Pritchard, 1937). Similarly, it was Rivers' *Medicine, Magic and Religion*, that enabled an understanding of the health systems in context of other socio-cultural systems. He believed that "*native medical practices and beliefs, taken together, were parts of culture and constituted a social institution*" (Rivers, 2013).

Ackerknecht, further brought to light that medical practices and beliefs were an integrated whole, yet isolated phenomenon in the social and cultural context, which pioneered a mainstreaming of anthropology of health, as an independent realm of discourse (Ackerknecht, 1962). This modernist paradigm was severely critiqued, yet it rested the plank for the debate of how anthropologists made a difference in perceiving health systems having strongly to do with a relation to other social institutions, that made them derive unique mechanisms to deal with medical issues. Through these anthropologists juggled the bridge between 'belief' and 'knowledge' of the people, that encapsulated this health system.

Interestingly, not alone were the structural articulation of health systems in socio-cultural locales highlighted by anthropologists, but also the way in which 'sickness' was explored through individual's agency of action, as per the 'sick role' ascribed, that was socially sanctioned and recognized, was an evidence of how care seeking was sought with this playout of defined roles (Parry, 2008).

The institutionalization of the realm of medical anthropology as a functional subset of anthropology, is accorded to Hunter which led to the documentation of early anthropological involvement in the international public health movement and began the use of a systems model in research of health practices. His 'strategic and integrating conceptual model' viewed medical institutions as a subsystem of cultural systems (Hunter, 1985; Torre,1958). It reeled in between the paradigmatic dictums of trending theories of the time, for instance how from often emphasizing the 'exotic' culture-bound syndromes (Van Loon, 1927) the studies on health moved to examining how disease, biomedically defined, was socially distributed between and within societies, especially societies being transformed by their increased dependency within international capitalist market systems (Dressler, 2001; Scotch, 1963). A decadal shift in how anthropologists went on to contribute to the study of health systems' thinking and research is perceived, as how it moved with the currents of theories, in vogue. The 1970s thus became a time for the Neo-Darwinian adaptationist viewpoint to take the centre stage. It was Alland's explicit structuralist model that took anthropology away from merely understanding 'beliefs' about health and illness to the ecological relations that determined the fate of health and specifications of illnesses in societies. Issues like population density, subsistence patterns, marriage and residence rules, and interactions with reservoirs of disease were the 'focal points in understanding disease as an outcome of adaptive efforts'(Dressler, 2001; Alland, 1970).

The same decade witnessed the meaning centred approach of Byrongood and Kleinman, being the forerunners in understanding health systems (Kleinman *et al.*, 1978). This approach took away disease from merely an object of scientific inquiry and advocated how the naturalistic and personalistic medical beliefs come together, when decisions are made about treatment, seeking healthcare or even defining a state as of 'ill' health. It brought to the fore that bio-medicinal practices existed in the societal framework, that were held together by symbolic and cultural constructs, as how the individual narrations of sufferings became encapsulated under the expression of the social suffering.

Traversing the journey of anthropology's contribution to health systems, further to the postmodernist era, wherein the intellectual poles shifted from belief and knowledge, to finding social, political and economic complexities of social space, that resulted in distribution of a disease (Dressler, 2001). It resonates well with Bourdieu's argument that cultural construction takes place within the constraints of social space, and thus the expressions of levels of suffering, severity of disease, triage of diagnosis, labelling of symptoms, comes down handy at the level of each social space (Bourdieu, 1985).

Capitalism, flexible accumulation and a time-space compression of the global world, has largely impacted the health systems largely in the past two decades (Moberg, 2018). The temporal and spatial standpoints of anthropology have enabled a reflection into how power, capital and inequity has seeped in the larger premise of an accessible health, that is a prominent development goal, both nationally as well as internationally. The political economic approach of anthropology discusses how the voices of subaltern such as disabled, women, people from lower economic status, non-white, who are thought to contribute less to the profit chains of the production cycles, are often marginalized from the mainstream dialogue of health and leading to their poorer health as a result (Estes & Linkins, 2000; Lupton, 2012). Thus, from the early 2000s, anthropologists, resolved a new meaning of health, as, 'good health is defined in political terms not only as a state of physical or emotional wellbeing but as access to and control over the basic material and non material resources that sustain and promote life at a high level of satisfaction', meaning that 'a key component of health is struggle' (Baer *et al.*, 1986).

Though, this approach was criticized for its nihilism and ignorance of how far the proficiency of health systems has reached in increasing life expectancy or through better contraceptive methods and a notion of health being localized. Yet, it remains at the fore to ensure that had the systems been inclusive, the need for healthcare inclusivity would not still be a goal on the bucket list!

Anthropology of the health systems over the past two decades has become more critical in the synthesis of its research to uncover the human body as a product of an interaction of both biological and social processes, that concerns with understanding the social production of medical knowledge; the functions of medicine and public health in social control; the importance of consciousness and agency in health-related behaviours and beliefs; the relation of health and medical language to power; the identification and labelling of disease; the contestable nature of medicine and disease as biomedical realities; and the meaning of the illness experience (Guarnaccia, 2001; Lupton, 2012).

Medicalization: The Social 'Iatrogenesis'

'From sex to food, from aspirins to clothes, from driving your car to riding the surf, it seems that under certain conditions or in combination with certain other substances or activities or if done too much or too little, virtually anything can lead to medical problems' (Zola, 1972).

Medicalization is referred to as the process by which 'some aspects of human life come to be considered as medical problems, whereas before they were not considered pathological. In sociology and anthropology, medicalization is not a "new" concept, yet the pressing capitalism, technology, consumer needs, globalization, engulfing of traditional health systems, has brought it to the fore of anthropological research in the past two decades (Maturo, 2012).

Illich brought to use the Greek term 'iatrogenesis' that refers to originating from a physician/treatment. Social iatrogenesis is the process of increase in the categorization of diseases through extension of medical categories in everyday life, which is not alone a tragedy of the increased use of biomedicine, but raging capitalism and thus rising needs of consumers, eventually ostracizing the use of traditional health systems (Illich, 1976). Conrad has proposed to consider medicalization in three respects (Conrad, 2009):

1. *Conceptual medicalization:* When medical framework is used to define entities out of non-medical realm for example, the natural drooping of breasts after pregnancy diagnosed as 'mammary ptosis'.
2. *Institutional medicalization:* When physicians have the power to steer non-medical personnel— what Freidson called 'professional dominance' (Freidson, 1974); for example, physicians being managers of hospitals without having any academic title in management or business administration).
3. *Interactional medicalization:* When the physician, in interaction with the patient, redefines a social problem into a medical one, for example homosexuality was listed as a pathology in the Diagnostic and Statistical Manual, of Mental Disorders until 1983 (Conrad, 2009; Maturo, 2012).

Due to a lack of attention given to the traditional ways of achieving optimal status of health, has led to a significant rise in medicalization. Anthropologists have noticed how even varied dietary patterns in different socio-cultural settings have been ignored by organizations like UNICEF, in promoting its health programme against malnourishment, by advocating the use of a single commodity by the name *Plumpy'Doz*. While introducing another Nutriset product, Plumpy'Doz to very young children in Somalia, UNICEF has asserted that, "The brown paste supplement is made from vegetable fat, peanut butter, sugar, milk, and other nutrients, and is designed to taste good to kids. Critically, it also has a longer shelf life than previous diet supplements and doesn't need to be mixed with water (just like Plumpy' Nut). Three teaspoons of Plumpy'Doz three times a day provides each young child with additional energy, including fats, high-quality protein and all the essential minerals and vitamins required to ensure growth and a healthy immune system." (UNICEF and the Medicalisation of malnutrition in children).

Plumpy'Doz is a branded product by UNICEF as a Ready to Use Therapeutic Foods (RUTF). This has led to a considerable critique of how medicalization has invaded nutrition of children, *via* completely ignoring the natural, cost effective and local derivatives that could be provided to them. A Health Ministry official in India critiqued its use and stated:

> 'RUTF is used in war-torn countries like Africa. We do not approve of the strategy as there are other low-cost alternatives available in the country itself' (*The Indian Express,* 2009).

This reflects how adversity is set up in issues that can be met through traditional knowledge. Though it calls for several pharma companies to have gained profits, by overriding the concept of food. The medicalization was at once challenged by traditional remedies in various countries.

A study in Bangladesh reported that 'F100'(Formula 100), a therapeutic milk product designed to treat severe malnutrition given along with home food resulted in an average weight gain of 7.7g/kg/day (Hossain *et al.*, 2009). In India, a Child in Need Institute in Kolkata has been using a rice/wheat and legume mix called Nutrimix with micronutrient supplementation in home settings. They report weight gains of 9g/kg/day. Nutrimix is prepared in the community by women's groups (Global Conference on Meeting Nutritional Challenges with Sustainability and Equity, 2009).

Anthropological research shows how in the past two decades this over commercialization and resulting consumption of biomedical prescriptions has led to an over medicalized premise by dragging health issues into its garb, which do not reflect the urgency (UNICEF and the Medicalisation of malnutrition in children).

Medicine and treatment have shifted from curative model to a preventive model through medicalization, that is selling on enhancing human life (Shim & Clarke, 2011), through the use of various biomedical devices to restore or safeguard the perceived 'normality'(Zola, 1983). The constant invasion of the human body by biomedicine is found in various conditions of psychological or physiological discomfort, where it was not even existing. It is not a serendipitous claim of rise in medicalization in the past two decades, but through various anthropological researches that demonstrate how social as well as biological factors such as advertisement, disease mongering, self-diagnosis, aesthetic benefits have led to a rampant invasion of human bodies by the biomedicine.

Childbirth: The Lost Agency of Women

The medicalization of childbirth with bringing 'delivery' to our discourse for narrating a birth, has drastically changed how culturally pregnancy was referred to as, this has set up expectations from women, solely owing to a hierarchy that runs deep into their feminine objective of existence, childbirth! This impedes a hierarchy into domination of women, who are though muted, in most patriarchal domains of the world. This brings a new dimension of silence to their lives (Johanson *et al.*, 2002). Mitchell calls this process as making women the *'living fetal monitors'* and rendering an alternative narrative of ascribing credentials to a woman being a mother. "Refusing prenatal diagnosis, giving birth at home, and even drinking coffee may be interpreted as signs that a woman has made the 'wrong' choices or lacks the 'right' information. ... Those who engage in these taboo activities risk being excluded from the category of 'good mothers' and maybe subject to increase surveillance, restriction, and instruction" (Mitchell, 2016).

The risk to maternal health and foetus health has led to an increased medicalization of childbirth (Parry, 2008). This process has eventually led to biomedicalization of the traditional healthcare mechanisms associated with childbirth, mostly jeopardizing the role of a midwife or *dai.* As Guha notes how medicalization impacted this practice of midwifery, "Whereas medicine was characterized by all the signs of professionalization, namely entry through merit (and not heredity) and specialized knowledge, dais clearly belonged to a pre-modern order of occupation" (Guha, 1998).

It has to be given to this medicalization that the child mortality due to negligence of proper care during childbirth, has largely reduced. But at the same time, it has romanticized itself as becoming indispensable in terms of a notion attached to safety during childbirth and has actually created a divide for those who cannot afford the medicalized superstructure in childbirth. Many women in India cannot afford institutional deliveries. "However, the emphasis on universal institutional delivery, as a key strategy has not only marginalized the role of the Traditional Birth Attendants (TBA–*dai*) in delivery but in all forms of health care provision" (The Role of Traditional Birth Attendants in National Rural Health Mission, 2008).

This eventually led to incentivization of childbirth, wherein the *dais* get financial incentives to enable women from rural households to access premises of institution delivery. The women are also encouraged through a sum of five hundred rupees, for choosing the institutional delivery over hole deliveries, under the *Janani Suraksha Yojana* programme (National Rural Health Mission). Traditions die hard and this incentivization could not play a larger role in making the institutional facilities available to all eligible women, due to factors like: their belief in reaching hospitals only if there is a complication, higher opportunity cost in comparison to home delivery, waiting till the last moment of delivery that often led to unavailability of vehicle or female health worker (Vellakkal *et al.*, 2017). Although the idea of the scheme was to prevent child and mother mortality, it fell to its own prey by how health workers exploited these women by making them wait till the last end, resulting in complications which usually went out of control for the rural health institution to handle (Chaturvedi *et al.*, 2015).

A Western predominance of rendering utmost trust on biomedicine, as almost equivalent to being miraculous has endangered women in the developing and underdeveloped countries mostly. It almost falls to the *Tylorean* ascription of a 'white man's job'(Tylor, 1871) to enable them to live a life of development, rightly according to how Kothari referred to this 'idea of development as a new form of colonialism'(Demaria & Kothari, 2017).

Inhorn sums up this perspective best when she states, "The technological excesses of biomedicine in the face of ongoing medicalization require constant surveillance and vigilance to prevent unnecessary medical control over women's lives" (Parry, 2008; Inhorn, 2006).

Mental illness: Over-Medicalized Yet Under-Stated

Anthropologists have strongly voiced Foucault's attempt at considering the process of indefinite medicalization to be one of the main features of society wherein, he stressed the role of doctors in 'deciding what was normal and what was pathological'(Foucault, 1976; Maturo, 2012). This has impacted the way how people with mental illness are handled. As the pace of life has increased to bounds, it has lowered levels of tolerance of psychological discomfort or sadness, has brought a steady increase of its diagnosis as depression (Horwitz & Wakefield, 2009; Illich, 1976; Maturo, 2012).

Many of the institutions in traditional societies had institutionalized ways of taking care of people with mental health problems. Many of the mental health problems were managed at community levels and did not call for institutionalized treatment and care in the form of asylums, as seen in urban and Western contexts. With this institutionalization is attached the idea of stigma, that eventually makes it difficult for the individual to heal with (Kleinman *et al.*, 1985). Biomedical psychiatry holds the folk mental health traditions to be regressive and obscure. Several ethnographic studies from India have depicted how plural mental health landscapes act efficiently in healing mechanisms of these afflictions. Hindu healing temple of *Balaji* in Rajasthan, is one of the prime sites for traditional treatment to restore healing in terms of mental health afflictions. One of the ethnographic studies of the site reveals how the global biomedical expectations have impacted its functioning and vehemently critiqued its practices. While the study denotes how participants attained a sense of betterment post getting treated at the site and sought it as a means to end their affliction, that primarily emerged from distress or evil eye (Sood, 2016). The trust into the agency of almighty, itself rendering an end to the affliction is the key aspect of this healing ritual, which is socially sanctioned. Of course, it can be critiqued on several grounds of the rational parachute of biomedicine, yet ascribing a certain form of deviant behaviour to a medical category is not viable in the diverse expanse of this global world (Cornard & Slodden, 2013). For example, the widespread over-diagnosis of conditions such as bipolar disorder, autism spectrum disorder, and attention deficit hyperactivity disorders (ADHD), especially among children, is now being documented—the US Centers for Disease Control recently estimated that 6.4 million children aged 4 to 17 had received an ADHD diagnosis at some point in their lives, amounting to 11 per cent of all US children, a 41 per cent increase in the last decade that has been met with alarm and concern by many doctors and parents" (Schwarz & Cohen, 2013).

This concern is alarming, as how a deviant child behaviour is being ascribed to a pathological problem. Further, the pharmaceutical agencies are 'selling sickness' through broadening the edges of categorizing mental health behaviours as a consequence of ill health through 'disease mongering'. The diagnosis has attached itself with the social stigma of curing the 'ill' to be back to normal, that affects the overall aspects of an individual's life (Moynihan *et al.*, 2012).

It has adsorbed into the social scenario as a mechanism of justifying the right kind of conduct 'mentally' in a society, and has a lot to do with power and its play attached to it. Medicalization of mental illness is becoming a tool in restricting people's reach of the divergence from the established sects of the society. In other words,

> "One could look back to Sigmund Freud, who over the course of a long career went from applying new ways of thinking to clinical encounters to grand statements on the nature of human civilization itself. In later decades, the international medical community was shocked by the use of psychiatric diagnoses such as 'sluggish schizophrenia' to invalidate political dissidence in the USSR; recently, the involvement of mental health professionals in such disparate issues as unemployment and terrorist radicalization has sparked intense debate in the UK" (Medicalisation and its discontents, 2016).

The medicalization of mental health has significantly benefited pharmaceutical companies, who answer the mental health problems with pseudo explanations in form of prescriptions that take the body to dormant stages, based on the patient's biology. "According to Health (IMS Health, 2010) antidepressants had about $10 billion in US sales in 2008, a major portion of pharmaceutical industry revenues. The expansion of the antidepressant market into bereavement would be a major boon for drug industry sales" (Conrad, 2007; IMS Health, 2010).

Thus, medicalization has invaded mental illness the most, with its roots in the Western biomedical psychiatry, with lesser answers and more questions, by still letting mental illness in any form be prime stigmas in society.

Conclusion

The advocacy of a utopian idea of health by World Health Organization, as a, "state of complete physical, mental and social wellbeing and not merely the absence of disease or infirmity" (World Health Organization, 1946), where it is often defined as a state rather than a course taken up by individuals at their own pace, in their own contexts and conditions, has led to humans competing in the race of this 'Edenic conception of health' (Maturo, 2012). Health, wellbeing, illness, disease and sickness are notions that are central to the embedded systems of varied socio-cultural settings, and the medicalization of them have resulted in disembarking from the traditional systems leading to an overconsumption of the biomedical services and a caused invasion in the attributes that were not referred to as pathological previously. It can be summed up as medicalization with its pathologization of everything is aiming at turning all human differences into medical conditions that is shaped by its creation of definitions of normality pertaining to behaviour, body shapes or other abilities (Conrad, 2007). An individual exercises its agency with the stakes resting on the social context of which he/she is a part of. Thus, the bio-medical premises which tend to overlook at the socio-cultural context and rather focus on tailor made solutions for problems that were not issues of health as such is a major concern.

REFERENCES

Ackerknecht, E.H. (1962). *Medicine and ethnology: Selected essays* (No. GN477. A24 1971.).

Adelson, N., Butt, L., and Kielmann, K. (Eds.). (2013). *Troubling natural categories: Engaging the medical anthropology of Margaret Lock*. McGill-Queen's Press-MQUP.

Alland, A. (1970). *Adaptation in cultural evolution: An approach to medical anthropology*. New York: Columbia University Press.

An innovative approach to prevent child malnutrition in Somalia. (2008). Retrieved February 06, 2021, from https://www.unicef.org/media/media_46991.html

Baer, H.A., Singer, M., and Johnsen, J.H. (1986). "Toward a critical medical anthropology". *Social science and medicine, 23*(2), 95-98.

Bourdieu, P. (1985). "The social space and the genesis of groups", *Theory and Society, 14*(6), 723-744.

Brotherton, P.S. and Nguyen, V.K. (2013). "Revisiting local biology in the era of global health", *Medical Anthropology, 32*(4), 287-290.

Chaturvedi, S., DeCosta, A., and Raven, J. (2015). "Does the Janani Suraksha Yojana cash transfer programme to promote facility births in India ensure skilled birth attendance? A qualitative study of intrapartum care in Madhya Pradesh", *Global health action, 8*(1), 27427.

Conrad, P. (2007). *The medicalization of society: On the transformation of human conditions into treatable disorders*. JHU Press.

Conrad, P. (2009). "The Shifting Engines of Medicalization, S. 480-492", In: Conrad, P., *The Sociology of Health and Illness. Critical Perspectives*. New York, NY: Worth Publishers.

Conrad, P., and Slodden, C. (2013). "The medicalization of mental disorder", In *Handbook of the sociology of mental health* (pp. 61-73). Springer, Dordrecht.

Demaria, F. and Kothari, A. (2017). "The Post-Development Dictionary agenda: paths to the pluriverse", *Third World Quarterly, 38*(12), 2588-2599.

Dressler, W.W. (2001). "Medical anthropology: toward a third moment in social science?" *Medical Anthropology Quarterly, 15*(4), 455-465.

Estes, C.L., and Linkins, K.W. (2000). "Critical perspectives on health and aging", *The handbook of social studies in health and medicine*, 154-172.

Evans-Pritchard, E.E. (1937). *Witchcraft, oracles and magic among the Azande* (Vol. 12). London: Oxford.

Foucault, M. (1976). La crisis de la medicina o la crisis de la antimedicina. *Educaciónmédica y salud, 10*(2), 152-170.

Freidson, E. (1974). *Professional dominance: The social structure of medical care*. Transaction Publishers.

Global Conference on Meeting Nutritional Challenges with Sustainability and Equity. (2009). International Baby Food Action network. www.ibfanasia.org/gc/conference-report.pdf (accessed 07 February, 2021).

Guarnaccia, P.J. (2001). "Introduction: the contributions of medical anthropology to anthropology and beyond", *Medical anthropology quarterly*, 423-427.

Guha, S. (1998). "From dais to doctors: The medicalisation of childbirth in colonial India", *Understanding Women's Health Issues: A Reader*, 145-161.

Horwitz, A. and Wakefield, J. (2009). "The medicalization of sadness", *Salute e Società*, *8*(2), 49-66.

Hossain, M.I., Dodd, N.S., Ahmed, T., Miah, G.M., Jamil, K.M., Nahar, B.,... and Mahmood, C.B. (2009). "Experience in managing severe malnutrition in a government tertiary treatment facility in Bangladesh", *Journal of health, population, and nutrition*, *27*(1), 72.

Hunter, S.S. (1985). "Historical perspectives on the development of health systems modeling in medical anthropology", *Social Science and Medicine*, *21*(12), 1297-1307.

Illich, I. (1976). Limits to medicine—Medical Nemesis: The expropriation of health, tr. it. *Nemesi medica—l'espropriazionedella salute.*

IMS Health. (2010). www.reuters.com/.../us-depression-drugs-idUSTRE 60454020100105 (accessed 05 February 2021).

Inhorn, M.C. (2006). "Defining women's health: A dozen messages from more than 150 ethnographies", *Medical anthropology quarterly*, *20*(3), 345-378.

Johanson, R., Newburn, M., and Macfarlane, A. (2002). "Has the medicalisation of childbirth gone too far?" *Bmj*, *324*(7342), 892-895.

Kleinman, A., and Good, B. (Eds.). (1985). *Culture and depression: Studies in the anthropology and cross-cultural psychiatry of affect and disorder*. University of California Press.

Kleinman, A., Eisenberg, L., and Good, B. (1978). "Culture, illness, and care: clinical lessons from anthropologic and cross-cultural research", *Annals of internal medicine*, *88*(2), 251-258.

Lupton, D. (2012). *Medicine as culture: Illness, disease and the body*. Sage.

Maturo, A. (2012). "Medicalization: Current concept and future directions in a bionic society", *Mens sana monographs*, *10*(1), 122.

Medicalisation and its discontents (2016). The Lancet Psychiatry. DOI:https:// doi.org/10.1016/S2215-0366(16)30120-1

Mitchell, L.M. (2016). *Baby's first picture*. University of Toronto Press.

Moberg, M. (2018). *Engaging anthropological theory: A social and political history*. Routledge.

Moynihan, R., Doust, J., and Henry, D. (2012). "Preventing overdiagnosis: How to stop harming the healthy", *Bmj*, *344*.

Parry, D.C. (2008). "We wanted a birth experience, not a medical experience: Exploring Canadian women's use of midwifery", *Health care for women international*, *29*(8-9), 784-806.

Pool, R. (1994). "On the creation and dissolution of ethnomedical systems in the medical ethnography of Africa", *Africa*, 1-20.

Rivers, W.H.R. (2013). *Medicine, magic and religion*. Routledge.

Schwarz, A. and Cohen, S. (2013). "ADHD seen in 11 per cent of US children as diagnoses rise", *New York Times*, 331.

Scotch, N.A. (1963). Sociocultural factors in the epidemiology of Zulu hypertension. *American Journal of Public Health and the Nations Health*, *53*(8), 1205-1213.

Shim, J.K. and Clarke, A.E. (2009). Medicalization and Biomedicalization Revisited: Technoscience and Transformations of Health, Illness and Biomedicine. *Medicalization and Biomedicalization Revisited*, 1000-1033.

Sood, A. (2016). The Global Mental Health movement and its impact on traditional healing in India: A case study of the Balaji temple in Rajasthan. *Transcultural psychiatry*, *53*(6), 766-782.

The Indian Express. (2009). Government stops Unicef from giving French protein paste to children. www.indianexpress.com/news/govt-stops-uniceffrom-giving-french-protein/496844/ (accessed 07 February, 2021).

The New York Times. (2013). A.D.H.D. Seen in 11 per cent of U.S. Children as Diagnoses Rise. https://www.nytimes.com/2013/04/01/health/more-diagnoses-of-hyperactivity-causing-concern.html (accessed 06 February, 2021).

The Role of Traditional Birth Attendants in National Rural Health Mission. (2008). Centre for Health and Social Justice. http://www.chsj.org/uploads/1/0/2/1/10215849/tbaconsulreport.pdf (Accessed: February 06, 2021).

Torre, M. (1958). "Health, Culture and Community: Case Studies of Public Reactions to Health Programmes," edited by Benjamin D. Paul (Book Review). *International Journal of Group Psychotherapy*, *8*(1), 346.

Tylor, E.B. (1871). *Primitive culture: Researches into the development of mythology, philosophy, religion, art and custom* (Vol. 2). J. Murray.

UNICEF and the Medicalisation of malnutrition in children. https://www.ghwatch.org/sites/www.ghwatch.org/files/D2_0.pdf (accessed 06 February, 2021).

Van Loon, F.H.G. (1927). Amok and Lattah. *The Journal of Abnormal and Social Psychology*, *21*(4), 434.

Vellakkal, S., Reddy, H., Gupta, A., Chandran, A., Fledderjohann, J., and Stuckler, D. (2017). "A qualitative study of factors impacting accessing of institutional delivery care in the context of India's cash incentive programme", *Social Science and Medicine*, *178*, 55-65.

World Health Organization. (1946). Preamble to the Constitution of the World Health Organization as adopted by the International Health Conference, New York, 19-22 June, 1946; signed on 22 July 1946 by the representatives of 61 States (Official Records of the World Health Organization, no. 2, p. 100) and entered into force on 7 April, 1948. *http://www. who.int/governance/eb/who_constitution_en.pdf*

Zola, I.K. (1972). "Medicine as an institution of social control", *The sociological review*, *20*(4), 487-504.

Zola, I.K. (1983). Socio-medical inquiries: Recollections, reflections, and reconsiderations.

PART III

Physical Health and Wellbeing

13
Culture Shapes Body Composition and Blood Pressure Levels
Reflections from Three Studies Conducted in Eastern India

Subho Roy, Nivedita Som, Anushka Ghosh, Priyanka Kanrar and *Swagato Pramanik*

Introduction

The study on cultural variability in adult body composition and blood pressure levels has been a topic of interest in anthropological research since a couple of decades (Lear *et al.*, 2007; Sarkar *et al.*, 2009; Carrol *et al.*, 2008; Mohamud *et al.*, 2011; Barreira *et al.*, 2012; Mungreiphy *et al.*, 2012; Carpenter *et al.*, 2013; Ghosh and Bandyopadhyay, 2013; Sabanayagam *et al.*, 2013; Wang *et al.*, 2017). But, how the cultural processes generate perception towards lifestyle, body image and health, further how they determine body composition and blood pressure levels is a novel arena of research. Dressler *et al.* (1996) conceptualized that an individual's reported behaviour corresponds to the culturally prototypical pattern that is referred to as 'cultural consonance'. For example, in Brazil, consumption of fresh fruits, vegetables, low fat chicken and sea foods are preferred as both healthy and prestigious. Individuals belonging to well off families in Brazil exhibit culturally valued status by consuming these foods. Thus, higher cultural consonance stimulates greater intake of healthy food that may prevent the risk of obesity and hypertension (Dressler *et al.*, 2008). On the other hand, lower cultural consonance in lifestyle was observed among African American group living in United States (US). In US, the popular culture is likely to prefer thin body shape, thereby emphasizing on low-fat diet. However, African American group living in US prefer to consume fat-based food items more, leading to an increase in the prevalence of hypertension (Dressler and Bindon, 2000). Here, cultural identification in one hand assimilates with culturally normative body ideals and lifestyle and on the other hand cultural identification contrasts with external cultural cues. For example, African-Americans, particularly women remain culturally identified with the thicker body ideals of the black culture, but they remain exposed to the White-American popular cultural cues that is related to a thinner body ideal (Sabik *et al.,* 2010).

Cross-cultural studies documented a higher incidence of larger body size and obesity in societies which are stratified, complex and are leading sedentary lifestyle (Brown and Konner, 1987; Lev-Ran, 2001; Gremillion, 2005). It seems that juxtaposition of two facts (like a species-wide metabolic adaptation to conserve energy resources during times of food scarcity and the cultural adaptations giving rise to a greater food security in complex societies) is likely to increase the incidence of overall adiposity among individuals. Furthermore, the pattern of body composition throughout the societies change with change in the indices of socio-economic development. For example, at the inception of industrialization, the level of adiposity among human populations was found to be high with increase in socio-economic status because of the inverse association between calorie intake and energy expenditure. However, with the advancement in modernization, the cultural expectation towards body image got changed and consequently the concept of thin body shape in women and the muscular body shape in men became popular as the 'ideal body type' particularly in Western societies (Martin, 2010; Prnjak *et al.*, 2019; Stojcic *et al.*, 2020). The affluent class chose to maintain this 'ideal body shape' as they had access to different cuisine and specialized physical training because of plenty of leisure time and adequate financial resources (Brown and Konner, 1987; Gremillion, 2005). Thus, it appears that in Western countries, an inverse association between the incidence of obesity and the socio-economic status was found with the rise in the popularity of the trend of being slim and trim (Monteiro *et al.*, 2004). On the contrary, the thinness is devalued and deemed to remain unattractive in many non-Western counties, including India. For example, in Arabic culture, thinness is considered as socially undesirable, while the fat body for women symbolizes fertility and womanhood (Musaiger, 2014; Khalaf *et al.*, 2015; Alhussaini *et al.*, 2018). In India, traditionally plump body shape is preferred. One colloquial statement 'look fat and fresh' implicates like a compliment among the Punjabi women of India for their physical beauty. However, in the contemporary time, the trend of being slim and trim is slowly creeping into the minds of the younger people in India (Som and Mukhopadhyay, 2015). Consequently, a shift in lifestyle (food consumption and physical activity) is observed among them and eventually it develops potential impact on body composition and blood pressure levels (Kaur, 2012). It appears from the above discussion that body composition and blood pressure are not only regulated by ethnicity, but are also induced by lifestyles perceived to be good and practiced by the members of an ethnic group (Paeratakul *et al.*, 2002; Gillum and Sempos, 2005; Dressler *et al.*, 2012). Thus, the members of an ethnic group have a shared understanding, embodied in their culture. For example, people of Western countries preferred thin body shape of females, while the plump body shape was traditionally preferred in Asian countries (Sakamaki *et al.*, 2005). Latino mothers believed obese children to be healthy and showed less concern about their child's weight. However, a few of them were likely to believe that obese children, in general, should be taken to a nutritionist or physician for seeking advice towards weight reduction (Pham and Harrison, 2007). There are examples where the process of modernization gradually shifted the perception of a community towards body shape and lifestyle (Becker, 2004) or has brought changes in the actual pattern of lifestyle among individuals which eventually causes adverse effects on body composition, blood pressure levels and health (Bardan and Laher, 2012).

In India, majority of the anthropological literature on body composition and blood pressure focused on socio-demographic and/or lifestyle correlates of body composition and blood pressure levels (Borah *et al.*, 2015; Chowdhury and Roy, 2016; Kaur and Kaur, 2018). This article attempts to delineate how culture influences on actual pattern of lifestyle and eventually shapes body composition and blood pressure levels. We hypothesized that cultural consonance intercedes the association of socio-demographic and lifestyle variables with body composition and blood pressure levels.

Method of Study

Three cross-sectional studies were conducted separately within a time frame of five years (2014-2019) on adult populations belonging to distinct ethnic groups residing in different areas of eastern India. The first two studies Study I (2014) and Study II (2016) were conducted in the cities of Kolkata and Howrah of the state of West Bengal respectively (Ghosh *et al.*, 2018; Kanrar *et al.*, 2021). The third one (Study III) was conducted in hilly areas of the East Sikkim in the year 2019 (Pramanik *et.al.*, 2021). In the present article, we presented the trend in the findings of these research works to draw a broad analytical framework of 'cultural consonance' model.

In each of these studies we compared how the perception towards, and the actual practice of lifestyle influence on body composition and blood pressure levels between ethnic groups inhabiting adjacently but representing distinct cultural milieu. For example, Study I included 150 individuals [80 Bengali-speaking Hindu (male = 38 and female = 42) and 70 Marwari Hindu (male = 29 and female = 41)] of age 30-40 years from three municipal wards (27, 38 and 63) of the Kolkata Municipal Corporation (KMC). Study II included 210 individuals [109 Bengali Hindu (male = 47 and female = 62) and 101 Santals (male = 43 and female = 58)] of age 18-50 years from the two municipal wards (26 and 50) of Howrah Municipal Corporation. Study III included160 males (80 each from the Rai and the Lepcha communities) aged 25-35 years from the Rai Gaon and the Phenzong villages of the Ranka *Gram Panchayat* unit of East Sikkim.

The cities of Kolkata and Howrah are numerically dominated by Bengali-speaking Hindu ethnic group. In Kolkata study area (Study I), both Marwari Hindu and Bengali Hindu peoples live in the same neighbourhood. The Marwari Hindus originally lived in Jodhpur region of southwest Rajasthan state of India and started migrating to different places of India after the decline of Rajput Kingdom. The Marwari Hindus recently living in Kolkata city started to colonize as the traders, bankers and financiers to the growing British power in Bengal since the second half of the nineteenth century (Strasser, 2013). In Howrah city (Study II), the Bengali Hindu and the Santal peoples reside in adjacent clusters within the study areas. Here, the Santals of this locality migrated from the districts of Bankura and Purulia of West Bengal around half a century ago. In Sikkim (Study III), the Nepalese caste group is numerically dominant, followed by Bhutia and Lepcha populations. The Rai is one of the major ethnic groups amongst the Nepalese Hindu living in Sikkim. The Rais have reportedly been settled in Sikkim from the 17th century (Subba, 2011). The Lepchas are thought to be the earliest inhabitants of Sikkim, but have adopted many elements of the culture of the Bhutia people, who entered Sikkim from Tibet during the 14th century and afterward (*ibid.*). The Lepchas usually live in the remotest valleys and speak in Tibetan dialect. Lepchas follow Buddhism, but still keep faith on their earlier pantheon of spirits and shamans for management of ailments, intercede with the gods, and preside over the rites accompanying birth, marriage, and death. The Lepchas, who were once hunters and gatherers, are presently engaged in farming economy.

In Study I, the participants were initially interviewed for their perception towards health and obesity, blood pressure problems and related health management. Data on socio-demographic characteristics and lifestyle pattern (food consumption and substance abuse, physical activities, and medical care) were collected. The participants were asked to report how often they consumed foods in the past one week starting from the date of interview. Duration of physical activities (in minutes) including physical exercise, sitting light work, sitting moderate work, standing light work, standing moderate work, standing heavy work were recorded for the past one week prior to the interview. Later, body composition and blood pressure levels were measured on each participant. The Student's t-test was used to compare the body composition and blood pressure levels between Bengali Hindu and Marwari Hindu groups for both males and females. Multivariate analysis of covariance (MANCOVA) was conducted to show the relationship of ethnicity with both the body composition and blood pressure levels. In Study II, the participants were interviewed about their beliefs and perception on the types of physical activities and consumption pattern. For example, the participants were asked whether they consider consumption of healthy foods and moderate physical activities necessary for reducing blood pressure and body fat and maintaining good health. Lifestyle information of the participants including their food consumption pattern and physical activities in the past one week starting from the date of interview were collected. Later, body composition and blood pressure levels were measured among the Bengali Hindu and the Santals. Our findings revealed how the perception/beliefs towards lifestyle and the actual pattern of lifestyle are related to body composition and blood pressure levels among these two groups. Principal component analyses were used to extract the components from the variables considered for estimating perception/beliefs towards lifestyle (including the possession of material goods, physical activities, food consumption and medical care). The first two components for each domain (including the possession of material goods, physical activities, food consumption and medical care) of perception/beliefs towards lifestyle were chosen to use in multiple linear regression analyses. Multivariate analysis of covariance (MANCOVA) was used to understand association of body composition and blood pressure levels with both the perception towards and actual lifestyle and ethnicity respectively. In Study III, initially the perception towards health and obesity, blood pressure problems and its management were compared between the Rai and the Lepcha groups. Case studies were collected on the perception towards health and obesity, blood pressure problems and its management from a subsample (a total of 12 case studies: 7 from the Rai group; 5 from the Lepcha group) of the study participants. Later, body composition and blood pressure levels were compared between these two ethnic groups. Lifestyle information of the participants included food consumption and substance use and physical activities (using a 24-hour recall method) and medical history. Later, body composition and blood pressure levels of the participants were compared between these two groups. Multiple linear regression analysis was performed to understand the association of the body fat patterning and blood pressure levels with socio-demographic and lifestyle variables. Multivariate analysis of covariance (MANCOVA) was conducted to show the relationship of ethnicity with both the body composition and blood pressure levels.

In each study, anthropometric measures (like stature, waist and hip circumferences, triceps, subscapular, suprailliac and medial calf skin fold thicknesses) were taken from each participant following the standard protocol (Lohman *et al.*, 1988). Body fat measures (like body mass index, percent body fat, fat mass, fat free mass, visceral fat, subcutaneous fat and skeletal muscle of whole body, trunk, arms and legs) were taken from each of the participants using Omron Body Composition Monitor (HBF-362). Blood pressure [systolic blood pressure (SBP) and diastolic blood pressure (DBP)] levels were measured on left arm of each participant using a blood pressure monitor (Omron M2 Manual Inflation Blood Pressure Monitor, Japan).

Results and Discussion

Study I

In Kolkata study, we observed that the incidence of hypertension and level of adiposity were greater among the Marwari Hindu group compared to the Bengali Hindu group. Moreover, body composition differed significantly between these two ethnic groups after controlling for lifestyle and age. Thus, it appears that ethnicity plays a significant role in determining the body composition and blood pressure level among individuals as observed in other studies (Lin *et al.*, 2004; Kumar *et al.*, 2006; Carrol *et al.*, 2008; Brummett *et al.*, 2012). Furthermore, we found a noticeable difference in the perception towards obesity, hypertension and its management strategies between the Marwari Hindu and the Bengali Hindu groups. The participants of the former group (irrespective of sex) were found to be contended with their perceived (present) health status and body weight; they did not consider that bringing dietary restriction would reduce the risk factors associated with obesity and hypertension. Further, the participants of the Marwari Hindu community did not consider the problem of obesity and hypertension as cardio-vascular risk factors at the age of 40 years of life. The Marwari Hindu participants preferred to undertake physical exercise, rather than dietary restriction, despite the males of this group were mostly engaged in sitting light type of work. Non-vegetarian foods (fish, egg and meat) were mostly consumed by the Bengali Hindu participants on the regular basis. Majority of the Marwari Hindu participants never or hardly ever preferred non-vegetarian foods. However, a very few of the Marwari Hindu participants reported to consume non-vegetarian foods on the occasion. Moreover, we found that the participants of Marwari Hindu group consumed dairy products (especially, butter, *ghee*) regularly without feeling bothered to become obese. Consequently, the higher incidence of hypertension along with greater level of adiposity was observed among Marwari Hindu group. This finding is consistent with other studies conducted in West Bengal (Majumder *et al.*, 1995; Das and Bose, 2006). Contrary to this, most of the participants from the Bengali Hindu group considered obesity to be associated with the increased risk of hypertension, which is disadvantageous for health. This type of attitude possibly developed concern among them to reducing the burden of obesity and hypertension by limiting the intake of carbohydrate and fat contents in their diet. Hence, cases of hypertension and the level of adiposity were found to be lower among Bengali Hindu group. One study in the same region showed how a group of Bengali Hindu adolescent girls attempted to reduce body fat by adopting unhealthy weight reduction measures (Som and Mukhopadhyay, 2015) perhaps because of the effect of modernization. The study remained short from concluding the effect of modernization on lifestyle variables owing to the paucity of data.

The consistency between the perception and the action was reflected among the participants of both the study groups. For example, despite being obese and hypertensive, the Marwari Hindu group remained satisfied with their own body weight and blood pressure levels, unlike their Bengali Hindu counterpart. The latter group adopted some measures of lifestyle to reduce body weight. This could be an effect of cultural consonance as suggested by William Dressler and co-researchers in several studies (Dressler *et al.*, 1991; Dressler *et al.*, 1996; Dressler *et al.*, 2004; Dressler *et al.*, 2005; Dressler, 2007; Dressler *et al.*, 2008; Dressler *et al.*, 2012). Study I epitomized that both the ethnic groups (the Bengali Hindu and the Marwari Hindu) had higher cultural consonance. However, such cultural consonance reflects a greater risk in the cardiovascular health of the Marwari Hindu than that of the Bengali Hindu.

Study II

The study showed that the perception towards lifestyle were similar between the participants of both Bengali Hindu and the Santals. Parallel to this, no conspicuous difference was observed between the participants of both these groups in their actual lifestyle pattern. The participants of both the ethnic groups, staying adjacently for generations, probably developed similar perception towards actual practices in their lifestyle pattern. Therefore, the difference between perception towards lifestyle and actual pattern of lifestyle for both the ethnic groups was not noticed. Descriptive statistics clearly revealed difference between the perception towards and the actual pattern of lifestyle between both the ethnic groups. For example, the participants, irrespective of ethnicity and sex, perceived that the consumption of healthy foods along with moderate level of physical activities could help in reducing the body fat and alleviate the problems of hypertension among them. But, in reality, these participants, irrespective of ethnic groups, hardly undertook physical exercise and other moderate activities. Further, they occasionally consumed healthy foods, like vegetables, fruits and pulses. From these findings, it is evident that the cultural consonance from the perspectives of healthy lifestyle remained low among the participants of both the ethnic groups. Participants, who perceived physical activity and consumption of healthy food as 'healthy lifestyle' showed inverse association with the measures of body fat, and blood pressure levels. On the other hand, the actual pattern of lifestyle of the study participants, which was quite dissimilar with their perception, also showed strong influences on body composition, and blood pressure levels.

The Study II epitomized that the Bengali Hindu and the Santals both signified the importance of moderate physical activities and consumption of nutritious food as the goal attainment for healthy life, but the members of both the groups often failed practicing such healthy lifestyle regularly. This gap, between beliefs and practices reflects lower cultural consonance that promotes a greater cardiovascular risk in both the study populations. Thus, it indicates that a shared knowledge and perception towards healthy lifestyle among individuals, perhaps encoded in own culture often fail to get translated in actual lifestyle pattern and eventually affects their physical health.

Study III

In our Sikkim study, a conspicuous difference in body composition was observed between the Rai and the Lepcha ethnic groups; the Lepchas were shorter and had higher BMI than the Rai. This finding is indicative of a higher level of overall adiposity among the Lepchas, which eventually made them hypertensive. Moreover, the association between body composition and blood pressure levels with ethnicity, after controlling lifestyle and age reinforces that ethnicity largely determines the body composition and blood pressure levels as observed in other studies (Lin *et al.*, 2004; Kumar *et al.*, 2006; Carrol *et al.*, 2008; Brummett *et al.*, 2012).

We also found a noticeable difference in the perception towards obesity, hypertension and its management between the Rai and the Lepcha participants. The Lepchas were least bothered of being hypertensive and they never considered it as cardiovascular risk. Rather, they considered hypertension as the adaptive development towards cold climatic condition at this high-altitude region. They preferred to consume salted tea with butter on a regular basis since they believed that this adaptive strategy could increase energy for performing strenuous physical activities at the high-altitude; and perceived that their regular involvement in tireless activities would keep them physically strong. In spite of their involvement in strenuous work (like agricultural activities and walking uphill and downhill), the higher incidence of hypertension along with greater level of adiposity was observed among the Lepchas. This finding is consistent with other studies conducted in different ethnic populations living in high altitude areas (Norbo *et al.*, 2015; Shen *et al.*, 2017).

In the Rai group, most of participants perceived obesity to be largely associated with increased risk of hypertension. They believed that obesity helps reducing physical energy and promotes health hazards. This type of attitude possibly developed concerns among them to lessen the burden of obesity and hypertension by following a healthy lifestyle (like moderate exercise and consumption of staple foods). However, cases of hypertension and the level of adiposity also remained high among the Rai. It appeared that the Rai participants, who are living in high-altitude areas, had the same problem of hypertension and greater level of adiposity like the Lepchas.

In this study, the consonance between the perception and the behaviours were reflected in both the Rai and the Lepcha ethnic groups.

For example, despite being hypertensive, the Lepchas remained unaware about their own body weight and blood pressure levels, unlike the Rai counterpart. They believed that the practice of religious rituals is protecting them from all the ailments. However, the Rai participants preferred to follow medical advice in managing obesity and hypertension, and adopted some measures in their lifestyle for health promotion. This might reflect the instance of cultural consonance as found in other studies (Dressler *et al.*, 1991; Dressler *et al.*, 1996; Dressler *et al.*, 2004; Dressler *et al.*, 2005; Dressler, 2007; Dressler *et al.*, 2008; Dressler *et al.*, 2012). Study III implied that the members of both the Rai and the Lepcha ethnic groups had higher cultural consonance; however, such cultural consonance promotes a greater cardiovascular health risk in both groups probably because of their abode in high altitude.

Conclusion

From the aforesaid discussion it appeared that ethnic diversity remains embedded in cultural behaviours and practices. Such kind of practices, rooted in the belief system of an ethnic group is likely to delineate the health condition of the group members. Members of ethnic group who closely approximate the prototypes for belief and behaviour, encoded in shared cultural model, are likely to reflect the higher cultural consonance and thereby a reduced health risk. On the contrary, the inconsistency between the perceptions and the behaviours reflects lower cultural consonance and increased health risk. Thus, cultural consonance intercedes the association between lifestyle and health.

India, being a culturally diverse country, similar type of research on other ethnic groups residing in different ecological settings is seriously required. This would help the policy makers to understand not only on how the actual lifestyle, embedded in cultural beliefs influence on physical health but to distinguish the changes occurred both in beliefs and behaviours among members of ethnic groups with modernization on physical health.

REFERENCES

Alhussaini, A.A., Alsuwedan, H.I., Alnefaie, H.F., Almubrek, R.A., Aldaweesh, S.A., Anitha, L., and Qassem, H. (2018). "Self-perception of body image among Saudi females at Princess Nourah University, Riyadh, Kingdom of Saudi Arabia", *Malaysian Journal of Nutrition*, *24*(1), 117-123.

Badran, M., and Laher, I. (2012). "Type II diabetes mellitus in Arabic-speaking countries", *International Journal of Endocrinology*, 2012 (s3), 1-11.

Barreira, T.V., Staiano, A.E., Harrington, D.M., Heymsfield, S.B., Smith, S.R., Bouchard, C., and Katzmarzyk, P.T. (2012). "Anthropometric correlates of total body fat, abdominal adiposity, and cardiovascular disease risk factors in a biracial sample of men and women", *Mayo Clinic Proceedings*, *87*(5), 452-460.

Becker, A.E. (2004). "Television, disordered eating, and young women in Fiji: negotiating body image and identity during rapid social change", *Culture, Medicine, Psychiatry*, *28*(4), 533-559.

Borah, P.K., Devi, U., Biswas, D., Kalita, H., Sharma, M., and Mahanta, J. (2015). "Distribution of blood pressure and correlates of hypertension in school children aged 5-14 years from North East India", *Indian Journal of Medical Research, 142*(3), 293–300.

Brown, P.J., and Konner, M. (1987). "An anthropological perspective on obesity", *Annals of the New York Academy of Sciences*, *499*, 29–46.

Brummett, B.H., Babyak, M.B., Siegler, I.C., Surwit, R., Georgiades, A., Boyle, S.H., and Williams, R.B. (2012). "Systolic blood pressure and adiposity: Examination by race and gender in a nationally representative sample of young adults", *American Journal of Hypertension*, 25(2), 140-144.

Carpenter, C.L., Yan, E., Chen, S., Hong, K., Arechiga, A., Kim, W.S., Deng, M., Li, Z., and Herber, D. (2013). "Body fat and body-mass index among a multiethnic sample of college-age men and women", *Journal of Obesity*, 1-7.

Carroll, J.F., Chiapa, A.L., Rodriquez, M., Phelps, D.R., Cardarelli, K.M., Vishwanatha, J.K., Bae, S., and Cardarelli, R. (2008). "Visceral fat, waist circumference, and BMI: Impact of race/ethnicity", *Obesity, 16*(3), 600-607.

Chowdhury, T.K., and Roy, S.K. (2016). "Blood pressure and body composition of rural Oraons of North 24 Parganas, West Bengal, India", *Anthropologischer Anzeiger*, *73*(2), 145-154.

Das, M., and Bose, K. (2006). "Presence of high rates of overweight and obesity among adult Marwaris of Howrah, West Bengal, India", *Collegium Antropologicum, 30*(1), 81-86.

Dressler, W.W. (1991). "Social support, lifestyle incongruity, and arterial blood pressure in a southern black community", *Psychosomatic Medicine, 53*(6), 608-620.

Dressler, W.W., Balieiro, M.C., Ribeiro, R.P., and Dos Santos, J.E. (2005). "Cultural consonance and arterial blood pressure in urban Brazil", *Social Science and Medicine*, *61*(3), 527-540.

Dressler, W.W., Balieiro, M.C., Ribeiroand, R.P., and Dos Santos, J.E. (2007). "Cultural consonance and psychological distress: examining the associations in multiple cultural domains", *Culture, Medicine, Psychiatry*, *31*(2):195-224.

Dressler, W.W., and Bindon, J.R. (2000). "The health consequences of cultural consonance: Cultural dimensions of lifestyle, social support, and arterial blood pressure in an African American community", *American Anthropologist*, *102*, 244–260.

Dressler, W.W., Dos Santos, J.E., and Balieiro, M.C. (1996). "Studying diversity and sharing in culture: An example of lifestyle in Brazil", *Journal of Anthropological Research*, *52*(3), 331–353.

Dressler, W.W., Oths, K.S., Balieiro, M.C., Ribeiro, R.P., and Dos Santos, J.E. (2012). "How culture shapes the body: Cultural consonance and body mass in urban Brazil", *American Journal of Human Biology, 24*(3), 325-331.

Dressler, W.W., Oths, K.S., Ribeiro, R.P., Balieiro, M.C., and Dos Santos, J.E. (2008). "Cultural consonance and adult body composition in urban Brazil", *American Journal of Human Biology, 20*(1), 15-22.

Dressler, W.W., Ribeiro, R.P., Balieiro, M.C., Oths, K.S., and Dos Santos, J.E. (2004). "Eating, drinking and being depressed: the social, cultural and psychological context of alcohol consumption and nutrition in a Brazilian community", *Social Science and Medicine, 59*(4),709-720.

Ghosh, A., Som, N., and Ray, S. (2018). "A comparative study on body composition and blood pressure levels between Marwari Hindu and Bengali Hindu groups living in West Bengal, India", In S. Ghosh and D.K. Limbu (Eds.) *Readings in Biological Anthropology*, B.R. Publishing Corporation: New Delhi.

Ghosh, J.R., and Bandyopadhyay, A.R. (2013). "Central adiposity and the risk of hypertension in Asian Indian girls", *World Journal of Pediatrics*, *9*(3), 256-260.

Gillum, R.F., and Sempos, C.T. (2005). "Ethnic variation in validity of classification of overweight and obesity using self-reported weight and height in American women and men: The Third National Health and Nutrition Examination Survey." *Nutrition Journal, 4*, 27.

Gremillion, H. (2005). "The cultural politics of body size", *Annual Review of Anthropology*, *34*,13–32.

Kanrar, P., Som, N., and Roy, S. (2021). A study on body composition, blood pressure and blood sugar levels among Bengali Hindu and Santals using cultural consonance model. *Journal of the Anthropological Survey of India,* 70(1), 26-61.

Kaur, G. (2012). Body composition, dietary intake and physical activity level of sedentary adult Indian women. *Food and Nutrition Sciences*, *3*(11), 1577-1585.

Kaur, M. and Kaur, R. (2018). "Body Composition, Blood Pressure Trends and Dietary Intake of Adult Males and Females of Bhil Tribe, Udaipur, Rajasthan (India)", *Anthropologie (Brno), 56*(1), 11-20.

Khalaf, A., Westergren, A., Berggren, V., Ekblom, Ö., and Al-Hazzaa, H. (2015). "Perceived and ideal body image in young women in south western Saudi Arabia", *Journal of Obesity, 2015*.

Kumar, B.N., Meyer, H.E., Wandel, M., Dalen, I., and Holmboe-Ottesen, G. (2006). "Ethnic differences in obesity among immigrants from developing countries, in Oslo, Norway". *International Journal of Obesity,* 30(4), 684-690.

Lear, S.A., Humphries, K.H., Kohli, S., Chockalingam, A., Frohlich, J.J., Birmingham, C.L. (2007). "Visceral adipose tissue accumulation differs according to ethnic background: results of the Multicultural Community

Health Assessment Trial (M-CHAT)". *American Journal of Clinical Nutrition, 86*(2), 353-359.

Lev-Ran, A. (2001). "Human obesity: an evolutionary approach to understanding our bulging waistline". *Diabetes Metabolism Research and Reviews, 17*(5), 347–362.

Lin, Y.C., Wang, M.J., and Wang, E.M. (2004). The comparisons of anthropometric characteristics among four peoples in East Asia. *Applied Ergonomics, 35*(2), 173-178.

Lohman, T.G., Roche, A.F., and Martorell, R. (1988). *Anthropometric Standardization Reference Manual*. Human Kinetics Books, Champaign, IL.

Majumder, P.P., Das, R.N., Nayak, S., and Bhattacharya, S.K. (1995). Genetic epidemiology of blood pressure in two Indian populations: Some lesson. *Human Biology, 67*(6), 827-842.

Martin, J. (2010). "The Development of Ideal Body Image Perceptions in the United States". *Nutrition Today, 45*(3), 98-110.

Mohamud, W.N., Musa, K.I., Khir, A.S., Ismail, A.A., Ismail, I.S., Kadir, K.A., Kamaruddin, N.A., Yaacob, N.A., Mustafa, N., Ali, O., Isa, S.H., and Bebakar, W.M. (2011). "Prevalence of overweight and obesity among adult Malaysians: an update". *Asia Pacific Journal of Clinical Nutrition, 20*(1), 35-41.

Monteiro, C.A., Moura, E.C., Conde, W.L., and Popkin, B.M. (2004). "Socioeconomic status and obesity in adult populations of developing countries: a review". *Bulletin of World Health Organization, 82*(12), 940–946.

Mungreiphy, N.K., Dhall, M., Tyagi, R., Saluja, K., Kumar, A., Tungdim, M.G., Sinha, R., Rongmei, K.S., Tandon, K., Bhardwaj, S., Kapoor, A.K., and Kapoor, S. (2012). "Ethnicity, obesity and health pattern among Indian population". *Journal of Natural Science, Biology, and Medicine, 3*(1), 52-59.

Musaiger, A.O. (2014). Body size preferences among young women in five Arab countries: a cross-cultural study. *International journal of adolescent medicine and health, 26*(3), 417-421.

Norboo, T., Stobdan, T., Tsering, N., Angchuk, N., Tsering, P., Ahmed, I., Chorol, T., Sharma, V.K., Reddy, P., Singh, S.B., Kimura, Y., Sakamoto, R., Fukutomi, E., Ishikawa, M., Suwa, K., Kosaka, Y., Nose, M., Yamaguchi, T., Tsukihara, T., Matsubayashi, K., Otsuka, K., and Okumiya, K. (2015). Prevalence of hypertension at high altitude: cross-sectional survey in Ladakh, Northern India, 2007-2011. *BMJ Open, 5*(4), e007026.

Paeratakul, S., White, M.A., Williamson, D.A., Ryan, D.H., and Bray, G.A. (2002). "Sex, race/ethnicity, socioeconomic status, and bmi in relation to self-perception of overweight". *Obesity Research, 10*(5), 345–350.

Pham, K.L., Harrison, G.G., and Kagawa-Singer, M. (2007). "Perceptions of diet and physical activity among California among adults and youths". *Preventing Chronic Disease, 4*(4), A93.

Pramanik, S., Som, N., and Roy, S. (2021). "Body fat patterning and blood pressure levels: a comparative study between the Rai and the Lepcha in Sikkim, *Anthropological Review*, 84(2), 131-147.

Prnjak, K., Pemberton, S., Helms, E., and Phillips J.G. (2020). "Reactions to ideal body shapes", *Journal of General Psychology, 147*(4), 361-380.

Sabanayagam, C., Teo, B.W., Tai, E.S., Jafar, T.H., and Wong, T.Y. (2013). "Ethnic differences in the association between blood pressure components and chronic kidney disease in middle aged and older Asian adults", *BMC Nephrology, 14*(1), 86.

Sabik, N., Cole, E.R., and Ward, L.M. (2010). "Ethnic identity as a moderator of the association between body image and disordered eating among Black and Asian American women", *Psychology of Women Quarterly, 34*, 139-154.

Sakamaki, R., Amamoto, R., Mochida, Y., Shinfuku, N., and Toyama, K. (2005). "A comparative study of food habits and body shape perception of university students in Japan and Korea", *Nutrition Journal, 4*, 31.

Sarkar, D., Mondal, N., and Sen, J. (2009). "Obesity and blood pressure variations among the Bengali Kayastha population of North Bengal, India", *Journal of Life Sciences, 1*(1), 35-43.

Shen, Y., Chang, C., Zhang, J., Jiang, Y., Ni, B., and Wang, Y. (2017). "Prevalence and risk factors associated with hypertension and prehypertension in a working population at high altitude in China: A cross-sectional study", *Environmental Health and Preventive Medicine, 22*(1), 19.

Som, N. and Mukhopadhyay, S. (2015). "Body weight and body shape concerns and related behaviours among Indian urban adolescent girls", *Public Health Nutrition, 18*(6), 1075-1083.

Stojcic, I., Dong, X., and Ren, X. (2020). "Body Image and Sociocultural Predictors of Body Image Dissatisfaction in Croatian and Chinese Women", *Frontiers in psychology, 11*, 731.

Strasser, S. (2013). *Commodifying everything: Relationships of the market*, Taylor and Francis: Hoboken.

Subba, J.R. (2011). *History, Culture and Customs of Sikkim*, Gyan Publishing House: New Delhi.

Wang, L., Southerland, J., Wang, K., Bailey, B.A., Alamian, A., Stevens, M.A., and Wang, Y. (2017). "Ethnic Differences in Risk Factors for Obesity among Adults in California, the United States", *Journal of Obesity,* 1-10.

14
Challenges and Prospects of Beta Thalassemia Screening
Global and Indian Scenario

Benrithung Murry and *Anand Kumar Gyanendra Singh Wahengbam*

Introduction

Thalassemia is a genetic blood disorder affecting the rate of hemoglobin production. In this disease condition the globin chains, involving α and β globin chains that make up the hemoglobin molecule are produced at a decreased rate or not produced at all. β-thalassemia is characterized by reduced synthesis of the hemoglobin subunit (beta chain) that results in microcytic hypochromic anemia, an abnormal peripheral blood smear with nucleated red blood cells, and reduced amounts of hemoglobin A (HbA) (Origa, 2000). Thalassemia has been associated with health burden which has been increasing on a global scale (Modell and Darlingson, 2008; Weatherall, 2010). As reported in the Global Burden of Disease (GBD), thalassemia was ranked 68th in 2010 in terms of disability-adjusted life years (DALYs), yet it ranked 24th when the 1-4 year age group was considered, indicating its important contribution to the under-5 mortality (Piel, 2016). High incidence of thalassemia is reported in the Mediterranean basin and parts of Africa, throughout the Middle East, the Indian subcontinent, Southeast Asia and Melanesia into the Pacific Islands which generally are known as the thalassemia belt (Kountouris *et al.*, 2014; De Sanctis *et al.*, 2017). However, thalassemia and sickle cell anemia have become global challenges of national health care systems which are due to global immigration (Hemminki *et al.*, 2015). It is reported that there is an overall carrier frequency of 4.05 per cent with the population of 1.2 billion, which estimates the additional 11,316 affected thalassemia births per year to the existing affected patients and also found that thalassemia is prevalent mostly among castes, religion and population groups (Petrou, 2010). Screening along with genetic counselling is shown to be an effective preventive strategy, thereby reducing the births of affected children through screening, counselling, prenatal diagnosis and selective termination of affected fetuses (Scriver *et al.*, 1984; Angastiniotis and Hadjiminas, 1991). However, in the absence of any follow up strategy, there are no significant changes in the incidence of thalassemia major as reported in some studies (Stamatoyannopoulos, 1974; Gamberini *et al.*, 1991). In Indian context, the screening strategy and approach needs to corroborate with the norms and practices of caste system, as castes are largely endogamous groups that invariably are governed by unique cultural milleu (Ray *et al.*, 2017). Therefore, the focus and strategy for prevention of β-thalassemia in India needs to address the low awareness level and a screening programme feasible in Indian society where such programmes should be better accepted, available and affordable to all sections of the society. In this chapter, an attempt has been made to discuss the challenges and prospects of the screening programmes on β-thalassemia around the world with special focus on the Indian context, as India is a multi-cultural and multi-ethnic nation.

Method

A comprehensive scoping searches were conducted with published literature from 1970s up to January 2019 using the electronic databases such as PubMed, ScienceDirect and Google Scholar with the following keywords 'β-thalassemia, carrier, screen, programmes, genetic counselling, national, health policy and effect or outcome'. This was followed by a search on the website of the World Health Organization (WHO), Ministry of Health and Family Welfare, Government of India and civil-society organizations such as Thalassemia International Federation (TIF), Indian Red Cross Society (IRCS) which were purposefully searched for studies and reports where relevant citations were selected to be included in the literature review. Those studies exclusively based on the programmes for screening of β-thalassemia carriers were included for this review while the rest have been excluded.

Discussion

Outcomes Emanating from the Existing Carrier Screening Programmes

β-thalassemia carrier screening programmes have been implemented in different countries across the world, where various approaches are adopted among different populations which include mandatory or voluntary, educating participants and screening at pre-pregnancy or during antenatal care (Cowan, 2009; Zlotogora *et al.*, 2009; Colah *et al.*, 2008; Armeli *et al.*, 2005). The main purpose of carrier screening programme is to identify asymptomatic carriers so that they are informed and educated for their reproductive risks and options available (Raffle, 2001). So far there is no attributed way to channelize genetic screening programme where the provisions of screening has not been influenced by cultural, social and religious beliefs (Marteau *et al.*, 2001).

Thalassemia screening programmes are of two types, such as mandatory and voluntary. When the screening is done before conception several options are available for a couple where they can opt for adopting a child, use artificial insemination and also consider egg or sperm donation, else by undergoing prenatal diagnosis they can decide to end the pregnancy if the fetus is found to have β-thalassemia major (Cousens *et al.*, 2010). As for mandatory programmes, World Health Organization published guidelines that stated genetic testing should not be made compulsory (WHO,1998). Iran, Saudi Arabia, Palestinian Territories and Cyprus are some of the countries that have laws allowing mandatory premarital screening for hemoglobinopathies to all the prospective couples willing to get married (Tarazi *et al.*, 2007; Cowan, 2009). Moreover in Iran, since 1991 thalassemia carrier screening was made a mandatory premarital blood test (Karimi *et al.*, 2007). However, this is subject to ethical issues as couples are restricted to decide on their own while exercising their choice on genetic screening (Samavat and Modell, 2004; Khorasani *et al.*, 2008). On the other hand, carrier couples are counselled and given advice which includes cancellation of marriage but they are given the choice to decide that marriage (Karimi *et al.*, 2007). Cyprus, a country with the highest carrier frequency in the world has developed a quasi-mandated premarital β-thalassemia carrier screening programme in the early 1980s (Cowan, 2009). A viable regulation has been introduced there where the Thalassemia Centre has to issue a certificate indicating the status of being screened and counselled (Cowan, 2009). Manadatory screening is being practiced with confidentiality in these countries, the prospective couples who are found to be carriers still could get married if they wish so and it is believed that the incidence of thalassemia is reduced with this method of screening (Al Hamdan *et al.*, 2007). Voluntary programmes have been conducted in high schools as well as before pregnancy and antenatally. Mitchell *et al.* (1996) described a β-thalassemia genetic screening programme that was conducted in high schools in Montreal. Prior to screening those high school students they were encouraged to provide individual consent for testing after a thorough education on thalassemia (Mitchell *et al.*, 1996). Many countries have adopted antenatal screening as a voluntary screening programme (Vallace and Ford, 2003). Subsequently, pregnant women were reported to provide informed consent and participate during a screening prior to blood test in their first ever antenatal visit (Colah *et al.*, 2008). In contrast, antenatal screening is provided in *ad hoc* mode in few countries where prevalence of thalassemia is lower (Locock and Kai, 2008). Screening programme is yet to be introduced in Continental Europe owing to the fact that there is the lack of awareness about hemoglobinopathies among policymakers, health professionals and groups at risk (Modell *et al.*, 2007). However, several South Asian at-risk countries such as Thailand, Taiwan, Singapore, Maldives and Sri Lanka have their own national screening programmes (Premawardhena *et al.*, 2004; Weatherall, 2005).

Reduction in the prevalence and prevention of the birth of thalassemia patients has been identified as the result of thalassemia carrier screening programme (Angastiniotis and Hadjiminas, 1991; Cao *et al.*, 1996). The reduction in disease incidence is attributed to proper prenatal diagnosis and widespread use of reproductive technologies that restricts affected childbirths, also marriages between carrier individuals are drastically low (Greengross *et al.*, 1999). Termination of a large number of affected fetuses after screening are reported in many countries thereby a reduction in the incidence of β-thalassemia is observed after implementing screening programmes (Mitchell *et al.*, 1996; Liao *et al.*, 2005; Colah *et al.*, 2008). The incidence of thalassemia in Sardinia in 1975 was one affected in every 250 births, but after the implementation of voluntary carrier screening programme the incidence as reported in 1995 was one affected in every 4000 births (Cao *et al.*, 1996). The incidence of thalassemia in Cyprus begins to decrease after the introduction of screening programme in the 1970s, which further developed into a mandatory screening in the early 1980s. By the beginning of the 21st century, i.e. 2002 and 2007 the country was able to achieve zero thalassemia status. Obtaining blood supply for treatment of thalassemia patients was a potential burden in Cyprus way before the implementation of carrier screening programme and this situation would have been aggravated if the programme had not existed when the incidence continued to rise simultaneously (Bate, 1975). Those affected with thalassemia were benefited with the decreased incidence of thalassemia as the demand for blood got reduced. This resulted in improving the management of treatment in Cyprus.

Prevalence and Preventive Strategies for β-Thalassemia in India

Numerous studies undertaken subsequently have shown that the prevalence of β-thalassemia varies from 1 to 17 per cent in different population groups with an overall frequency of 3-4 per cent, which amounts to 35-45 million carriers in our multi-ethnic and culturally and linguistically diverse population of 1.3 billion people. Community wise β-thalassemia carrier frequencies have been reported by different scholars in different regions of India. Communities that belong to Western and Northern India such as the Sindhis, Kutchhi Bhanushalis and Punjabis are reported to have high prevalence, i.e. 5-10 per cent of β-thalassemia in the country (Mehta *et al.,* 1972; Sukumaran, 1975). The prevalence of hemoglobinopathies in India is estimated to be 1.2 per 1000 live births (Christianson *et al.,* 2006). According to Population Reference Bureau (2010), this estimation yielded approximately 27 million births per year which translated to annual births of 32,000 babies with hemoglobinopathies. Within this overall disease classification, a WHO Working Group (1989) on guidelines for the control of hemoglobin disorders estimated a 3.9 per cent carrier frequency for β-thalassemia in India, encompassing all types of β-thalassemia trait. This particular estimate was a derivative from data collected prior to 1984 which rely on basic hematological methods of analysis (Livingstone, 1985).

A WHO update on β-thalassemia in India indicated a similar overall carrier frequency of 3-4 per cent, which would translate to around 35.1 to 46.8 million carriers of the disorder nationwide (WHO, 2008). Simultaneously, a screening project based on 56,814 college students and pregnant women recruited in the states of Maharashtra, Gujarat, Punjab, Karnataka, West Bengal and Assam indicated a carrier rate of 2.78 per cent (Mohanty *et al.*, 2008). These variable carrier frequency estimates have been used to approximate numbers of new affected births per year, which when calculated gave a range from 10,000 to 15,000 cases (Sheth *et al.*, 2008; Tamhankar *et al.*, 2009), of which 8,000 to 10,000 would present with a severe form of the disease (Colah *et al.,* 2009). If accurate, the figures would indicate a cumulative total of 100,000 children with thalassemia major in India (WHO, 2008). Unfortunately, there are no adequately representative data sets to confirm or deny these approximations, and with 50,000 to 60,000 strictly endogamous communities in India (Gadgil *et al.*, 1998), and is dubious whether the average disease prevalence estimate could readily be applied to each and every community and sub-population. The carrier frequency for β-thalassemia ranges from 0.3 to 17 per cent in different local communities (Weatherall and Clegg, 2001). The prevalence of β-thalassemia in India was highest in the Sindhi and Punjabi communities, and it was only towards the end of the twentieth century that reports from other Indian states demonstrated the wide distribution and extensive heterogeneity of β-thalassemia mutations in different Indian sub-populations (Varawalla *et al.*, 1991; Varawalla *et al.*, 1992).

The need for prevention of β-thalassemia is obvious due to high frequency of the condition, the great expense and difficulties in providing optimal treatment for patients, and the innumerable fatalities from untreated β-thalassemia. Prevention would not only be a good public health practice, as envisioned in Alma Ata Declaration (Kravitz, 2019), but it would also be cost-effective. It would be of tremendous help in reducing the burden of the disease for patients, families and the health services. The chief elements of a control programme were developed in the 1970s by a team of experts at the World Health Organization (WHO, 1994). These include prenatal diagnosis in couples who have given birth to an affected child, as well as those identified to be at risk, prospective antenatal screening, community carrier screening, and counselling and prenatal diagnosis.

β-thalassemia screening has been considered to be very successful in many parts of the world where the disease was highly prevalent. (Cousens *et al.*, 2010) *Preventive* programmes based on heterozygote detection, counselling and fetal diagnosis have been very effective in reducing birth of thalassemia major infants in Sardinia, Cyprus, Greece and Italy (Cao *et al.*, 1998). The strategy of identifying carriers and asking carriers not to marry carriers without providing fetal diagnosis does not have any significant impact in the actual practice of marriages between heterozygotes. The Montreal Thalassemia Screening Programme as described by Mitchell *et al.* (1996) comprises educational activities, screening of potential carriers, diagnostic procedures, counselling resources and finally, procedures for fetal diagnosis. All the identified carriers happened to remember their carrier status ever since their screening was done in high school, then later on their partners were tested too and also performed prenatal diagnosis if required (Mitchell *et al.*, 1996). The newly diagnosed cases of thalassemia were found to be fallen by 90 per cent since the beginning of this screening programme (Capua, 1998). The practice of within caste endogamy which is not only central to the institution of caste, but is also one of the most resilient caste based practices till date (Patel *et al.*, 2012).

Different methods and levels of β-thalassemia screening programmes are adopted worldwide. In India several studies have attempted to assess the impact of these screening activities and they are being discussed here. Screening of high school and college students with one-time counselling is found to have insufficient impact towards prevention (Colah *et al.*, 2007). Cascade screening is a vital approach in identifying β-thalassemia carrier which is most cost-effective (Gorakshakar and Colah, 2009). Premarital screening is practiced successfully in Middle East countries where the prevalence of thalassemia is high; the reason being the religious objection to prenatal diagnosis and medical termination of pregnancy (Samavat and Modell, 2004; Guler *et al.*, 2007). A study in India reported the cancellation of prospective marriage after premarital screening where they cited the reason as religious and personal objection to prenatal testing and the consequent abortion (Tamhankar *et al.*, 2009). A hospital based study reported that antenatal screening is not ideal in India due to two reasons. One of them is late screening which was done after the first trimester of pregnancy. And the other is the inappropriate time to inform women about the risk of producing a child with a genetic disease during pregnancy (Colah *et al.*, 2001).

> *A strong male child preference is seen in the Indian society where the birth of a male child surmounts the status of a woman. For instance, Reena (name changed), a 32 year old pregnant woman visited the Division of Genetics, Department of Pediatrics, All India Institute of Medical Sciences (AIIMS), New Delhi and had a prenatal test for thalassemia. The doctors found that she carried a thalassemia baby and advised her to undergo abortion. But she refused and urged the doctors to reveal the sex of the baby as she was willing to give birth to the baby if it is a boy, else she can terminate her pregnancy.*

The Indian Red Cross Society has done a remarkable work on thalassemia thereby conducting the largest screening programme as per record (IRCS, 2010) which was organized in Ahmedabad and some other cities in Gujarat. The Prime Minister's Jai Vigyan Thalassemia Control Programme, a national level project on thalassemia screening covered six major Indian cities where the prevalence of hemoglobinopathies is very high (Colah *et al.*, 2008; Mohanty *et al.*, 2008). The Working Group on the Disease Burden for the 12th Five-Year Plan recommends for prevention and management of genetic blood disorders with emphasis on carrier detection in the community and prenatal diagnosis (Ministry of Health and Family Welfare, 2012). Additionally, the National Health Mission (2016) had also introduced policy for prevention and control of hemoglobinopathies in India which is in accordance to the guidelines of WHO (1989). However, the process of screening and counselling programme being implemented in rural and tribal areas were found to have lesser good practice (Patra and Sleeboom-Faulkner, 2010; Mohanty and Das, 2011). Extensive work on molecular characterization of hemoglobinopathies and β-thalassemia in West Bengal, and also sickle cell anemia in Maharashtra from Human Genetics Extension Programme of Anthropological Survey of India (ASI) throws light on the recent growing awareness of the problem of β-thalassemia as also addressed by many disciplines and studies done by numerous scholars. Consequently, anthropologists are able to earmark a number of populations with exclusive cultural specifications where they identified high risk populations for the hemoglobin disorders. In spite of this, there is a lack of follow up studies in terms of intervention or post-intervention evaluation, which is crucial to reduce the incidence of hemoglobinopathies and β-thalassemia in India (ASI, 2008).

Existing Problem of Screenings in India

Premarital screening has been available for decades in India. The scheme of identifying carriers and advising them not to marry another carrier has not been successful with the existing level of knowledge and awareness of thalassemia (Pallikadavath *et al.*, 2004; Colah *et al.*, 2007). This is supported by the fact that blood is considered to be deeply valued in the Bengali kinship system, and a genetic mutation is understood to corrupt the blood (Chattopadhyay, 2006). Eventually, people refused to undergo screening for fear of being exposed of any impurity in the blood. Carriers have obstacle in marriage as it is a means for continuity of the lineage which is much influenced by culture (Bandopadhyay, 2004). Parents are much hesitated to get their daughters tested for the fear of losing eligible suitors if daughters are carriers (Uberoi, 1993). Thalassemia minor status is being associated with stigma thus people are reluctant to undergo testing and reveal the status (Chattopadhyay, 2006). While some are of the opinion that over-emphasis on premarital screening should be avoided in India, it is equally imperative that the prevalence of this disease in the country is controlled. The policy should determine the carrier status of subjects before reproduction, or during early pregnancy, so that prenatal diagnosis can be done among the at risk couples. Screening programmes for β-thalassemia should aim to sensitize the community to the problem, establish hematological technologies for screening, and molecular and obstetric techniques for prenatal diagnosis.

Cascade screening identifies many more carriers than general population screening, as was shown in studies in India and Pakistan (Gorakshakar and Colah, 2009; Ahmed *et al.*, 2002). Information on the attitudes towards screening for thalassemia was collected among 200 families of index cases residing around Mumbai, where 20 per cent of these families had expressed an unfavourable reaction from their relatives (Sangani, 1990). Hence, in order to avoid social stigmatization, these parents were secretive about their child having thalassemia major. In a follow up study from previously screened and counselled high-risk communities, it was found that 46 per cent of the carriers had got all their siblings tested while, 42 per cent had not informed their siblings about their carrier status (Yagnik, 1997). Another study highlighted the issues related to non-available screening centres, high costing for the test and lack of assistance and support (Saxena and Phadke, 2002).

Recently, the Government of India has formulated a policy for prevention and control of hemoglobinopathies which include β-thalassemia, sickle cell disease and variant hemoglobins in the country to address the issue of the rising prevalence of hemoglobinopathies and creating awareness in the community for better participation in carrier screening. Carrier screenings could be undertaken among high school and college students, premarital and preconception carrier screening are to be in hospitals with appropriate genetic counselling. A card to identify the status through colour codes, indicating carrier or diseased would be provided to all the screened individuals. In the rural areas, accredited social health activist (ASHA) workers would be trained in identifying anemic individuals who would be distinguished from hemoglobinopathies and referred to the primary health centre for further investigation. Nevertheless, this is likely to create an undesirable circumstance in the identification of carrier individuals in the rural areas. A similar incident occurred in Taiwan, where the birth of thalassemia children was reported and was related to problems in the screening procedure (Chern *et al.*, 2007).

For those people who migrated and settled in urban areas leaving their social and cultural roots seemed to pay less attention to caste system (Mosse, 2018). However, caste is vital to those in rural, village and is exhibited in the socio-economic activities (Sharma, 2012). Endogamy as a product of caste system has maintained the founder effect contributed to an excess of heritable diseases in India in subsequent generations ramified different recessive diseases (Sivasubbu and Scaria, 2019). Moreover, a high reproductive rate within few individuals caused the increased frequency of rare mutations to be inherited to subsequent generations (Reich *et al.*, 2009). This ultimately demands the need for consideration of caste system in India at the time of carrier screening for β-thalassemia. Caste-based carrier screening programme needs to be encouraged as similar caste populations are distributed across different regions in the country so that the targeted population should not be missed out as screenings done so far are very much polarized.

Conclusion

Globally, the lack of proactive stance of the governments where the incidence of thalassemia is high and lesser commitment of the community to prioritize thalassemia screening have been the pertinent challenges. These can be addressed by intensifying the existing health care services with clear objectives and motives, raising awareness and providing education to the health professionals and populations at large. In India, there has been a nationwide effort to promote education and awareness with intensification of β-thalassemia carrier screening being initiated by the government and non-governmental organizations since 1970s as thalassemia posed a burden to the health care practices. However, genetic counselling to the detected carriers has not been effectively implemented except in a few private institutions, which led to the burgeoning burden of the disease leaving behind a vast majority of the carriers in ignorance. Numerous screening programmes have already been completed without adequate follow ups. A long term follow up post-screening programme could reduce the incidence of thalassemia. Awareness programmes should be formulated and carried out with the help of parent-patient organizations so that the disease burden could be well perceived. There is undoubtedly a need for greater attention to provide proper education which can break cultural and emotional barriers in mate selection. Given the present scenario of thalassemia in India, it can be concluded that screening programmes should cater three criteria. First, it should adapt to the cultural practices for better acceptability; second, genetic counselling strategies by trained professionals need to be formulated; and third, ensure affordable and easily accessible testing facility such as necessary laboratory equipment and staff for accurate diagnosis.

REFERENCES

Ahmed, S., Saleem, M., Modell, B., Petrou, M. (2002). "Screening extended families for genetic hemoglobin disorders in Pakistan", *N Engl J Med*, *347*:1162–8.

Al Hamdan, NA., Al Mazrou, YY., Al Swaidi, FM., *et al.* (2007). "Premarital screening for thalassemia and sickle cell disease in Saudi Arabia", *Genetics in Medicine*, *9*:372-377.

Al Swaidi, FM., *et al.* (2007). "Premarital screening for thalassemia and sickle cell disease in Saudi Arabia", *Genetics in Medicine*, *9*:372-377.

Amreli, C., Robbins, SJ., Eunpu, D. (2005). "Comparing knowledge of β-thalassemia in samples of Italians, Italian-Americans, and non-Italian-Americans", *Journal of Genetic Couseling*, *14*:365-376.

Angastiniotis, MA., Hadjiminas, MG. (1991). "Prevention of thalassaemia in Cyprus", *Lancet*, *1*:369-70.

Anthropological Survey of India. (2008). Human Genetics Extension Programme. <https://ansi.gov.in/human-genetics-extension-programme/> [accessed 27/6/2019].

Bandopadhyay, S. (2004). *Caste, culture, and hegemony: Social domination in colonial Bengal*. New Delhi, Thousand Oaks, CA: Sage Publications.

Bate, CM. (1975). "Thalassemia in Cyprus", *Proc Roy Soc Med*, *68*:514-516.

Cao, A., Galanello, R., Rosatelli, MC. (1998). "Prenatal diagnosis and screening of the haemoglobinopathies", *Baillieres Clin Haematol*, *11*:215–38.

Cao, A., Rosatelli, M.C., Galanello, R. (1996). "Control of β-thalassemia by carrier screening, genetic counselling and prenatal diagnosis: The Sardinian experience", *Ciba Found Symp*, *197*: 137–151; discussion 151–135.

Capua, A. (1998). "The Montreal Thalassemia Screening programme", *Ann NY Acad Sci*, *850*, 401-403.

Chattopadhyay, S. (2006). *'Rakter dosh'—Corrupting blood: The challenges of preventing thalassemia in Bengal, India. Soc Sci Med*, *63*:2661–73.

Chern, J.P., Lin, K.H., Lu, M.Y. (2007). Beta-thalassemia major births after National Screening Programme in Taiwan. *Pediatr Blood Cane*, *50*: 58-61

Christianson, A., Howson, C.P., Modell, B. (2006). *March Dimes global of report on birth defects: The Hidden Toll of Dying and Disabled Children*. March of Dimes Birth Defects Foundation.

Colah, R., Gorakshakar, A., Nadkarni, A., Phanasgaonkar, S., Surve, R., Sawant, P., Mohanty, D., Ghosh, K. (2009). "Regional heterogeneity of β-thalassemia mutations in the multi-ethnic Indian population", *Blood Cells Mol Dis*, *42*:241–246.

Colah, R., Surve, R., Wadia, M., Solanki, P., Mayekar, P., Thomas, M., *et al.* (2008). "Carrier screening for beta-thalassemia during pregnancy in India: A 7-year evaluation", *Genet Test*, *12*:181-185.

Colah, R., Thomas, M., Mayekar, P. (2007). "Assessing the impact of screening and counseling high school children for β-thalassaemia in India", *J Med Screening, 14*:3.

Colah, R., Surve, R., Wadia, M., *et al.* (2008). "Carrier screening for β-Thalassemia during pregnancy in India: A 7-year evaluation", *Genet Test, 12*: 181–186.

Colah, RB., Gorakshakar, A., Surve, R., Wadia, M., Ghosh, K., Mohanty, D. (2001). "Feasibility of antenatal screening of β-thalassaemia in Mumbai, India", *Acta Haematol, 105*:105-252.

Cousens, N.E., Gaff, C.L., Metcalfe, S.A., Delatycki, M.B. (2010). "Carrier screening for beta-thalassemia: A review of international practice". *Eur J Hum Genet, 18*:1077–1083.

Cowan, R.S. (2009). "Moving up the slippery slope: Mandated genetic screening on Cyprus", *Am J Med Genet Part C Semin Med Genet, 151C*:95–103.

De Sanctis, V., Kattamis, C., Canatan, D., *et al.* (2017). "β-Thalassemia Distribution in the Old World: An Ancient Disease Seen from a Historical Standpoint", *Mediterr J Hematol Infect Dis, 9*(1):e2017018. doi:10.4084/MJHID.2017.018. doi: 10.1016/j.bcmd.2008.12.06.

Gadgil, M., Joshi, NV., Manoharan, S., Patil, S., Prasad, U.V.S. (1998). "Peopling of India", In Balasubramanian D., Appaji Rao N., editors. *The Indian human heritage*. Hyderabad: Universities Press, pp. 100–129.

Gamberini, M.R., Lucci, M., Vullo, C., Anderson, B., Canella, R., Barrai, I. (1991). "Reproductive behaviour of families segregating for Cooley's anaemia before and after the availability of prenatal diagnosis", *J Med Genet, 28*:523–9.

Gorakshakar, A.C., and Colah, R.B. (2009). "Cascade Screening for β-thalassaemia: A practical approach for identifying and counselling carriers in India", *Indian J Community Med, 34*:354-6.

Gorakshakar, A.C., Colah, R.B. (2009). "Cascade screening for beta-thalassemia: A practical approach for identifying and counseling carriers in India", *Indian J Community Med, 34*:354–6.

Government of India. (2012). Prevention and Control of Non Communicable Diseases (Report of the Working Group on Disease Burden for 12th Five Year Plan). (WG-3: Non Communicable Diseases). New Delhi: Ministry of Health and Family Welfare. Retrieved from: https://niti.gov.in/planningcommission.gov.in/docs/aboutus/committee/wrkgrp12/health/WG_3_2non_communicable.pdf

Government of India. (2016). Prevention and Control of Haemoglobinopathies in India: Thalassaemias, Sickle Cell Disease and other Variant Haemoglobins (National Health Mission Guidelines on Hemoglobinopathies in India). New Delhi: Ministry of Health & Family Welfare. Retrieved from: https://nhm.gov.in/images/pdf/in-focus/NHM_Guidelines_on_Hemoglobinopathies_in_India.pdf.

Greengross, P., Hickman, M., Gill, M. *et al.* (1999). "Outcomes of universal antenatal screening for haemoglobinopathies", *J Med Screen, 6*:3-10.

Guidelines for control of hemoglobin disorders. (1994). World Health Organization hereditary disease programme. Geneva: WHO; WHO/HDP/HB/gl/94.1.

Guler, E., Karacan, M. (2007). "Prevalence of beta thalassemia and sickle cell anemia trait in premarital screening in Konya Urban area, Turkey". *J PediatrHematol Oncol, 29*: 783–785.

Hemminki, K., Li, X., Forsti, A., Sundquist, J., Sundquist, K. (2015). "Thalassemia and sickle cell anemia in Swedish immigrants: Genetic diseases have become global", *SAGE Open. Med*, 3:2050312115613097.

Indian Red Cross Society. (2010). Gujarat State Branch. *Annual Report 2009-2010*. Ahmedabad: IRCS, Gujarat State Branch.

Karimi, M., Jamalian, N., Yarmohammadi, H., *et al.* (2007). *Premarital screening for β-thalassaemia in Southern Iran: Options for improving the programme. J. Med Screen, 14*:62-66.

Khorasani, G., Kosaryan, M., Vahidshahi, K., *et al.* (2008). "Results of the national programme of prevention of Thalassemia major in the Iranian Province of Mazandaran", *Hemoglobin, 32*:263-271.

Kountouris, P., Lederer, C.W., Fanis, P., Feleki, X., Old, J., Kleanthous, M. (2014). "IthaGenes: An interactive database for haemoglobin variations and epidemiology", *PLoS One, 9*(7): e103020. Published 2014, July 24. doi:10.1371/journal.pone.0103020.

Kravitz, J.D. (2019). "Redefining Global Health; Integrating an Alma Ata Declaration Retrospective", *J Community Med Public Health Care, 6*: 046.

Liao, C., Mo, Q., Li, J., *et al.* (2005). "Carrier screening for α- and β-thalassemia in pregnancy: The truth of an 11-year prospective programme in Guangshou Maternal and Neonatal Hospital", *Prenat Diagn, 25*:163-171.

Livingstone, F.B. (1985). *Frequencies of hemoglobin variants: Thalassemia, the glucose-6-phosphate dehydrogenase deficiency, G6PD variants, and ovalocytosis in human populations*. New York: Oxford University Press.

Locock, L., Kai, J. (2008). "Parents' experiences of universal screening for haemoglobin disorders: Implications for practice in a new genetics era", *Br J Gen Pract, 58*:161-168.

Marteau, TM., Dormandy, E., Michie, S. (2001). "A measure of informed choice", *Health Expect, 4*:99-108.

Mehta, B.C., Dave, V.B., Joshi, S.R., Baxi, A.J., Bhatia, H.M., Patel, J.C. (1972). "Study of hematological and genetical characteristics of Cutchi Bhanushali community". *Indian J Med Res, 60*:305–311.

Mitchell, J.J., Annie, C., Carol, C., and Charles R. Scriver. (1996). Twenty-Year outcome analysis of Genetic Screening Programmes for Tay-Sachs and β-thalassemia Disease Carriers in High Schools. *Am.J.Hum.Genet, 59*: 793-798.

Modell, B., Darlison, M., Birgens, H., Cario, H., Faustino, P., Giordano, P.C., Gulbis, B., Hopmeier, P., Lena-Russo, D., Romao, L., *et al.* (2007). "Epidemiology of haemoglobin disorders in Europe: An overview". *Scand J Clin Lab Invest, 67*: 39–69

Modell, B. and Darlingson, M. (2008). "Global epidemiology of haemoglobin disorders and derived service indicators", *Bull World Health Organ*, *86*(6): 480-487.

Mohanty, D., and K. Das. (2011). "Genetic Counselling in Tribals in India." *Indian Journal of Medical Research*, *134* (4): 561–571.

Mohanty, D., Colah, R., Gorakshakar, A. (2008). *Jai Vigyan S. & T mission project on community control of thalassaemia syndromes—awareness, screening, genetic counselling and prevention*. A national multicentric task force study of ICMR (2000–2005), (eds.) Indian Council of Medical Research, New Delhi.

Mohanty, D., Colah, R., Gorakshakar, AC. (2008). *Jai Vigyan S & T Mission Project on community control of thalassemia syndromes—Awareness, screening, genetic counselling and prevention.* New Delhi: Indian Council of Medical Research.

Mosse, D. (2018). Caste and development: Contemporary perspectives on a structure of discrimination and advantage. *World Development*, *110*: 422-436.

National Health Mission. (2016). *Prevention and Control of Hemoglobinopathies in India – Thalassemias, Sickle Cell Disease and Other Variant Hemoglobins (Guidelines on hemoglobinopathies in India).* New Delhi: Ministry of Health and Family Welfare.

Origa, R. (2000). "Beta-Thalassemia". In: Adam, M.P., Ardinger, H.H., Pagon, RA, *et al*., (eds.) *Gene Reviews* [Internet]. Seattle: University of Washington. (https://www.ncbi.nlm.nih.gov/books/ NBK1426/).

Pallikadavath, S., Foss, M., & Stones, W. (2004). "Antenatal care: Provision and inequality in rural north India", *Social Science & Medicine*, *59*(6), 1147-1158.

Patel, A., Naik, P., Shah, M., Sharma, N., Narmadeshwar, P., Parmar, P. (2012). "Prevalence of common hemoglobinopathies in Gujarat: an analysis of a large population screening programme". *Nat J Commun Med*, *3*:112–116.

Patra, P.K., and Sleeboom-Faulkner, M. (2010). "Population Genetic Screening for Sickle Cell Anaemia Among Rural and Tribal Communities in India: The Limitations of Socio-ethical Choice." In *Frameworks of Choice: Predictive and Genetic Testing in Asia,* edited by M. Sleeboom-Faulkner, 65–90. Amsterdam: Amsterdam University Press.

Petrou, M. (2010). "Screening for beta thalassaemia", *Indian J Hum Genet*, *16*(1):1–5. doi:10.4103/0971-6866.64934.

Piel, F. (2016). "The present and future Global Burden of the inherited disorders of haemoglobin". *Hematol. Oncol. Clin. N. Am*, *30*, 327–341.

PRB. (2010). *World population data sheet.* Population Reference Bureau, Washington DC.

Premawardhena, A., De Silva, S., Arambepola, M., Olivieri, N., Merson, L., Muraco, J., Allen, A., Fisher, C., Peto, T., Vichinsky, E., *et al.* (2004). Thalassemia in Sri Lanka: A progress report. *Hum Mol Gene*, *13*: R203–R206

Raffle, AE. (2001). "Information about screening—Is it to achieve high uptake or to ensure informed consent?", *Health Expect.* *4*:92-98.

Ray, T. Chaudhuri, A. Sahai, K. (2017). *Whose education matters? An analysis of intercaste marriage in India. Technical Report,* Indian Statistical Institute, Delhi Economics and Planning Unit.

Reich, D., Thangaraj, K., Patterson, N., Price, AL., Singh, L. (2009). "Reconstructing Indian population history", *Nature, 461*: 489–94.

Samavat, A., Modell, B. (2004). "Iranian national thalassemia screening programme", *BMJ, 329*: 1135–1137.

Sangani, B., Sukumaran, P.K., Mahadik, C., Yagnik, H., Telang, S., Vas, F., *et al.* (1990). "Thalassemia in Bombay: the role of medical genetics in developing countries", *Bull World Health Organ, 68*:75–81.

Saxena, A., Phadke, S.R. (2002). "Feasibility of thalassaemia control by extended family screening in Indian context", *J Health PopulNutr, 20*:31–5.

Scriver, CR., Bardanis, M., Cartier, L., Clow, C.L., Lzancaster, G.A., Ostrowsky, J.T. (1984). "Beta-thalassemia disease prevention: Genetic medicine applied". *Am J Hum Genet, 36*:1024-38. 17.

Sharma, K.L. (2012). "Is there Today Caste System or there is only Caste in India?" *Polish Sociological Review, 1*(78), 245-263.

Sheth, J.J., Sheth, F.J., Pandya, P., Priya, R., Davla, S., Thakur, C., Vaz, F. (2008). "β-thalassemia mutations in Western India", *Ind J Pediatr, 75*:567–570. doi: 10.1007/s12098-008-0109-3.

Sivasubbu, S. and Scaria, V. (2019). "Genomics of rare genetic diseases – experiences from India", *Human Genomics, 13*(1).

Stamatoyannopoulos, G. (1974). "Problems of screening and counseling in the hemoglobinopathies", In: Motulsky A.G, Lenz, W, editors. *Birth defects. Amsterdam: Excerpta Medica*, pp. 268–276.

Sukumaran, P.K. (1975). "Abnormal hemoglobins in India", In: Sen N.N., Basu, A.K. (eds.) *Trends in hematology*. Saraswati Press, Calcutta. pp. 225–236.

Tamhankar, P.M., Agarwal, S., Arya, V., Kumar, R., Gupta, U.R. and Agarwal, S.S. (2009). "Prevention of homozygous beta thalassemia by premarital screening and prenatal diagnosis in India", *Prenat Diagn, 29*:637–638. doi: 10.1002/pd.2176.

Tarazi, I, A.l. Najjar, E., Lulu, N. and Sirdah, M. (2007). "Obligatory premarital tests for beta-thalassemia in the Gaza Strip: evaluation and recommendations", *Int J Lab Hematol, 29*: 111–118.

Uberoi, P. (1993). *Family, kingship & marriage in India*. New Delhi: Oxford University Press.

Vallance, H., Ford, J. (2003). "Carrier testing for Autosomal-Recessive disorders". *Critical Reviews in Clinical Laboratory Sciences, 40*:473-497.

Varawalla, N.Y., Fitches, A.C., Old, J.M. (1992). "Analysis of β-globin gene haplotypes in Asian-Indians: origin and spread of β-thalassemia on the Indian subcontinent", *Hum Genet, 90*:443–449. doi: 10.1007/BF00220475.

Varawalla, N.Y., Old, J.M., Sarkar, R., Venkatesan, R., Weatherall, D.J. (1991). "The spectrum of β-thalassemia mutations on the Indian subcontinent: the basis for prenatal diagnosis", *Brit J Haemat*, *78*:242–247. doi: 10.1111/j.1365-2141.1991.tb04423.x

Weatherall, D.J. (2010). "The inherited diseases of haemoglobin are an emerging global health burden", *Blood*, *115* (22): 4331-4336.

Weatherall, D.J., Clegg, J.B. (2001). "Inherited haemoglobin disorders: An increasing global health problem", *Bull WHO*, *79*:704–712.

Weatherall, D.J. (2005). "Keynote address: the challenge of thalassemia for the developing countries". *Ann N Y Acad Sci*, 1054:11-17.

WHO. (1989). Guidelines for the control of hemoglobin disorders: Report of the VIth Annual Meeting of the WHO Working Group on Hemoglobinopathies, Cagliari, Sardinia, 8–9 April, Geneva, World Health Organization.

WHO. (2008). Joint WHO-TIF meeting on management of haemoglobin disorders (2nd: 2008: Nicosia, Cyprus) Geneva, World Health Organization. (NLM classification: WH 190).

Yagnik, H. (1997). "Post counseling follow up of thalassemia in high risk communities", *Indian Pediatr*, *34*:1115–8.

Zolotogora, J., Carmi, R., Lev, B. *et al.* (2009). A targeted population carrier screening programme for severe and frequent genetic diseases in Israel, *Eur J Hum Genet*, *17*:591-597.

15

Current Status of Beta Thalassemia in India

Challenges and Road Map Ahead

Roumi Deb and *Ratika Samtani*

Introduction

Thalassemia are hemoglobinopathies which are a result of inherited genetic conditions that originate from a lack or malfunction of the adult haemoglobin protein. Hereditary haemoglobin disorders, particularly Beta Thalassemia and Sickle cell disease are the most common single gene disorders globally and are also one of the important causes of genetic mortality and morbidity. They represent one of the most common monogenic disorders in India rendering a heavy economic burden on the families and nation. In their severe forms, they are associated with chronic, life impairing and life threatening diseases that can lead to disability or death. Considering Beta Thalassemia, unfortunately many children in and across the globe continue to be born and suffer from it mainly due to lack of awareness and lack of comprehensive programmes and strategies to prevent them.

The term thalassemia comes from the Greek word "Thalassa," which according to the Greek mythology represents the "spirit of the sea". Even though Thalassemias are prevalent across diverse geographies, the name thalassemia was coined so as a very high frequency of thalassemia was first observed in the Mediterranean Basin with many families passing the mutations through generations. Thalassemia's basically involves changes or alterations in the globin chains (alpha or beta chains) that make up the haemoglobin molecule. The disease is classified as either alpha or beta thalassemia depending on whether the alpha or beta haemoglobin gene harbours a mutation. Four genes (two from each parent) are needed to make enough alpha or beta globin protein chains of the haemoglobin molecule.

The severity of thalassemia is determined by how many of these genes are affected—higher the number, more severe the symptoms.

Beta Thalassemia, caused by mutations in the Human Beta-Globin gene, is more diverse as compared to Alpha Thalassemia (which is caused by the reduction of alpha globin chains) and is characterised by a quantitative reduction of Beta globin chains. Different types of Beta-thalassemia include Beta-Thalassemia minor/Beta-thalassemia carrier/Beta-thalassemia trait, Beta-thalassemia intermediate and Beta Thalassemia major. The HBB gene directs the production of a protein known as beta-globin. As mentioned earlier, haemoglobin contains beta-globin as a component (subunit) and is made up of four protein subunits, two of which are beta-globin subunits and two of which are alpha-globin subunits. The generation of Beta-globin chains is decreased or absent when the Beta-globin gene is mutated. Point mutations which account for the vast majority of mutations in the Beta globin gene causing Beta Thalassemia are unique to geographic populations. These genetic mutations cause a range of reduction and severity in the expression of Beta globin gene—from a minor reduction (mild β+ thalassemia alleles) to a total loss (β0 thalassemia). In other words, some mutations in the HBB gene block beta-globin development entirely. Beta-zero (0) thalassemia is characterised by the lack of beta-globin. Other HBB gene mutations enable some beta-globin production but at a lower level.

Of all the types of Beta Thalassemia, Beta thalassemia major is the most severe and Beta thalassemia intermedia is milder than thalassemia major. Beta Thalassemia major occurs when two mutated copies of the Human Beta Globin gene are inherited resulting in absence of beta-globin thereby leading to reduced amount of functional hemoglobin. Red blood cells do not grow normally without enough haemoglobin, resulting in a lack of mature red blood cells. The signs and symptoms of the disease appear in the first two years of life. This condition causes severe anaemia which can make one feel exhausted and frail. Additionally, beta thalassemia major slows development in infants and young children. This condition requires regular blood transfusions for the management of severe anaemia. Furthermore, too much iron may build up in one's body as a result of frequent transfusions, causing damage to liver, heart, and endocrine system of the affected. Due to an accumulation of damaged red blood cells, the spleen and liver can develop to an abnormally large size from childhood to adulthood. Since the disease causes the bone marrow (i.e. the spongy part of the bones) to expand, the bones can also become brittle and thin.

The symptoms of beta thalassemia intermedia are milder than those of beta thalassemia major, due to which frequent blood transfusions may not be required if at all they are needed. Thalassemia intermedia symptoms may occur in early childhood or later in life. People who are affected have mild to severe anaemia as well as sluggish growth and bone defects. Patients with TI who do not receive care have a higher rate of morbidity and a lower health-related quality of life. Patients with TI can develop severe symptoms that affect almost every organ system. Some of the complications seen in TI patients include pulmonary hypertension, osteoporosis, 25-hydroxy vitamin D deficiency, gallstones, and thromboembolic disease.

Individuals who have Beta Thalassemia minor (also referred to as Beta Thalassemia trait) are phenotypically normal, with very fewer symptoms and mild anaemia. They carry one copy of the mutated gene which is recessive in nature and therefore, not expressed in the heterozygous state. They have both normal hemoglobin A and the abnormal beta thalassemia (β) hemoglobin in their red blood cells. In other words, people with beta thalassemia trait do not have beta thalassemia disease and also cannot develop the diseases later in life. However, they can pass beta thalassemia trait to their children.

Thalassemia major and intermedia are autosomal recessive diseases, meaning both copies of the HBB (Human Beta globin) in each cell are mutated. The parents of a person with Beta Thalassemia have one copy of the mutated gene but they usually do not display any signs or symptoms of the disease.

Epidemiology of β-thalassemia

World Scenario

According to the WHO report published in 2008, more than 40,000 infants each year are born with β-thalassemia, of whom about 25,500 are transfusion-dependent β-thalassemia (Modell *et al*, 2008). Worldwide, Beta Thalassemia has been observed to be in the highest frequency in the Mediterranean region, the Middle East, and Southeast Asia and lowest in Northern Europe and North America (Colah *et al.*, 2010). It is estimated that 1.5 per cent of the individuals are β-thalassemia carriers (Colah *et al.*, 2010). The prevalence of carrier rates of β-thalassemia is relatively high in Southeast Asia, with the reported prevalence ranges from 1.25 per cent to 1.66 per cent in India (Mondal, 2016) and is 2.21 per cent in China (Huan,

2016). It is very high in the middle east region of the world; one of the reasons for this is increase in the cultural preference for consanguineous mating (De Sanctis, 2017). In the recent past, Northern, Western, and Southern Europe has witnessed a heavy increase in the frequency of hemoglobinopathies. Many people have also migrated from regions where β-thalassemia is endemic, such as Syria, Afghanistan, and Myanmar to countries such as Italy, Turkey, U.S. etc. where the incidence and prevalence of β-thalassemia has increased significantly in the recent years.

There exist multiple factors for the changing epidemiology of Beta Thalassemia in the world today. Furthermore, with the rise in knowledge and general awareness, comprehensive prevention programmes which include public education, genetic counselling and population screening accompanied by prenatal diagnostics have been extremely fruitful. Public awareness and education is the backbone for all the prevention programmes. Massive Screening programmes have been effectively developed in multiple countries and have been tailored to local needs and customs (Colah *et al.*, 2010). In many European countries where β-thalassemia has been historically endemic, for example Greece, Italy, and Cyprus, screening programmes have been well established and that they receive an enormous number of immigrants from endemic countries, such as the United Kingdom and France. Italy's prevention programme has been a major success due to an increase in awareness among the general population which has lead to acceptance of screening in the population. Since 1970s, in Italy, there has been policies and planning for prevention of Haemoglobinopathies in place. Cyprus is one success story, where a thalassemia preventive initiative began in the year 1973 and has resulted in a substantial reduction in the incidence of Beta Thalassemia. Similarly, the Greek National Prevention Programme for Thalassemia and Other Hemoglobinopathies, which began in the year 1974 and involved education and prenatal diagnosis, has resulted in a substantial reduction in the number of affected new-borns, from 150 to 200 cases per year prior to the screening programme to less than 5 cases per year by 2010 (Voskaridou *et al*, 2010). The national programme for the prevention and control of thalassemia major and thalassemia/Hb E in Thailand, which was developed in the year 1994 has proven to be very beneficial because it provides complete reimbursement for carrier screening in pregnant women and their partners. Since the Thai government requires women who have a molecularly confirmed compromised foetus with extreme thalassemia syndromes, including thalassemia major and thalassemia/Hb E to terminate their pregnancy before 24 weeks of pregnancy, this policy has largely resulted in a substantial decline in Beta Thalassemia major (Wanapirak, 2004).

However, there is a great deal of variation in how these preventive programmes are accepted and used around the world. Acceptance rates in European countries, such as the United Kingdom, were over 90 per cent in couples of Mediterranean descent, but just 20 per cent in couples of Asian (mostly Pakistani) origin (Modell *et al.*, 2001). Consanguineous relationships, religious values, and low socio-economic status are all barriers to the effectiveness of these screening systems. Consanguineous marriages, which are widespread in many areas where thalassemia is prevalent, such as North Africa and the Middle East, have played a role in raising the risk of autosomal recessive diseases, such as Beta Thalassemia. A prospective study in Turkey observed that 48 per cent of beta thalassemia major or intermedia babies were born to consanguineous parents (Aydınok *et al.*, 2018). Similarly, a study from Egypt consisting of 44 patients with β-thalassemia reported that 60.6 per cent had consanguineous parents (Hussein *et al.*, 2007). It is important to define the disease's prevalence in each country in order to better coordinate health-care services.

Indian Scenario

With a population of 1.21 billion people, India is home to 4,693 communities, including 427 tribal groups, according to the 2011 Census. While all states have Beta-thalassemia and other haemoglobinopathies, the incidence varies greatly from region to region. Thalassemia and structural haemoglobin variants are extremely common in India, but only a small percentage of patients are properly treated, and prolonged care is out of reach for most families. In our multi-ethnic, culturally and linguistically diverse population of 1.21 billion people, the estimated prevalence of Beta thalassemia carriers is 3-4 per cent, which corresponds to 35 to 45 million carriers (Madan *et al.*, 2010). Every year, 10,000-12,000 children are born with thalassemia major in India (Aggarwal *et al.*, 2014). It is the commonest single gene disorder in India accounting for highest incidence of offspring mortality. The average prevalence of Beta-thalassemia trait was 2.78 per cent, ranging from 1.48 to 3.64 per cent in different nations, while Beta-thalassemia trait prevalence in 59 ethnic groups ranged from 0 to 9.3 per cent (Mohanty *et al.*, 2013). Very limited information is available on the prevalence of β-thalassemias and other haemoglobinopathies among various ethnic communities/groups across India. Previous research has shown that some populations in Western and Northern India, such as the

Sindhis, Kutchhi Bhanushalis, and Punjabis, have a high prevalence of Beta-thalassemia (Sukumaran, 1975; Mehta *et al.*, 1972; Balgir, 2005). The prevalence of the Beta-thalassemia trait was 16.81 per cent among Sindhis in Nagpur, Maharashtra, according to a survey (Mulchandani *et al.*, 2008). The highest prevalence of the Beta-thalassemia phenotype was observed in Jains from Bangalore (9.6%) followed by Buddhists from Mumbai (5.9%) and Sikhs from Ludhiana (3.7%) (Mohanty *et al.*, 2013). According to Patel *et al.*, the Bhanushalis (8.1%), Bhaktas (7.9%) and Lohanas (6.5%) have a high prevalence of Beta-thalassemia trait (Patel *et al.*, 2012). Thalassemia has also been found to be prevalent in tribal communities. Rao and Gorakshakar (1990) found a prevalence of Beta-thalassemia trait of 1.6 to 5.6 per cent among tribal groups in Maharashtra, while the prevalence of Beta-thalassemia trait was also high (6.3 to 8.5%) among tribal groups in Orissa (Balgir, 2005, 2006) and non-tribal populations in Madhya Pradesh in Central India (Chatterjee *et al.*, 2010). According to Colah *et al.*, 2017; overall, the communities with a high frequency of Beta Thalassemias are: "*Sindhis, Lohanas, Bhanushalis, Vellalas (8–17%); Vasava, Chaudhry, Gamit, Kokana tribes from Surat, south Gujarat (12–15%); Aroras, Khatris, Jaths, (6–10%); Prajapatis, Banias, Jains, Patels, Mayavanshis (6–8%); Bhuyan, Pik, Dudh Kharia tribes from Sundargarh, Odisha and Rohit tribe from Surat, south Gujarat (6–8%); Kayastha, Mandols (5–9%); Menons, Shiyas, Fakirs (5–7%); Neo Buddhists, Mahars (4-6%)*".

Various government and non-government organisations have worked hard in the past three to four decades to achieve the goal of Thalassemia free society, but community regulation in such a large and diverse country is extremely difficult. Beta-Thalassemia condition is life threatening causing immense suffering to the patient as well as the family. In the Indian context, the treatment of a thalassemia major child necessitates daily blood transfusions and iron chelation therapy, both of which are costly and time-consuming, putting a significant and growing demand on the family as well as already limited health services available. India has numerous population groups which are stratified based on socio-cultural mileu. Anthropological research will help to explain and analyse the socio-cultural barriers that exist in genetic diseases such as thalassemia. As a result, the need of the hour is to place a greater emphasis on preventing the birth of such children in the future. Therefore, preventing thalassemia is the only practical way to achieve rapid reduction in the frequency of the disorder. Countries like Cyprus, Greece and Sardinia could achieve a 90 per cent reduction in thalassemia by creating prevention strategies rather than looking into treatment alternatives.

Various projects, such as the Indian Council of Medical Research's Multicentre Jai Vigyan programme, the West Bengal State Thalassemia Control Programme, the Gujarat State Thalassemia Control Programme, and Punjab's "Project Rainbow have all aided in developing screening programmes and determining the prevalence of Beta-thalassemia and other hemoglobinopathies. These programmes have had a significant impact and thalassemia control programmes have now been developed in many states, with screening being conducted in various target groups. However, these programmes must be implemented at regular intervals, and a strict follow-up should be made a practice. Promoting community education and understanding, intensifying screening in all states with micro-mapping to determine the true burden and developing appropriate facilities for genetic counselling and prenatal diagnosis in public sector institutions are all worthwhile options for thalassemia control.

Molecular Characterization of Beta Thalassemia in Indian Population

Molecular Characterization of Beta thalassemia of either the patients with Beta thalassemia major and their families or individuals from different geographic regions is very much needed in order to devise better management and diagnostic strategies. The beta-globin chain of Haemoglobin molecule is encoded by the HBB gene, which spans 1.6 kb on the short-arm of chromosome 11 (Bunn *et al*, 1986). The genomic sequence of HBB contains three exons, two intervening sequences (IVS1 and IVS2) and the 5' and 3' untranslated regions (UTRs). The beta-globin locus harbours, in addition to the HBB gene, the -globin (HBE) gene, the two -globin (HBG) genes (HBG-G and HBG-A), and the -globin (HBD) gene. Most genes at this locus are expressed at specific time points in development (Bunn *et al.*, 1986).

As defined by various population studies, there exist more than 200 HBB gene mutations with a sub-set of ~40 mutations responsible for the majority of beta-thalassemia cases globally (Flint *et al.*, 1998). The various classes of mutations which cause beta-thalassemia include missense/nonsense, splicing, regulatory, deletions, insertions. Out of over 200 causal β-globin gene mutations, 11 have been shown to be common in India, which are mainly community specific and this can be instrumental in identification, diagnosis and curtailing the propagation of the disease. Among these 11, six account for about 94 per cent of all positive cases in India (Kazazian *et al.*, 1984) which includes— "*619 bp deletion at 3' end of beta-globin gene, IVS-1 nt 5 (G-C), IVS-1 nt 1 (G-T), frame shift mutations FS 8/9 (+G), codon 41/42 (-CTTT) and nonsense codon 15*". The spectrum of mutations varies and are different in different population groups of India.

Molecular characterization of Beta Thalassemia in patients with Beta thalassemia major and their families as well as individuals from various geographic regions was previously studied in Indian populations by various scholars (Verawalla *et al.,* 1991, 1992; Garewal *et al.*, 1994; Verma *et al.*, 1997; Madan *et al.*,1998; Vaz *et al.*, 2000; Chakrabarti *et al.*, 2005; Nadkarni *et al.*, 2009; Tamhankar *et al.*, 2009; Munshi *et al.*, 2009). Such research has been extremely beneficial in terms of gaining a better understanding of the disease's prevalence and subsequent management. According to these authors, of the 6 most prevalent mutations of Beta thalassemia in India, IVS 1-5 G-C is the most common Indian mutation in most states of India whereas among the migrants from Pakistan, 619 bp del is found to be most frequent. There exists vast regional differences or disparities in the prevalence of the mutation across north, east and south India, which has also been demonstrated by various scholars. Mutations which are less frequent and observed in the Indian populace, which are: "*codon 15 (G-A), codon 16 (-C), codon 30 (G-C), IVS-1-110 (G-A), -88 (C-T), CAP+1 (A-C), codon 5 (-CT), FS 41/42 (-CTTT), codon 88 (+T), 25 bp deletion, IVS-2nt1 (G-A) and IVS-1 minus 1 (G-A)*".

The frequency of different mutations varies significantly in different regions of India. The IVS-1-5 mutation, which is the most common in India and ranges from 22.8 to 81.4 per cent in different parts of the country, with Tamil Nadu in south-eastern India having the highest rate. The 619 bp deletion mutation has been identified as the most common beta-thalassemia mutation in patients from the north-western part of India (including the states of Punjab, Haryana, Uttar Pradesh, and Rajasthan, adjoining Delhi), Sindh, and Gujarat. Study by Shah in 2017 revealed IVS 1-5 G-C mutation exhibited higher incidence followed by 619 bp deletion in Rajasthan, Gujarat, and Maharashtra (Western India) populations as compared to West Bengal and Assam populations of Eastern India (Shah *et al.*, 2017).

There exists an ethnic and genetic variation in prevalence of DNA mutations in beta-thalassemia among individuals from different parts of India. Documenting community specific mutations for beta thalassemia in various communities of India can be extremely beneficial in diagnosis, prevention and management of the disorder. Thus, it becomes a matter of grave concern to screen more populations groups for the disease as there are about 25-30 million people carrying the beta-thalassemia trait in India and about 8000 children homozygous for this trait are born every year. Molecular characterization among high risk communities and screening for more communities for Beta Thalassemia in India can ensure a cost effective diagnosis programme for that population. For example, 619 bp del which is prevalent among the Sindhi community can be used as a diagnostic marker for carrier detection of Beta thalassemia among Sindhi community (India) followed by codon 41/42 (-TCTT) and codon 8/9 especially in northern India. The most commonly used methods for molecular diagnosis are reverse dot blot analysis or primer-specific amplification, ARMS PCR, real-time PCR or microarray technology. Sequencing of the HBB coding region can also detect and analyse mutations in the HBB coding region and associated flanking regions.

Challenges and Way Forward: Road Map for India

The enormous burden of Beta Thalassemia in India emphasizes on creating strategies for reducing the burden of the disease among the vast and varied population. Over the past decades, management of the disease has been possible to an extent with regular blood transfusions and iron chelation therapy, however the complications associated with the disease are always on a rise. Emerging developments in micro array technology, newer methods in mutation detection are leading to genetic identification and control of the disorder specifically at the population level, but these methods are still at its early stage and largely unreachable by the majority of the Indian population. Research into gene therapy is still ongoing and may emerge as one of the treatment options available for Beta Thalassemia. The prospect of curing Beta Thalassemia holds a great potential for the future for alleviating human suffering in India.

In spite of the steps taken by the Government, control of Thalassemia has been difficult in India due to lack of awareness of the disease among people and adequate planning and management for prevention of disease and due to social and cultural taboos. As India is a vast country with about 4635 ethnic communities, it becomes extremely necessary to know the spectrum of mutations of Beta Thalassemia gene in different regions among different ethnic groups for prenatal diagnosis and Genetic counselling. Thus, the first step in the prevention of Beta Thalassemia is the identification of the carrier. To reach the goal of "Thalassemia free society", a control programme is needed involving Community Specific

Screening, Awareness and Counselling Programme for Beta-Thalassemia Prevention and a detailed comprehensive strategy must be adopted to know the exact magnitude of genetic health load.

The road map for reducing the burden of Beta Thalassemia needs a systematic effort which includes education and awareness generation among the diverse communities of India as well as both urban and rural populations; micro mapping of various ethnic groups across diverse geographies as well as creating state-wise registries will give an indication of the true burden of the disease since most studies available today are reports from hospital records; extensive screening centres need to be established that will be instrumental in screening and providing genetic counselling services. Since majority of Indian population lives in rural areas, a robust concentrated effort is required specially aimed at populations residing in these areas for awareness generation and sensitization. Other steps include educating health professionals, schools and colleges students, pregnant mothers and the general public as well as developing prenatal diagnosis centres in various parts of the country along with developing cost-effective treatment facilities across the country. A concerted effort with the involvement of universities, hospitals and institutions along with the medical fraternity, non-government organizations working in the area of thalassemia reduction can aid in successfully reducing thalassemias.

In conclusion, need of the hour is that the emphasis must shift from treatment to the prevention of birth of such children in future. Therefore, preventing thalassemia is the only practical way to achieve rapid reduction in the frequency of the disorder. Countries like Cyprus, Greece and Sardinia could achieve a 90 per cent reduction in Thalassemia by creating prevention strategies rather than looking into treatment alternatives. There is a pressing need to raise public knowledge about Beta Thalassemia, which necessitates awareness generation and mobilisation programmes, as well as proper health education and sensitization of individuals, families, and communities to embrace these preventive remedial steps. Carrier screening and antenatal screening with inductive programme can be very fruitful strategy in containing the disease. High cost of Bone Marrow transplant, regular blood transfusions and iron chelation therapies, all point out to a single fact that prevention of this disorder is better than cure in every aspect.

REFERENCES

Aggarwal, R., Prakash, A., Aggarwal, M. (2014). "Thalassemia: An overview", *J Sci Soc*, *41*,3-6. doi: 10.4103/0974-5009.126696

Aydınok, Y., Oymak, Y., Atabay, B. *et al.* (2018). "A national registry of thalassemia in Turkey: Demographic and disease characteristics of patients, achievements, and challenges in prevention", *Turk J Haematol*, *35*,12 18. doi: 10.4274/tjh.2017.0039

Balgir, R.S. (2006). "Genetic heterogeneity of population structure in 15 major scheduled tribes in central & eastern India: a study of immuno-hematological disorders", *Indian J Hum Genet*, 12, 86–92.

Balgir, R.S. (2005). "Spectrum of hemoglobinopathies in the state of Orissa, India: a ten years cohort study", *JAPI*, *53*,1021-1026.

Bunn, H.F., Forget, B.G. (1986). *Hemoglobin: Molecular, genetic and clinical aspects,* W.B. Saunders Company, Philadelphia, PA.

Chakrabarti, P., Gupta, R., Mishra, A., Rai, M., Singh, V.P., Dash, D. (2005). "Spectrum of Beta thalassemia mutations in North Indian States: A Beta thalassemia Trait with two mutations in cis", *Clin Biochem*, *38*, 576-578.

Chatterjee, N., Mishra, A., Soni, R., Kulkarni, H., Mantani, M., Shrivastava, M. (2010). "Bayesian estimates of the prevalence of β-thalassemia trait in voluntary blood donors of central India: A survey", *Hemoglobin*, *34*, 548-560.

Colah, R., Gorakshakar, A., Italia, K.(2017). "Burden of thalassemia in India: The road map for control". *Pediatric Hematology Oncology Journal*, *2*(4), 79-84.

Colah, R., Gorakshakar, A., Nadkarni, A. (2010). "Global burden, distribution and prevention of β thalassemias and hemoglobin E disorders". *Expert Rev Hematol*, *3*, 103-117.

De Sanctis, V., Kattamis, C., Canatan, D. *et al.* (2017). "β thalassemia distribution in the Old World: an ancient disease seen from a historical standpoint". *Mediterr J Hematol Infect Dis*, *9*(1), e2017018. doi: 10.4084/MJHID.2017.018

Flint, J., Harding, R.M., Boyce, A.J., Clegg, J.B. (1998). "The population genetics of the haemoglobinopathies". *Bailliere's Clin Haematol*, *11*(1), 1-51.

Garewal, G., Fearon, C.W., Warren, T.C., Marwaha, N., Marwaha, RK., Mahadik, C., Kazazian, H.H. (1994). "The molecular basis of Beta Thalassemia in Punjabi and Maharashtrian Indians includes a multilocus aetiology involving triplicated α-globin loci", *Br J Haematol*, 86, 372-376.

Huang, S., Xu, Y., Liu, X., Zhou, M., Wu, X., Jia, Y. (2016). "Molecular newborn screening of four genetic diseases in Guizhou Province of South China", *Gene*, *591*,119-122. doi: 10.1016/j.gene.2016.07.019

Hussein, G., Fawzy, M., Serafi, T.E. *et al.* (2007). "Rapid detection of beta Thalassemia alleles in Egypt using naturally or amplified created restriction sites and direct sequencing: A step-in disease control. Hemoglobin", *31*, 49-62. doi: 10.1080/03630260601057088

Kazazian, H.H. Jr., Orkin, S.M., Antonarakis, S.E., Sexton, J.P., Boehm, C.D., Goff, S.C., Waber, P.G. (1984). "Molecular characterization of seven b-thalassemia mutations in Asian Indians", *EMBO J, 3*, 593-596.

Madan, N., Sharma, S., Rusia, U., Sen, S., Sood, S.K. (1998). "Beta- Thalassemia mutations in northern India (Delhi)", *Ind J Med Res, 107*, 134-141.

Madan, N., Sharma, S., Sood, S.K., Colah, R., Bhatia, H.M. (2010). "Frequency of β-thalassemia trait and other hemoglobinopathies in northern and western India", *Indian J Hum Genet, 16*(1), 16-25.

Mehta, B.C., Dave, V.B., Joshi, S.R., Baxi, A.J, Bhatia, H.M., Patel, J.C. (1972). "Study of hematological & genetical characteristics of Cutchi Bhanushali community", *Indian J Med Res, 60*, 305–311.

Modell, B., Darlison, M. (2008). "Global epidemiology of haemoglobin disorders and derived service indicators", *Bull World Health Organ, 86*, 480-487. doi: 10.2471/blt.06.036673

Modell, B., Khan, M., Darlison, M., King, A. *et al.* (2001). "A national register for surveillance of inherited disorders: β-thalassaemia in the United Kingdom", *Bull World Health Organ, 79*(11), 1006-1013.

Mohanty, D., Colah, R.B., Gorakshakar, A.C. *et al.* (2013). "Prevalence of β-thalassemia and other haemoglobinopathies in six cities in India: A multicentre study", *J Community Genet, 4*(1), 33-42. doi:10.1007/s12687-012-0114-0

Mondal, S.K. and Mandal, S. (2016). Prevalence of thalassemia and hemoglobinopathy in eastern India: A 10-year high performance liquid chromatography study of 119,336 cases. *Asian J TransfusSci, 10*, 105-110.

Mulchandani, D.V., Fulare, M.B., Zodpey, S.P., Vasudeo, N.D. (2008). "Prevalence and some epidemiological factors of beta thalassemia trait in Sindhi community of Nagpur city, India", *Indian J Public Health, 52*,11–15

Munshi, A., Anandraj, M.P.J.S., Joseph, J., Shafi, G., Anila, A.N., Jyothy, A. (2009). "Inherited hemoglobin disorders in Andhra Pradesh, India: A population study", *Clinica Chemica Acta, 400*:117-119.

Nadkarni, A., Gorakshakar, A., Surve, R., Sawant, P., Phanasgaonkar, S., Nair, S., Ghosh, K., Colah, R.B. (2009). "Hematological and molecular analysis of novel and rare beta-thalassemia mutations in the Indian population", *Hemoglobin, 33*(1), 59-65.

Patel, A., Naik, P., Shah, M., Sharma, N., Narmadeshwar, P., Parmar, P. (2012). "Prevalence of common hemoglobinopathies in Gujarat: an analysis of a large population screening programme", *Nat J Commun Med, 3*, 112-116.

Rao, V.R., Gorakshakar, A.C. (1990). "Sickle cell hemoglobin, β-thalassemia and G6PD deficiency in tribes of Maharashtra, India", *Gene Geogr, 4*, 131-134.

Shah, P.S., Shah, N.D., Ray, H.S.P., Khatri, N.B., Vaghasia, K.K., Raval, R.J., Shah, S.C., Rao, M.V. (2017). "Mutation analysis of β-thalassemia in East-Western Indian population: A recent molecular approach", *ApplClin Genet, 10*, 27-35.

Sukumaran, P.K. (1975). "Abnormal hemoglobins in India", In: Sen N.N., Basu A.K. (eds.) *Trends in hematology*. Saraswati Press, Calcutta, pp. 225-236.

Tamhankar, P.M., Agarwal, S., Arya, V., Kumar, R., Gupta, U.R., Agarwal, S.S. (2009). "Prevention of homozygous beta thalassemia by premarital screening and prenatal diagnosis in India", *Prenal Diagn*, 29, 83-88.

Vaz, F.E.E., Thakur, C.B., Banerjee, M.K., Gangal, S.G. (2000). "Distribution of β-Thalassemia Mutations in the Indian Population Referred to a Diagnostic Centre", *Hemoglobin*, *24*(3): 181-194.

Verawalla, N.Y., Old, J.M., Sarkar, R., Venkatesan, R., Weatherall, D.J. (1991). "The spectrum of Beta-Thalassemia mutations on the Indian Subcontinent: the basis for prenatal diagnosis", *Br J Haematol*, *78*, 242-247.

Verma, I.C., Saxena, R., Thomas, E., Jain, P.K. (1997). "Regional distribution of β-thalassemia mutations in India", *Hum Genet*, *100*, 109-113.

Voskaridou, E., Ladis, V., Kattamis, A. *et al.* (2012). "A national registry of haemoglobinopathies in Greece: deducted demographics, trends in mortality and affected births", *Ann Hematol*, *91*,1451-1458. doi: 10.1007/s00277-012-1465-7.

Wanapirak, C., Muninthorn, W., Sanguansermsri, T., Dhananjayanonda, P., Tongsong, T. (2004). "Prevalence of thalassemia in pregnant women at Maharaj Nakorn Chiang Mai Hospital", *J Med Assoc Thai*, *87*, 1415-1418.

16

A Review of Musculoskeletal Disorders and Psychosocial Stress Among Farmers

Current Gaps and Roadmap for Future Research

Shivani Chandel and *Chonsing Shimrah*

Introduction

Musculoskeletal disorders (MSDs) are one of the leading contributors of disability and chronic illness worldwide (WHO, 2019; Storheim and Zwart, 2014). "Musculoskeletal disorders comprise a wide scale of degenerative and inflammatory conditions that cause distress to joints, muscles, ligaments, tendons, supporting blood vessels and peripheral nerves", (Punnett and Wegman, 2004). These conditions result in pain and discomfort of various body parts such as the neck, shoulders, elbows, forearms, wrists, and hands (Buckle and Jason Devereux, 2002). The pain and discomfort in joints, bones, muscles, and connective tissues may develop into chronic illnesses such as osteoarthritis, osteoporosis, sarcopenia, and lupus erythematosus, respectively at later stages (WHO, 2019). According to the National Institute for Occupational Safety and Health (NIOSH), MSDs are the second most severe occupational disorder after respiratory disease (Putz *et al.,* 1997). Globally, the prevalence of MSDs ranges from 14 per cent to 42 per cent (Sharma, 2012). In developing countries like India, the prevalence of MSDs among adult population ranges from 6.92 per cent - 76.8 per cent (Kishore, 2019).

MSDs are results of pathological effects (Bongers *et al.*, 1993) and various lifestyle factors such as inadequate physical activity, obesity, smoking, and malnutrition (WHO, 2019). Incidents like fractures, injuries, and aging processes can lead to the development of MSDs (Briggs *et al.*, 2016). Work-related musculoskeletal disorders (WMSDs) occur due to adverse working environments such as high task repetition, forceful exertion, repetitive or sustained awkward postures (David, 2005). Many studies have reported that individuals in certain industries and occupations such as industrial work, construction workers in manufacturing factories, migrant workers (Soe *et al.*, 2015), and farmers (Dessein and Nevens, 2007; Furey *et al.*, 2016) have three to four times higher risk for developing MSDs as compared to the general population (Punnett and Wegman, 2004). Farming, being strenuous and complex in nature, falls under the category of risk occupations (Lee *et al.*, 2002). Farmers are particularly at high risk because they are involved in performing hard labour throughout the year, including digging the ground, carrying seeds, uprooting plants, planting and sowing, harvesting, sheafing, carrying harvested crops, threshing, sweeping, and winnowing (Das, Ghosh and Gangopadhyay, 2013). In some rural areas, despite advancements in farming tools and technologies farming is practice usir g traditional tools and techniques. This traditional farming method demands physically exhausting tasks such as repetition of awkward working positions, static posture, long working hours, and rigorous work routine (Walker-Bone and Palmer, 2002; Davis and Kotowski, 2007; Osborne *et al.*, 2010).

MSDs have become a major burden on individuals, health systems, and social care systems (Woolf and Pfleger, 2003). MSDs are a perfect example of chronic diseases with low mortality, but high morbidity rates (Bevan, 2015). Further, MSDs also lead to mental distress due to low productivity at the workplace and home, absenteeism, early retirement from work, and reduced ability to participate in social activities (Alexopoulos *et al.*, 2004; Bevan, 2015). This mental distress over time can develop into complicated mental health issues such as anxiety and depression. MSDs have a high impact on both individual and country economies as the treatments of MSDs are expensive. Individuals lose their accumulated wealth and at a global level, every country spends millions on MSDs healthcare services (Morse *et al.*, 1998). For example, in countries like The Netherland, Canada, and USA the total direct cost for musculoskeletal disorders health services was 0.7 per cent, 1.0 per cent, and 1.2 per cent of the gross national product, respectively (Lawrence *et al.*, 1998; Woolf and Pfleger, 2003; Ekpenyong and Inyang, 2014). In Asian countries like Korea, the economic cost of musculoskeletal disorder was $6.89 billion, which represents 0.7 per cent of the country's gross domestic product (Oh *et al.*, 2011). All these countries are non-dominant agricultural societies and less dependent on farm production in comparison to agrarian countries like India where almost 75 per cent of the population live in rural areas and practicing agricultural activity

(Fazal, 2001). Moreover, the agriculture sector in India contributes about 27 per cent of the nation's gross domestic product (GDP). Therefore, it is expected that the likely financial cost of MSDs treatment will be more in countries that still have a high farmer population. Generally, people go for treatment only when the conditions become severe and MSDs at its later stage can be treated only by undergoing major surgeries using invasive technology (Katz, Earp and Gomoll, 2010) such as therapeutic ultrasound, joint, total knee replacement (W-Dahl, Robertsson, and Lidgren, 2010), hip replacement (Learmonth, Young, and Rorabeck, 2007), Oxygen-ozone (O_3), injecting unprocessed bone marrow aspirate (BMA) to treat bone defects. However, to date, only a few countries have the report on the MSDs prevalence rate of the total population and the allocated budget for MSDs treatment. Individuals with MSDs are prone to developing additional illnesses due to the side effects of drugs and medicine intake for relieving pain and discomfort to go back to work. Long-term use of narcotic painkillers and NSAIDs (Non-Steroidal Anti-Inflammatory Drugs) can cause gastrointestinal problem, renal failure, liver failure, and heart failure (Voaklander *et al.*, 2006).

A considerable amount of studies on farmers have reported that environmental stressors have a significant impact on the development and exacerbation of MSDs. However, some researchers have stated that MSDs are the result of not only physical risk factors alone (Dionne *et al.*, 2001) rather psychosocial aspects are important to be considered to understand the epidemiology of MSDs. Although psychosocial factors may not directly cause MSDs, rather they may influence muscle tension or other physiological processes and decrease muscle activity (Vignoli *et al.*, 2015). It is high time to shift focus and give emphasis on other variables that are associated with MSDs. For farmers, mental disorders have been identified as one of the key risk factors for suicide attempts (Liu and Zhang, 2018). In rural areas, psychosocial stress is not considered a serious health concern; people generally go for treatment only when the conditions become severe. This is why there are high suicide rates among farmers, farm managers, and agricultural labourers (McPhedran and de Leo, 2013). Both psychosocial stress and MSDs are reported to be highly prevalent among farmers. However, there is less research on their co-existence and association of these two common conditions among farmers.

Most of the existing studies on the association between MSDs and psychosocial stress are confined to white-collar occupational groups (Lachowski *et al.*, 2017), (Ng, Voo, and Maakip, 2019). It is important to understand the association between these two common health issues, i.e. MSDs and psychosocial stress in the context of farmers. Farmers support millions of livelihoods by supplying essential goods and products throughout the year. Any endangerment in their physical and mental health will not only deteriorate farmers' lives but may increase poverty as farming is still a major occupation in many countries (Morton, 2007). Thus, it is important to focus on both the farmer's physical and mental health. The present review tries to understand the association of psychosocial stress and musculoskeletal disorders among farmers.

Methods

Literature Search Strategies

This review was conducted using the principles of PRISMA (Preferred Reporting Items for Systematic Reviews and Meta-Analyses). The literature search to be included in the current review was carried out across the following search engine: Scopus, Pub med, and Google scholar. Following Keywords and Medical Subject headings "musculoskeletal disorders"or "chronic pain" and "psychosocial stress" or "mental health" and ("farmers" or "farmer") were used to extract papers. The papers identified through various search engines were managed by Microsoft excel and Mendeley software. Further, title and abstract reviews were performed to find studies that seemed appropriate for the study. The final decision for inclusion was made only after reading the full paper.

Inclusion criteria: Any relevant cross-sectional, longitudinal, and observational study was included for the review. Papers with full text available and written only in the English language were included. For this review, only those papers which were original research articles published in the last five years were included. Studies on the association between MSDs and psychosocial stress were only included.

Exclusion criteria: Any review paper, poster presentation abstract, conference lecture, full-text unavailable paper were excluded from this study. Articles that were written other than the English language were also excluded. Studies that report only the prevalence of MSDs and psychosocial stress independently were excluded, studies focusing solely on intervention and validation of tools and techniques were also excluded. Association studies of MSDs and stress in occupations other than farmers were excluded from this review.

Results

Identification and Selection of the Included Studies

At the initial stage of the literature search using multiple keywords, the search engine produced 129 results. After filtering duplicate records, 123 papers were left and from these 123 papers after reading the title and abstract, those papers which were on occupations other than farming were excluded. Types of studies such as review, lecture, commentary, book chapter were also excluded. Paper written in any language other than English was excluded. After excluding all the papers based on exclusion criteria 59 records were selected for further screening. 59 full-text articles were screened out of which 34 papers were excluded because they did not meet the inclusion criteria (intervention studies and studies solely focused on the validation of methods and techniques for assessing MSDs) and only 25 papers were left. Out of this 25, 11 papers were excluded as they reported prevalence of MSDs or psychosocial stress among farmers independently. Finally, only 14 papers that meet the inclusion criteria were selected to be included in the current review.

In the selected papers, prevalence and risks factors for musculoskeletal disorders, chronic pain, and injuries were assessed by using various techniques and questionnaires, namely the Standardized Nordic questionnaire, Ovako Working Posture Analysis System (OWAS), Rapid Entire Body Assessment (REBA) technique, Multi-method ergonomic review technique (MMERT), Quick Exposure Check (QEC), Rapid Upper Limb Assessment (RULA) and Structural Equation Modelling (SEM). Psychosocial factors were assessed by using questionnaires which mainly consisted of questions about job satisfaction, working hours, speed of work, nature of the work, and overall quality of life. They were assessed using various scales such as Symptoms Checklist anxiety, and depression subscales (SCL-25), Center for Epidemiologic Studies Depression Scale Short Form (CES-D 10), Depression Scale Short Form (CES-D 10), the 22-item Thai version of the job content questionnaire, SF-36 questionnaire, 9-Questions depression rating scale, self-reported questionnaire (SRQ-20), Migrant Farmworker Stress Inventory, The Suanprung stress test. Socio-demographic variables such as age, sex, socio-economic status were collected using a modified questionnaire.

MSDs Leading to Psychosocial Stress

A cross-sectional study among farmers in Victoria, Australia reported that those who had an injury experience post-traumatic thoughts which make them anxious in the recovery period. They also grief over the loss of their pre-injury life on the farm (Murray *et al.*, 2019; Murray *et al.*, 2019). A study in Northeast Thailand reported that the farmers who suffer from MSDs were reported to have a low quality of life, and those farmers with poor quality of life are in turn experience severe levels of stress and were more prone to depression (Prommawai, Laohasiriwong, and Nilvarangkul, 2019). A cross-sectional study among Iranian farmers reported that MSDs, mental disorders, and injuries (e.g., cuts and fractures) were the main determinants of the farmers' quality of life (Rostamabadi *et al.*, 2019a).

Psychosocial Stress Leading to MSDs

Cross-sectional studies among farmers in Iran and Rajasthan, India reported that Older individuals and less educated farmers were reported to be more prone to MSDs (Momeni *et al.*, 2020; Mishra and Satapathy, 2019). A study among farmers from Thailand showed that their surrounding environmental threat and loss of crops due to pests were their major concern making them feel depressed and in turn more prone to the development of MSDs (Saksorngmuang *et al.*, 2020). They also reported that farmers with depressive symptoms (OR 3.40) were more likely to report shoulder disorders compared to those farmers who did not have these factors (Saksorngmuang *et al.*, 2020). A longitudinal study among Latino manual labourers reported that depression was associated with significantly higher odds of reporting neck-shoulder pain (OR3.30 CI 1.3500,8.07) or wrist/hand pain (OR 2.69, 95% CI 1.00-7.10) (Trible *et al.*, 2016). In India, the financial burden was the major force of farmers' exposure to the risk of MSDs, such as working at high speed and less break during working hours as farmers were paid per unit of land they harvest/cut (Jain *et al.*, 2018).

From these various reports, it can be inferred that there is a bidirectional association between MSDs and psychosocial stress among farmers. In some studies, it has been reported that MSDs lead to psychosocial stress whereas in others *vice versa*. However, in contrast to these bidirectional association findings, a cross-sectional study among Thai rubber farmers reported that there was no association between psychosocial stress and lower back pain (Udom, Janwantanakul and Kanlayanaphotporn, 2016).

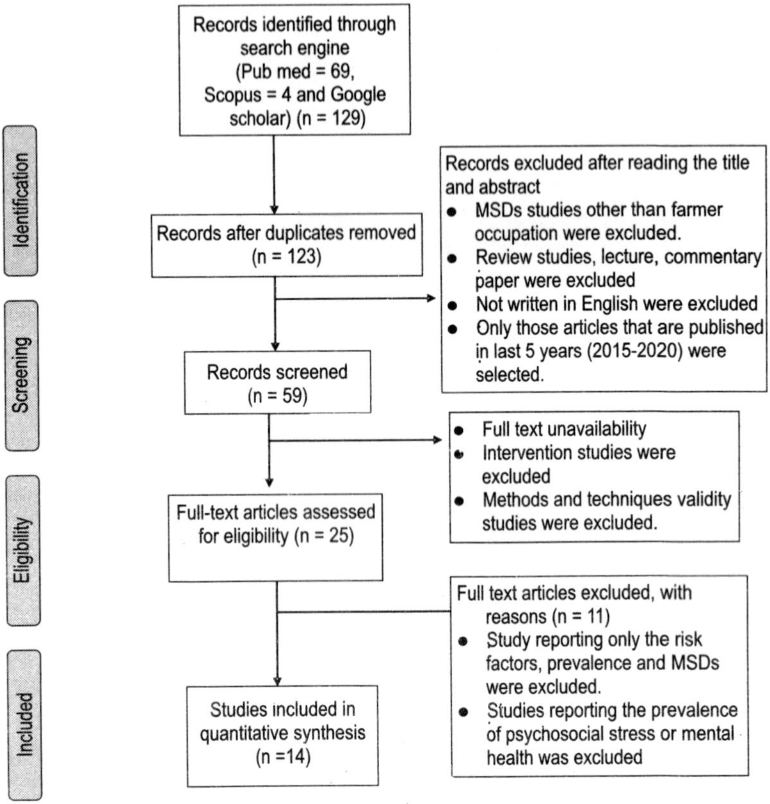

Fig. 16.1: Stages of review investigating the role of psychosocial stress on musculoskeletal disorders

Discussion

This review aimed to understand the association between MSDs and psychosocial stress among farmers. The present review shows a lack of literature and population-based study on the association between psychosocial and MSDs among farmers. MSDs have been reported to have multiple risk factors and over time these factors interact with each other to create an elevated risk for one another. This review showed that the presence of either MSDs or psychosocial stress becomes a risk factor for one another. Both work-related stress and non-work-related stress gave rise to the development of MSDs. On the other hand, the outcome of MSDs such as loss of productivity, enduring body pain, increased dependency on others and family members and financial burden lead to psychosocial stress among farmers. Literature shows that the co-occurrence of psychosocial stress and pain is more frequent than exceptions (Asmundson and Katz, 2009). The presence of chronic pain has been reported as a strong indicator of severe depression and *vice versa* (Maletic and Raison, 2009). Previous studies have reported that the prevalence of anxiety disorder and major depressive disorder increased up to 54 per cent and 32 per cent, respectively when patients experience pain in more than one area (Manchikanti *et al.*, 2001). There are various theories and models which discuss the association of MSDs and psychosocial stress.

Multiple models have explained that psychosocial factors influence directly or indirectly and lead to musculoskeletal pain. Some of the model and theories includes *Hyperventilation theory* (Schleifer, Ley, and Spalding, 2002), *Dysfunction of the Hypothalamic-Pituitary-Adrenal (HPA) Axis* (McBeth *et al.*, 2007; McFarlane, 2007), *Somatizing* (Lipowski 1998). All these theories explain the likelihood of MSDs development in the human body due to increasing stress levels when one encounters psychosocial stress. When an individual is exposed to the adverse situation they respond by bringing physiological changes such as increased production of cortisol hormone in the body's muscles and cells, which cause muscle tension, loss of bone net, increased sensitivity to pain (somatizing) (Lipowski, 1998) and susceptibility to muscle injuries (Melin and Lundberg, 1997). In contrast to this explanation given by various theories, population, and clinical-based studies have reported the other way round by reporting MSDs to give rise to psychosocial stress (Rostamabadi *et al.*, 2019b). High rates of chronic pain and disability are reported to have contributed to pain-related fear and anxiety leading to interaction-avoidance due to chronic pain which results in jeopardizing day-to-day activity and deteriorate the overall quality of life (Tüzün, 2007; Poleshuck and Green, 2008).

All the farmers are not exposed to similar types of factors. There are varied kinds of factors responsible for the development of both MSDs and psychosocial stress. These factors vary depending on the age, sexes, socio-demographic variables, regional variation among farmers. Farmers in lower and middle-income countries with slower diffusion of technology still operate using conventional tools (e.g. knife, sickle, traditional plough, harrow, spade etc.) and still practice farming by doing manual labour.

Table 16.1: Studies that examine the association of psychosocial stress and MSDs among farmers

Sl. No.	Author and Year	Study design and Sample size	Measurement tools		Major findings
			MSDs assessment tools	Stress Scale/Tools	
1.	(Saksorngmuang *et al.*, 2020)	A cross-sectional study of 370 rubber farmers of Thailand	Nordic Musculoskeletal Disorders, Rapid Upper Limb Assessment (RULA)	The 22-item Thai version of the job content questionnaire, Epidemiologic Studies Depression Scale (CES-D)	Depression symptom (OR 3.40) were also more likely to report shoulder disorder compared with the rubber farmers who did not have these factors.
2.	(Rostamabadi *et al.*, 2019)	A cross-sectional study was conducted among 736 Iranian male farmers	A modified questionnaire was used to collect the prevalence of chronic pain and injuries	The SF-36 questionnaire was used to obtain information on the quality of life	Many chronic diseases and injuries showed an inverse correlation with the quality of life, but the strongest association was found between MSDs and mental disorders.
3.	(Momeni *et al.*, 2020)	A cross-sectional study among 1501 Iran agricultural workers	Nordic Musculoskeletal Disorders Quick Exposure Check (QEC) technique	Modified questionnaire	Work-related stress such as Working Posture, Hand Tools, and Manual Material Handling (MMH) Work Organization (WO) were risk factors for MSDs. More number of older individuals and less educated farmers were found to be more prone to MSDs.
4.	(Jain, Meena, & Dangayach, 2018)	A cross-sectional study among 138 Rajasthan agriculture workers	Multi-method ergonomic review technique (MMERT) Nordic musculoskeletal disorders	Modified demographic questionnaire	74.6% farmers were having MSDs. Non-Work-related factors (age, gender, smoke, education, income, and tool satisfaction) were found to contribute to the development of MSDs among this group of workers.
5.	(Mishra & Satapathy, 2019)	A cross-sectional Study among 25 Farmers of five villages of South Odisha in India	The standardized Nordic questionnaire, Ovako Working Posture Analysis System (OWAS), and the "Rapid Entire Body Assessment (REBA)" technique.	Socio-demographic questionnaire	Socio-demographic variables along with adverse work environment were affecting different body parts like neck, shoulder, upper back, lower back, elbow, wrist/hand, thigh, knees, and ankles.
6.	(Jain, Meena, Dangayach, *et al.*, 2018)	A cross-sectional study among selected villages of Eastern Rajasthan 140 farmers (114 Males, 26 Females)	The multi-method ergonomic review technique (MMERT) rapid upper limb assessment (RULA) method	Demographic questionnaire	Farmers with MSDs were having low salary satisfaction as compare to those without MSDs.

(contd.)

contd.

7.	(Lachowski *et al.*, 2017)	A cross-sectional study of 396 employees of the State Forests from 8 regions of Poland	Modified Nordic Questionnaire for assessment of musculoskeletal disorders	Questionnaire about job satisfaction	There was a significant relationship between lower levels of job satisfaction and the occurrence of MSDs.
8.	(Chatterjee & Kumar Acharya, 2020)	A cross-sectional study of 90 farm women of the village Boinchigram, West Bengal	Interview on their Diet, nature of their work	Equation to measure the Psycho-social hazard	Disorganized and improper work due to routine-heavy workload, infrequent rest breaks, longer working hours, hectic and routine work are the most important causes of work-related stress.
9.	(Logstein, 2016)	A cross-sectional study of 926 farmer participants	Structural Equation Modelling (SEM)	Symptoms Checklist Anxiety and Depression Subscales (SCL-25)	Higher work demands in agriculture led to more mental health problems.
10.	(Murray *et al.*, 2019)	A cross-sectional study among 31 farmers in the state of Victoria, Australia	Semi-structured telephone interviews, which focused on their experiences since the injury	Demographic data, extracted from (Victorian State Trauma Registry) VSTR database for all eligible participants	Farmers experience lack of independence, post-trauma after injuries, and grief about their lost of pre-injury life on farm.
11.	(Prommawai *et al.*, 2019)	A cross-sectional analytical study among 529 samples selected through multistage random sampling from 3 provinces of the Northeast (NE) of Thailand	Standardized Nordics questionnaire	Depression was assessed using a 9-Questions depression rating scale. The 9 items covered frequency of depressive symptoms [bored, sleeping, tired, and suicide etc.,) during the past 2 weeks	Farmers with MSDs have low quality of life, and those farmers with poor quality were more prone to depression (Adjusted OR=2.09; 95% CI: 1.41-3.10; p-value<0.001), they were also reported to have high and severe levels of stress (Adjusted OR=2.11; 95% CI: 1.43-3.13; p-value<0.001).
12.	(Tribble *et al.*, 2016)	A longitudinal studies among Latino manual labourer in North Carolina	Self-reported musculoskeletal pain was measured using 11 specific pain locations on the body.	CES-D 10 for depression and shortened scale derived from the Migrant Farm worker Stress Inventory Stress was used to measure depression and stress, respectively	Depression was associated with significantly higher odds of reporting neck-shoulder pain (OR3.30 CI 1.3500,8.07) or wrist/hand pain (OR 2.69, 95% CI 1.00,7.10)
13.	(Udom *et al.*, 2016)	A cross-sectional survey was conducted among 450 Thai rubber farmers using cluster random sampling	Modified Nordic questionnaire	The Suanprung stress test contains 20 items rated on a 5-point Likert scale with item responses ranging from "1" (no stress) to "5" (extremely high stress)	Only individual and occupational factors, but no psychosocial factors, were found to be associated with Lower back pain.
14.	(Meucci *et al.*, 2015)	A cross-sectional study conducted in southern Brazil. A random sample of tobacco farmers was interviewed	Standardized Nordic questionnaire for Musculoskeletal symptoms	Minor psychiatric disorders were measured according to the self-reported questionnaire (SRQ-20)	This study reported that those farmers with minor psychiatric disorders had nearly four times more Chronic lower back pain than those without minor psychiatric disorders.

Hence, they are more vulnerable to physical stressors (Kumaraveloo and Lunner Kolstrup, 2018; Mishra and Satapathy, 2019). In some region, farmers are often exposed to external stressors that are beyond their control such as unpredictable weather, pesticide exposure, climate variability/ drought (Dessein and Nevens, 2007; Yazd *et al.*, 2019) job strain, job dissatisfaction (Chatterjee and Kumar Acharya, 2020), poor task control (Jain *et al.*, no date). Same farmers are exposed to personal factors such as a lack of financial and social support (Lachowski *et al.*, 2017; Duffield *et al.*, 2017). Despite the majority of farmers being exposed to a variety of physical and psychological stressors, these problems are often ignored and take preventive measures only when it reaches its peak of severity. This is why there is a high rate of suicide among farmers in countries like India, Sri Lanka, Canada, England, and Australia as compared to their general population (Fraser *et al.*, 2005). Previous studies have reported farming as an occupation with the highest risk for committing suicide predominantly due to adverse socio-economic and psychosocial circumstances (Merriott, 2016). Especially in agrarian countries like India, where more than 75 per cent of individuals are agriculturalists, there is a high rate of farmer's suicide as much as 12,602 suicide cases in 2015 (NCRB in Accidental deaths and suicides in India, Ministry of Home Affairs, New Delhi, 2015). Psychosocial stress arises mainly due to perceived debt, addiction, environmental problems, poor prices for farm produce, family responsibilities, government lack of concern, poor irrigation, increased cost of cultivation, private money lenders, expensive chemical fertilizers, and crop failure due to climate change and pest were reported to be the major reasons for farmers' stress (Dongre and Deshmukh, 2012). On the other hand, in developed countries, time pressure, financial problems, loneliness due to geographical and social isolation are frequently cited as major psychosocial risk factors affecting the health of farmers (Gregoire, 2002). Apart from the physical and mental health risk, MSDs also lead to additional health problems, especially among farmers. Farmers need to be free from physical discomfort and pain to work efficiently. As a result, it is very common for farmers to take available instant relief medicine and drugs which will give rise to additional illness due to side effects of the pain killers and drugs. For example, the commonly used drug Opioids to relieve chronic pain are known to have side effects which include delayed gastric emptying, hyperalgesia, immunologic and hormonal dysfunction, muscle inflexibility, and myoclonus (Benyamin *et al.*, 2008).

It is not possible to introduce and implement uniform intervention for all farmers. It is important to address that there are variations of both physical stressors and psychosocial stressors due to the heterogeneity of cultural, environmental, and socio-economic background of farmers around the world. Therefore, future researchers should try to bring forward the cultural-regional specific intervention to tackle the problem of farmers.

Conclusion

Farmers not only ensure the food and nutritional security of the nation but also contribute a large scale to the country's economy. Hence, any danger to the well-being of farmers is a cause of national concern. It is evident that farmers are prone to both MSDs and psychosocial stress and together it may lead to severe co-morbidities. The most effective method to prevent the development of chronic MSDs and psychosocial stress is the management of the risk factors at their early stages. There is a need to develop and promote farmer's specific psycho-ergonomic interventions especially in rural areas as people generally tend to neglect psychosocial stress symptoms and it remains undetected until it reaches the severe stage. Moreover, it is important to create awareness among farmers regarding the side effects of drugs and medication that they consume for temporary relief. Further, there should be an allocation of a budget specifically for MSDs healthcare services at the national level. The treatment and intervention should be cost-effective to reach those farmers who are at the bottom of the socio-economic hierarchy of the countries. Also, there is a need to develop standardized and validated intervention tools at the community level specifically developed for farmers.

REFERENCES

Alexopoulos, E.C., Stathi, I.C., and Charizani, F. (2004). *Prevalence of musculoskeletal disorders in dentists. BMC Musculoskeletal Disorders*. https://doi.org/10.1186/1471-2474-5-16

Asmundson, G.J.G., and Katz, J. (2009). "Understanding the co-occurrence of anxiety disorders and chronic pain: State-of-the-art", In *Depression and Anxiety*. https://doi.org/10.1002/da.20600

Benyamin, R., Trescot, A.M., Datta, S., Buenaventura, R., Adlaka, R., Sehgal, N., Glaser, S.E., and Vallejo, R. (2008). "Opioid complications and side effects", In *Pain Physician*.

Bevan, S. (2015). "Economic impact of musculoskeletal disorders (MSDs) on work in Europe", In *Best Practice and Research: Clinical Rheumatology* (Vol. 29, Issue 3, pp. 356–373). Bailliere Tindall Ltd. https://doi.org/10.1016/j.berh.2015.08.002

Bongers, P.M., De Winter, C.R., Kompier, M.A.J., and Hildebrandt, V.H. (1993). "Psychosocial factors at work and musculoskeletal disease", In *Scandinavian Journal of Work, Environment and Health*. https://doi.org/10.5271/sjweh.1470

Briggs, A.M., Cross, M.J., Hoy, D.G., Sànchez-Riera, L., Blyth, F.M., Woolf, A.D., and March, L. (2016). Musculoskeletal Health Conditions Represent a Global Threat to Healthy Aging: A Report for the 2015 World Health Organization World Report on Ageing and Health. In *Gerontologist*. https://doi.org/10.1093/geront/gnw002

Buckle, P.W., and Jason Devereux, J. (2002). "The nature of work-related neck and upper limb musculoskeletal disorders", In *Applied Ergonomics*. https://doi.org/10.1016/S0003-6870(02)00014-5

Chatterjee, R. and Kumar Acharya, S. (2020). "Perception of Biophysical Stresses Confronted by the Farm Women: The Socio-economic and Ecological Interpretation", *Original Research Article Chatterjee and Acharya, AJAEES* (4), 51–63. https://doi.org/10.9734/AJAEES/2020/v38i430337

Das, B., Ghosh, T. and Gangopadhyay, S. (2013). "Prevalence of musculoskeletal disorders and occupational health problems among groundnut farmers of West Bengal, India", *Journal of Human Ergology*, *42*(1–2), 1–12. https://doi.org/10.11183/jhe.42.1

David, G.C. (2005). "Ergonomic methods for assessing exposure to risk factors for work-related musculoskeletal disorders". *Occupational Medicine*, *55*(3), 190–199. https://doi.org/10.1093/occmed/kqi082

Davis, K.G., and Kotowski, S.E. (2007). "Understanding the ergonomic risk for musculoskeletal disorders in the United States Agricultural Sector", In *American Journal of Industrial Medicine*. https://doi.org/10.1002/ajim.20479

Dessein, J., and Nevens, F. (2007). "I'm sad to be glad". An analysis of farmers' pride in Flanders. *Sociologia Ruralis*. https://doi.org/10.1111/j.1467-9523.2007.00437.x

Dionne, C.E., Von Korff, M., Koepsell, T.D., Deyo, R.A., Barlow, W.E., and Checkoway, H. (2001). "Formal education and back pain: A review", In *Journal of Epidemiology and Community Health*. https://doi.org/10.1136/jech.55.7.455

Dongre, A.R., and Deshmukh, P.R. (2012). "Farmers' suicides in the Vidarbha region of Maharashtra, India: A qualitative exploration of their causes", *Journal of Injury and Violence Research*. https://doi.org/10.5249/jivr.v4i1.68

Duffield, S.J., Ellis, B.M., Goodson, N., Walker-Bone, K., Conaghan, P.G., Margham, T., and Loftis, T. (2017). "The contribution of musculoskeletal disorders in multimorbidity: Implications for practice and policy", In *Best Practice and Research: Clinical Rheumatology*. https://doi.org/10.1016/j.berh.2017.09.004

Ekpenyong, C.E., and Inyang, U.C. (2014). "Associations between worker characteristics, workplace factors, and work-related musculoskeletal disorders: A cross-sectional study of male construction workers in Nigeria",

International Journal of Occupational Safety and Ergonomics. https://doi.org/10.1080/10803548.2014.11077057

Fazal, S. (2001). "The need for preserving farmland. A case study from a predominantly agrarian economy (India)", *Landscape and Urban Planning*. https://doi.org/10.1016/S0169-2046(00)00134-1

Fraser, C.E., Smith, K.B., Judd, F., Humphreys, J.S., Fragar, L.J., and Henderson, A. (2005). "Farming and mental health problems and mental illness", *International Journal of Social Psychiatry*. https://doi.org/10.1177/0020764005060844

Furey, E.M., O'Hora, D., McNamara, J., Kinsella, S., and Noone, C. (2016). *The Roles of Financial Threat, Social Support, Work Stress, and Mental Distress in Dairy Farmers' Expectations of Injury. Frontiers in Public Health*. https://doi.org/10.3389/fpubh.2016.00126

Gregoire, A. (2002). "The mental health of farmers", In *Occupational Medicine*. https://doi.org/10.1093/occmed/52.8.471

Jain, R., Lal Meena, M., Sharan Dangayach, G., and Kumar Bhardwaj, A. (n.d.). "Risk factors for musculoskeletal disorders in manual harvesting farmers of Rajasthan", In jstage.jst.go.jp. Retrieved July 17, 2020, from https://www.jstage.jst.go.jp/article/indhealth/56/3/56_2016-0084/_article/-char/ja/

Jain, R., Meena, M.L., Dangayach, G.S., and Bhardwaj, A.K. (2018). "Risk factors for musculoskeletal disorders in manual harvesting farmers of Rajasthan", *Industrial Health*. https://doi.org/10.2486/indhealth.2016-0084

Katz, J.N., Earp, B.E., and Gomoll, A.H. (2010). "Surgical management of osteoarthritis", In *Arthritis Care and Research*. https://doi.org/10.1002/acr.20231

Kishore, J. (2019). "Prevalence of Musculoskeletal Disorders Amongst Adult Population of India", *Epidemiology International, 04*(03), 22–26. https://doi.org/10.24321/2455.7048.201915

Kumaraveloo, K.S., and Lunner Kolstrup, C. (2018). "Agriculture and musculoskeletal disorders in low- and middle-income countries", *Journal of Agromedicine*. https://doi.org/10.1080/1059924X.2018.1458671

Lachowski, S., Choina, P., Florek-Łuszczki, M., Goździewska, M., and Jezior, J. (2017). "Dissatisfaction with work as a risk factor of musculoskeletal complaints among foresters in Poland", *Annals of Agricultural and Environmental Medicine*. https://doi.org/10.26444/aaem/80985

Lawrence, R.C., Helmick, C.G., Arnett, F.C., Deyo, R.A., Felson, D.T., Giannini, E.H., Heyse, S.P., Hirsch, R., Hochberg, M.C., Hunder, G.G., Liang, M.H., Pillemer, S.R., Steen, V.D., and Wolfe, F. (1998). Estimates of the prevalence of arthritis and selected musculoskeletal disorders in the United States. *Arthritis and Rheumatism*. https://doi.org/10.1002/1529-0131(199805)41:5<778::AID-ART4>3.0.CO;2-V

Learmonth, I.D., Young, C., and Rorabeck, C. (2007). "The operation of the century: Total hip replacement", In *Lancet*. https://doi.org/10.1016/S0140-6736(07)60457-7

Lee, E., Burnett, C.A., Lalich, N., Cameron, L.L., and Sestito, J.P. (2002).

"Proportionate mortality of crop and livestock farmers in the United States, 1984-1993", *American Journal of Industrial Medicine*. https://doi.org/10.1002/ajim.10131

Liu, Y., and Zhang, J. (2018). "The Impact of Negative Life Events on Attempted Suicide in Rural China", *The Journal of Nervous and Mental Disease*. https://doi.org/10.1097/NMD.0000000000000727

Maletic, V., and Raison, C.L. (2009). "Neurobiology of depression, fibromyalgia and neuropathic pain", *Frontiers in Bioscience*. https://doi.org/10.2741/3598

Manchikanti, L., Singh, V., Pampati, V., Damron, K.S., Barnhill, R.C., Beyer, C., and Cash, K.A. (2001). "Evaluation of the relative contributions of various structures in chronic low back pain", *Pain Physician*.

McBeth, J., Silman, A.J., Gupta, A., Chiu, Y.H., Ray, D., Morriss, R., Dickens, C., King, Y., and Macfarlane, G.J. (2007). "Moderation of psychosocial risk factors through dysfunction of the hypothalamic-pituitary-adrenal stress axis in the onset of chronic widespread musculoskeletal pain: Findings of a population-based prospective cohort study", *Arthritis and Rheumatism*. https://doi.org/10.1002/art.22336

McFarlane, A.C. (2007). "Stress-related musculoskeletal pain", In *Best Practice and Research: Clinical Rheumatology*. https://doi.org/10.1016/j.berh.2007.03.008

McPhedran, S., and de Leo, D. (2013). "Risk factors for suicide among rural men: Are farmers more socially isolated?" *International Journal of Sociology and Social Policy*. https://doi.org/10.1108/IJSSP-03-2013-0038

Melin, B., and Lundberg, U. (1997). "A biopsychosocial approach to work-stress and musculoskeletal disorders", *Journal of Psychophysiology*.

Merriott, D. (2016). "Factors associated with the farmer suicide crisis in India", In *Journal of Epidemiology and Global Health*. https://doi.org/10.1016/j.jegh.2016.03.003

Mishra, D. and Satapathy, S. (2019). "Ergonomic risk assessment of farmers in Odisha (India)", *International Journal of Systems Assurance Engineering and Management*, *10*(5), 1121–1132. https://doi.org/10.1007/s13198-019-00842-5

Momeni, Z., Choobineh, A., Razeghi, M., Ghaem, H., Azadian, F., and Daneshmandi, H. (2020). "Work-related Musculoskeletal Symptoms among Agricultural Workers: A Cross-sectional Study in Iran". *Journal of Agromedicine*, 1–10. https://doi.org/10.1080/1059924X.2020.1713273

Morse, T.F., Dillon, C., Warren, N., Levenstein, C., and Warren, A. (1998). "The economic and social consequences of work-related musculoskeletal disorders: The Connecticut Upper-extremity Surveillance Project (CUSP)". *International Journal of Occupational and Environmental Health*. https://doi.org/10.1179/oeh.1998.4.4.209

Morton, J.F. (2007). "The impact of climate change on smallholder and subsistence agriculture", In *Proceedings of the National Academy of Sciences of the United States of America*. https://doi.org/10.1073/pnas.0701855104

Murray, M., Beattie, J., McLeod, C., Pedler, D., Brumby, S.A., and Gabbe,

B. (2019). "It could have been a lot worse: The psychological effects of farm-related serious injury in Victoria". *Rural and Remote Health*. https://doi.org/10.22605/RRH5323

Ng, Y.M., Voo, P., and Maakip, I. (2019). "Psychosocial factors, depression, and musculoskeletal disorders among teachers". *BMC Public Health*. https://doi.org/10.1186/s12889-019-6553-3

Oh, I.H., Yoon, S.J., Seo, H.Y., Kim, E.J., and Kim, Y.A. (2011). "The economic burden of musculoskeletal disease in Korea: A cross-sectional study", *BMC Musculoskeletal Disorders*. https://doi.org/10.1186/1471-2474-12-157

Osborne, A., Blake, C., McNamara, J., Meredith, D., Phelan, J., and Cunningham, C. (2010). "Musculoskeletal disorders among Irish farmers", *Occupational Medicine*, *60*(8), 598–603. https://doi.org/10.1093/occmed/kqq146

Poleshuck, E.L., and Green, C.R. (2008). "Socioeconomic disadvantage and pain", In *Pain*. https://doi.org/10.1016/j.pain.2008.04.003

Prommawai, N., Laohasiriwong, W., and Nilvarangkul, K. (2019). "Musculoskeletal Disorders and Quality of Life of Sugarcane Farmers in the Northeast of Thailand: A Cross-sectional Analytical Study", *Journal of Clinical and Diagnostic Research*. https://doi.org/10.7860/jcdr/2019/41844.12924

Punnett, L. and Wegman, D.H. (2004). "Work-related musculoskeletal disorders: The epidemiologic evidence and the debate", *Journal of Electromyography and Kinesiology*. https://doi.org/10.1016/j.jelekin.2003.09.015

Rostamabadi, A., Jahangiri, M., Naderi Mansourabadi, B., Javid, M., Ghorbani, M., and Banaee, S. (2019a). "Prevalence of Chronic Diseases and Occupational Injuries and their Influence on the Health-Related Quality of Life Among Farmers Working in Small-Farm Enterprises", *Journal of Agromedicine*. https://doi.org/10.1080/1059924X.2019.1592047

Rostamabadi, A., Jahangiri, M., Naderi Mansourabadi, B., Javid, M., Ghorbani, M., and Banaee, S. (2019b). "Prevalence of Chronic Diseases and Occupational Injuries and their Influence on the Health-Related Quality of Life Among Farmers Working in Small-Farm Enterprises", *Journal of Agromedicine*, *24*(3), 248–256. https://doi.org/10.1080/1059924X.2019.1592047

Saksorngmuang, P., Kaewboonchoo, O., Ross, R., and Boonyamalik, P. (2020). "Working hazards and health problems among rubber farmers in Thailand". *Walailak Journal of Science and Technology*. https://doi.org/10.14456/vol17iss10pp

Schleifer, L.M., Ley, R., and Spalding, T.W. (2002). "A hyperventilation theory of job stress and musculoskeletal disorders". *American Journal of Industrial Medicine*, *41*(5), 420–432. https://doi.org/10.1002/ajim.10061

Sharma, R. (2012). *Epidemiology of Musculoskeletal Conditions in India,* ICMR Task Force Project.

Soe, K.T., Laosee, O., Limsatchapanich, S., and Rattanapan, C. (2015). "Prevalence and risk factors of musculoskeletal disorders among Myanmar migrant workers in Thai seafood industries", *International Journal of Occupational Safety and Ergonomics*. https://doi.org/10.1080/10803548.2015.1096609

Storheim, K. and Zwart, J.A. (2014). "Musculoskeletal disorders and the Global Burden of Disease study", In *Annals of the Rheumatic Diseases*. https://doi.org/10.1136/annrheumdis-2014-205327

Tribble, A.G., Summers, P., Chen, H., Quandt, S.A., and Arcury, T.A. (2016). "Musculoskeletal pain, depression, and stress among Latino manual labourers in North Carolina", *Archives of Environmental and Occupational Health*, *71*(6), 309–316. https://doi.org/10.1080/19338244.2015.1100104

Tüzün, E.H. (2007). "Quality of life in chronic musculoskeletal pain", In *Best Practice and Research: Clinical Rheumatology* (Vol. 21, Issue 3, pp. 567–579). https://doi.org/10.1016/j.berh.2007.03.001

Udom, C., Janwantanakul, P., and Kanlayanaphotporn, R. (2016). "The prevalence of low back pain and its associated factors in Thai rubber farmers", *Journal of Occupational Health*. https://doi.org/10.1539/joh.16-0044-OA

Vignoli, M., Guglielmi, D., Balducci, C., and Bonfiglioli, R. (2015). "Workplace bullying as a risk factor for musculoskeletal disorders: The mediating role of job-related psychological strain", *BioMed Research International*. https://doi.org/10.1155/2015/712642

Voaklander, D.C., Kelly, K.D., Rowe, B.H., Schopflocher, D.P., Svenson, L., Yiannakoulias, N., and Pickett, W. (2006). "Pain, medication, and injury in older farmers", *American Journal of Industrial Medicine*. https://doi.org/10.1002/ajim.20292

W-Dahl, A., Robertsson, O. and Lidgren, L. (2010). "Surgery for knee osteoarthritis in younger patients", *Acta Orthopaedica*. https://doi.org/10.3109/17453670903413186

Walker-Bone, K., and Palmer, K.T. (2002). "Musculoskeletal disorders in farmers and farm workers", *Occupational Medicine*, *52*(8), 441–450. https://doi.org/10.1093/occmed/52.8.441

Woolf, A.D., and Pfleger, B. (2003). Burden of major musculoskeletal conditions. In *Bulletin of the World Health Organization*. https://doi.org/10.1590/S0042-96862003000900007

Yazd, S.D., Wheeler, S.A., and Zuo, A. (2019). "Key risk factors affecting farmers' mental health: A systematic review", In *International Journal of Environmental Research and Public Health* (Vol. 16, Issue 23). MDPI AG. https://doi.org/10.3390/ijerph16234849

17

Effect of Gender, Residence and Ethnicity on Anthropometric Parameters

P. Venkatramana, S.A.A. Latheef and *P. Annaiah*

Introduction

Measurement of human body consisting of bones, muscles and adipose tissues by recording lengths, widths, heights or diameters is termed as anthropometry (NHNESIII, 1988). These measurements are useful to estimate size, composition and proportion of the human body (Latheef *et al.*, 2018). Nutrition and family health survey include the measurement of body mass index and mid upper arm circumference to assess the chronic energy deficiency (BMI<18.5 Kg/m^2), nutritional status and general obesity. Height and weight are components used for estimating general obesity and waist alone and in combination with hip circumference [waist-hip ratio (WHR)] are used for deriving central obesity. Besides waist circumference, WHR, waist-height ratio, conicity index, neck circumference, abdominal volume index, per cent of body fat, intra abdominal adipose tissue and body fat are used as indices of central obesity in which anthropometric parameters are important components (Latheef *et al.,* 2018). Waist circumference and WHR are used as components for detection of metabolic syndrome. The aforementioned description suggests that anthropometric variables serve as important components of indices employed in evaluating the nutritional and disease conditions of the populations.

Anthropometric variables like waist-height ratio, waist circumference, per cent body fat, WHR and body fat index were found to be influenced by ethnicity (Lutoslawska *et al.,* 2014; Frignania *et al.,* 2015; Goh *et al.,* 2014). Effect of gender and residence on few anthropometric variables was reported in the heterogenous populations (Shaik *et al.,* 2020; Mohan *et* *al.*2016; Adediran *et al.,* 2013) and only in a few endogamous populations (Mohan Reddy, 2019; Venkatramana *et al.,* 2002; Reddy, 1998). It is not known the effect of gender, residence and ethnicity on the remaining anthropometric variables are caused by alone or in combination. Caste populations share common gene pool and similar environment. Therefore, in this study the effect of gender, residence and ethnicity were studied on 38 anthropometric variables/indices involving three endogamous populations, namely *Reddy, Golla* and *Madiga* from Andhra Pradesh.

Material and Methods

A total of 900 subjects from Reddy, Golla and Madiga Caste populations belonging to the urban and rural areas were drawn from Chittoor District of Andhra Pradesh. In each caste population, 75 subjects of each sex (total=150) from either urban or rural were recruited for the study. The data for the urban sample were collected from Tirupati city of Chittoor District while the rural samples were drawn from eight villages of Chittoor District, namely Ramapuram, Nadimuru, Diguvaramapuram, Diguvaramapuram Harijanawada, Kammapalli Harijanawada, Gollapalli, Venkataramapuram, and Panakam.

A Brief Description on the Investigated Endogamous Populations

Reddy: The Reddy is one of the forward Castes in Andhra Pradesh. They are also called as 'Kapu' in Rayalaseema. A total of 88 sub-castes are reported in this Caste. The dominant Sub-Castes of Reddis are Panta, Pedakanti, Akuthota, Pokanati, Desuri, Kodithe, Motati, Bhumanchi, Morasu and Palle. For the present study, the data were collected from Akuthota Reddy only. They Speak and write Telugu language. Consanguineous marriages are common among the Reddis. Occupationally they are engaged in agriculture, business, government jobs, animal husbandry and cattle rearing.

Madiga: They are one of the largest Scheduled Caste groups in India. The Madiga are known as 'Mang' in Maharashtra; the 'Chakkaliya' in Tamil Nadu and the 'Matang' in North India. In Ancient times they were engaged in hunting and gathering and presently involved in leather works, and as agricultural labours. About 25 sub-Castes in Madigas are reported and among the predominant Sub-Castes are Dappu Madiga, Mashti Madiga, Jogi Madiga, Penda Madiga, Telugu Madiga, Arava Madiga and Periki Madiga. In the present study data on the Telugu Madiga were included. They speak and write Telugu language. In this Caste also consanguineous marriages are common.

Golla: The Golla is a pastoral and Backward community. This Caste population is distributed throughout India and known by different names. The Gollas of Andhra Pradesh speak and write Telugu language. The Sub-Castes of Gollas include Erra, Ala, Pooja, Gangeddu, Gauda, Karma, Pakanati, Racha, Peddeti and Krishna. Each Sub-Caste is strictly an endogamous unit. The present study has been carried out on Krishna Gollas. The Gollas were traditionally sheep and cattle herders and involved in dairy activities. Now they are engaged in agriculture, government jobs and business.

Variables included in the Study: A total of 20 anthropometric variables (height, weight, sitting height, diameters of biacromial, biiliac wrist, elbow and ankle, circumferences of forearm, upper arm, waist, abdominal, hip and calf, skin folds of biceps, triceps, subscapular, suprailiac, abdominal and calf) in three endogamous populations were measured following Lohman *et al.* (1998) and 18 indices [body mass index (BMI)] (Weight in Kgs/height in m^2), waist-hip ratio (WHR), height index (HI) (sitting height/height), height-weight ratio (HWR), ponderal index (PI) $\left(\text{height}/\sqrt[3]{\text{weight}}\right)$, arm muscle circumference (AMC) (Ca – (π×St), arm muscle area (AMA) $\left(\frac{\text{Ca} - (\text{À} \times st)^2}{4\text{À}}\right)$, fat free weight (FFW) $\frac{\%\,\text{bodyfat}}{100} \times \text{Actual Body Weight}$, bone mineral content (BMC) $(3.9 \times T^2 \times H \times [10^{-4}])$; sum of three trunk skinfolds (TSF3) (abdominal + sub-scapular + suprailiac), sum of six skinfolds (SF6) (abdominal + sub-scapular + suprailiac + calf + triceps + biceps), the trunk extremity ratio (TE) (TSF3/[calf + triceps + biceps]), and the relative fat pattern index (RFPI) (sub-scapular/ [sub-scapular + suprailiac] were calculated according to Hasstedt *et al.* (1989). Body density (Durnin and Rahman, 1967), per cent of body fat (%BF) (Siri, 1956), total body water (TBW) (Allen *et al.,* 1959) and body fat (BF) (Siri, 1961) were estimated as per the recommendations of the authors. Height, sitting height, biacromial and biiliac diameter with anthropometer; knee, elbow and ankle diameters with sliding caliper and wrist diameter with sliding caliper; circumferences of forearm, upper arm, waist, abdominal, hip and calf with tape; skin folds of biceps, triceps, subscapular, suprailiac, abdominal and calf with Lange skin fold caliper, were measured.

Statistical analyses: Continuous variables were presented in mean and standard error of mean. Means of the groups were compared with student *'t'* test and one way analysis of variance. Effect of gender, ethnicity and residence on anthropometric variables/indices and interactions of gender, ethnicity and residence on anthropometric variables/indices were investigated using two-way multivariate analysis of variance.

Results

The descriptive statistics of Anthropometric variables described below in terms of gender, residence and ethnicity.

Gender

Significantly higher averages of height, weight, sitting height, diameters of biacromial, wrist, elbow and ankle and circumference of forearm and arm muscle, TSF3, TSF6, TE ratio, PI, body density, BMC, TBW, WHR and FFW were observed in males against females ($p<0.01$), whereas averages were significantly higher in variables such as age, biceps, triceps, subscapular, suprailiac and abdominal skin folds, circumferences of hip and calf, BMI, RFPI, AMA, %BF in women against men ($p<0.01$) in urban Reddy subjects (Table 17.1).

In rural Reddy, significantly higher averages of skin folds of biceps, triceps, subscapular and calf, TSF3, RFPI, %BF and FFW were found in females against males ($p<0.01$). In men, averages were significantly higher in variables such as weight, height, sitting height, diameters of biacromial, wrist, elbow and ankle, circumferences of waist, forearm, abdominal and calf, WHR, height index, AMC, AMA, height-weight ratio (HWR), PI and BMC ($p<0.01$) than women (Table 17.1).

Golla men in urban areas showed significantly higher averages of weight, height, sitting height, diameters of biacromial, wrist, elbow and ankle, circumferences of waist, upper arm, forearm and abdominal, WHR, AMC, AMA, BMC, HWR, FFW, TBW ($p<0.01$) and body fat (BF) ($p<0.05$) against women ($p<0.01$). In women significantly higher averages of skin folds of biceps, triceps ($p<0.01$), and subscapular ($p<0.05$), hip circumference, TSF6, %BF ($p<0.01$), BMI and TSF3 ($p<0.05$) were found when compared to men (Table 17.1).

In rural Golla men, significantly higher averages of weight, height, sitting height, diameters of biacromial, biilliac, wrist, elbow and ankle ($p<0.01$) and knee ($p<0.05$); circumferences of waist, upper arm, forearm and abdominal, WHR, AMC, AMA, HWR, PI, FFW, BMC and TBW

Table 17.1: Mean and standard error of mean of anthropometric parameters among studied ethnic groups

Variable	*Reddy*				*Golla*				*Madiga*			
	Urban		*Rural*		*Urban*		*Rural*		*Urban*		*Rural*	
	Male (*n* = 75)	*Female* (*n* = 75)	*Male* (*n* = 75)	*Female* (*n* = 75)	*Male* (*n* = 75)	*Female* (*n* = 75)	*Male* (*n* = 75)	*Female* (*n* = 75)	*Male* (*n* = 75)	*Female* (*n* = 75)	*Male* (*n* = 75)	*Female* (*n* = 75)
Age (years)	39.84±1.31	46.30 ±1.70**	37.69 ±1.43	39.46 ±1.28	42.40±1.27	42.33 ±1.27	40.12 ±1.37	38.60 ±1.19	34.56 ±1.45	34.80 ±1 38	38.06 ±1.44	37.26 ±1.18
Weight (kg)	62.30 ±1.17	56.20±1.21**	60.48 ±0.99	50.78 ±0.95**	63.16 ±0.90	54.25 ±0.87**	59.94 ±0.86	51.36 ±0.79**	57.46 ±1.09	48.53 ±1.22**	51.20 ±0.88	47.18 ±0.84**
Height (cm)	166.99±5.83	151.63±6.79**	167.39 ±0.66	152.0.65±0.60**	165.76±0.47	150.31 ±0.58**	165.65±0.61	152.93 ±0.51**	165.32±0.71	151.93 ±0.45**	164.61 ±0.44	152.57 ±0.57**
Sitting Height	86.50 ±0.43	78.63 ±0.37**	85.38±0.36	79.70±0.40**	85.28 ±0.28	76.79 ±0.29**	85.04 ±0.33	78.47 ±0.25**	85.20 ±0.42	77.88 ±0.30**	82.75 ±0.30	78.00 ±0.36**
Biceps SF (mm)	4.36±0.26	8.05 ±0.41**	3.22 ±0.20	5.33 ±0.25**	4.66 ±0.22	6.42 ±0.40**	4.28±0.17	5.49 ±0.22**	4.49 ±0.32	6.38±0.40**	2.36 ±0.13	4.54 ±0.23**
Triceps SF (mm)	13.50±0.48	21.09 ±0.79**	11.14±0.49	15.24±0.49**	13.52 ±0.43	16.09 ±0.64**	12.57 ±0.34	14.89 ±0.35**	13.29 ±0.51	18.38 ±0.75**	8.88 ±0.44	14.26 ±0.51**
Subscapular SF (mm)	16.84 ±0.59	22.40 ±0.77**	15.65±0.67	18.01±0.58**	17.40 ±0.53	19.29 ±0.61*	15.72 ±0.54	17.69 ±0.41*	16.93 ±0.64	18.86± 0.86	11.70 ±0.55	16.97 ±0.48**
Suprailiac SF (mm)	21.12 ±0.77	24.04 ±0.79**	18.58±0.87	18.65±0.62	20.02 ±0.57	21.64 ±0.66	17.97 ±0.63	18.73 ±0.42	21.32 ±0.76	20.45 ±0.79	12.61±0.74	18.73 ±0.47**
Abdominal SF (mm)	22.72 ±0.80	25.81 ±0.79**	20.61 ±0.92	19.94 ±0.71	21.69 ±0.65	23.34 ±0.69	20.22 ±0.73	20.42 ±0.46	22.94 ±0.82	21.16 ±0.85	14.30 ±0.77	20.30 ±0.56**
Calf SF (mm)	14.50 ±0.41	15.53 ±0.51	11.49±0.45	15.92± 0.35**	14.74 ±0.35	15.21 ±0.37	13.46 ±0.32	14.64 ±0.24*	14.25 ±0.46	16.33 ±0.50**	10.18 ±0.45	13.61 ±0.34**
Biacromial Dia (cm).	37.60 ±0.24	33.14±0.18**	35.91±0.28	33.26±0.22**	37.68 ±0.20	34.00 ±0.20**	37.33 ±0.13	33.56 ±0.20**	37.47 ±0.21	32.75 ±0.17**	36.05 ±0.19	33.17 ±0.28**
Biiliac Dia (cm).	31.66 ±0.22	31.63 ±0.24	30.00±0.20	30.07 ±0.24	31.94 ±0.20	31.41 ±0.24	31.64 ±0.14	30.39 ±0.17**	30.32 ±0.21	30.32 ±0.24	29.82 ±0.18	29.57 ±0.16
Wrist Dia (cm).	5.23 ±0.31	4.79 ±0.03**	5.36 ±0.03	4.85 ±0.02**	5.28±0.03	4.85 ±0.03**	5.33±0.27	4.87±0.02**	5.22 ±0.03	4.77 ±0.02**	5.31±0.03	4.79 ±0.02**
Elbow Dia (cm).	6.30±0.04	5.89 ±0.04**	6.57± 0.06	5.76 ±0.03**	6.15±0.05	5.54±0.05**	6.43±0.04	5.58 ±0.03**	6.37±0.04	5.89±0.04	6.30±0.03	5.66 ±0.03**
Knee Dia (cm).	9.80±0.07	9.83±0.06	9.75 ±0.07	9.57±0.07	9.91 ±0.05	9.60 ±0.06	9.64 ±0.05	9.46±0.05*	9.47 ±0.08	8.93 ±0.11**	9.23 ±0.07	9.00 ±0.06*
Ankle Dia (cm).	6.48±0.03	6.02±0.04**	6.72 ±0.05	5.98±0.03**	6.57 ±0.04	5.84 ±0.04**	6.70 ±0.04	6.03 ±0.02**	6.51 ±0.04	5.97±0.03**	6.41 ±0.03	6.00 ±0.03**
Waist Cir (cm).	80.13±0.94	78.08 ±0.93	80.38±0.99	76.73±0.79**	81.21 ±0.79	76.07 ±1.68**	79.64 ±0.94	75.93 ±0.75**	77.56 ±1.06	72.64 ±1.08**	73.18 ±0.75	72.21±0.89
Hip Cir (cm).	92.06 ±0.92	97.34 ±0.99**	90.75±0.84	92.45±0.92	93.19 ±0.66	96.54 ±0.92**	90.49 ±0.78	92.80 ±0.74**	89.09 ±0.77	90.43 ±1.09	84.07 ±0.69	88.60 ±0.85**
Upperarm Cir (cm).	26.83 ±0.26	27.19 ±0.30	27.24±0.31	26.44±0.33	27.94 ±0.28	26.41 ±0.33**	28.58 ±0.22	25.83 ±0.25**	26.53 ±0.26	25.50 ±0.37*	25.43 ±0.21	24.72 ±0.25*
Forearm Cir (cm)	25.70±0.16	24.13 ±0.25**	26.70±0.24	24.59± 0.23**	26.40 ±0.19	23.70 ±0.21**	27.12 ±0.19	24.39 ±0.16**	25.77 ±0.21	23.61 ±0.28**	25.18 ±0.16	23.31 ±0.15**
Chest Cir (cm).	87.41 ±0.74	87.36 ±0.99	87.71±0.73	85.79± 0.80	87.61 ±0.56	87.24 ±0.76	86.25 ±0.72	84.25 ±0.77	86.70 ±0.83	82.86 ±0.96**	81.78 ±0.61	80.89 ±0.82
Abdominal Cir (cm).	84.31 ±1.13	81.98 ±1.11	84.99 ±1.10	80.22±1.13**	86.72 ±1.08	82.40 ±0.99**	83.76±1.15	79.69 ±0.97**	81.84 ±1.30	77.32 ±1.28*	75.72 ±0.96	76.08 ±1.11
Calf Cir (cm).	33.42±0.32	34.45 ±0.30*	33.65±0.29	32.22 ±0.31**	32.85 ±0.28	32.76 ±0.27	31.70 ±0.22	33.08 ±0.20**	32.72 ±0.28	31.40 ±0.37**	30.41 ±0.22	30.95 ±0.30
BMI (Kg/m^2)	22.32 ±0.36	24.41 ±0.48**	21.58 ±0.33	21.72 ±0.33	22.96 ±0.28	24.03 ±0.39*	21.82 ±0.28	21.93 ±0.29	21.03 ±0.38	20.99 ±0.49	18.85 ±0.28	20.26 ±0.34**
WHR	0.87±0.005	0.80±0.006**	0.88 ±0.00	0.83±0.00**	0.87 ±0.00	0.80 ±0.00**	0.87 ±0.01	0.81 ±0.00**	0.86 ±0.00	0.80±0.05**	0.87 ±0.00	0.81 ±0.00**
Height Index	0.51±0.001	0.51± 0.001	0.51 ±0.00	0.52 ±0.00**	0.51 ±0.00	0.51±0.00	0.51 ±0.00	0.51 ±0.00	0.51±0.00	0.51±0.00	0.50 ±0.00	0.51 ±0.00**
TSF3	60.68±2.05	72.25 ±2.27**	54.85±2.34	56.61 ±1.85	59.12 ±1.66	64.28 ±1.91*	53.92 ±1.86	56.85 ±1.23	61.20 ±2.02	60.48 ±2.41	38.62 ±2.01	56.01 ±1.42**
TSF6	93.06 ±2.94	116.93 ±3.60**	80.72±3.25	93.10±2.70**	92.05 ±2.37	102.01 ±3.04**	84.24 ±2.54	91.80 ±1.81*	93.24 ±2.96	101.59 ±3.76	60.00 ±2.80	88.44 ±2.22**

(Contd.)

Contd.

TE Ratio	1.88±0.03	1.65 ±0.03**	2.16±0.06	1.55±0.028	1.80 ±0.03	1.73 ±0.03	1.76 ±0.03	1.63 ±0.02	1.94 ±0.04	1.48 ±0.03**	1.80±0.04	1.76 ±0.03
RFPI	0.44±0.006	0.48 ±0.005**	0.46±0.00	0.49±0.00**	0.46±0.00	0.47±0.00	0.46±0.00	0.48±0.00**	0.44±0.00	0.47 ±0.00**	0.49 ±0.00	0.47±0.00*
AMC	22.58 ±0.19	20.56 ±0.26**	23.74±0.24	21.65±0.26**	23.69 ±0.23	21.35 ±0.28**	24.63 ±0.20	21.15 ±0.22**	22.35 ±0.22	19.72 ±0.26**	22.64 ±0.17	20.24 ±0.22**
AMA	0.56±0.09	1.69±0.24**	1.04±0.07	0.13 ±0.11**	0.67 ±0.07	0.17±0.67**	0.96±0.066	0.24 ±0.08**	0.56 ±0.11	0.95 ±0.21**	1.29 ±0.05	0.21±0.13**
H W Ratio	0.37±0.006	0.37±0.007	0.36±0.00	0.33 ±0.00**	0.38±0.00	0.36 ±0.00**	0.36 ±0.00	0.33 ±0.00**	0.34±0.00	0.31 ±0.00**	0.31 ±0.00	0.30 ±0.00
Ponderal Index	42.31±0.23	39.85 ±0.26**	42.81±0.24	41.42±0.21**	41.74 ±0.18	39.86 ±0.23**	42.44 ±0.18	41.27 ±0.18**	43.06 ±0.27	42.03 ±0.31*	44.52 ±0.21	42.44 ±0.24**
Body Density	1.05 ±0.00	1.04 ±0.00**	1.05 ±0.00	1.05 ±0.00	1.05 ±0.00	1.05 ±0.00	1.05 ±0.00	1.05 ±0.00	1.05 ±0.00	1.05±0.00	1.06 ±0.00	1.05 ±0.00**
%B F	19.70±0.43	23.29 ±0.55**	17.60±0.60	20.07±0.40**	19.74 ±0.41	21.30 ±0.42**	18.58 ±0.38	20.23 ±0.26**	19.72 ±0.44	21.13 ±0.54*	13.76 ±0.58	19.62 ±0.32**
FFW	49.77±0.72	42.79 ±0.76**	49.52±0.62	40.42±0.66**	50.52 ±0.60	42.48 ±0.54**	48.63 ±0.58	40.87 ±0.55**	45.85 ±0.69	37.91 ±0.76**	43.85 ±0.54	37.78 ±0.58**
Bone Mineral content	3.16±0.04	2.61 ±0.03**	3.31±0.04	2.55 ±0.03**	3.16 ±0.03	2.45 ±0.03**	3.20 ±0.03	2.51 ±0.02**	3.07 ±0.04	2.43 ±0.03**	2.98 ±0.02	2.41 ±0.02**
TBW	36.54 ±0.54	31.49 ±0.58**	36.23±0.46	29.68±0.50**	37.13 ±0.45	31.38 ±0.41**	35.61± 0.43	30.07 ±0.42**	33.53 ±0.52	27.81 ±0.58**	32.03 ±0.41	27.72 ±0.44**
Body Fat	12.58±0.48	13.40 ±0.50	10.95±0.48	10.35±0.34	12.64 ±0.37	11.44 ±0.43*	11.30 ±0.36	10.49 ±0.27	11.60 ±0.44	10.62 ±0.49	7.35±0.40	9.39 ±0.29**

SF: Skinfold; TE: trunk extremity ratio; AMC: Arm-muscle circumference; AMA: Arm-muscle area; HW ratio: Height-Weight ratio; %BF: Percent of body fat; TBW: Total body water; C: Cholesterol; FFW: Fat free weight.

**p<0.01 *p<0.05.

($p<0.01$) were observed against women. In contrast to men, rural women showed significantly higher averages of skin folds of biceps, triceps ($p<0.01$), subscapular and calf ($p<0.05$), hip circumference ($p<0.01$), TSF6 ($p<0.05$) and %BF ($p<0.01$) (Table 17.1).

Urban Madiga men showed significantly higher averages of weight, height, sitting height, diameters of biacromial, wrist, knee, and ankle ($p<0.01$) and ($p<0.05$); circumferences of waist, calf, forearm, chest ($p<0.01$), upper arm and abdominal ($p<0.05$), WHR, TE ratio, AMC, HWR, BMC and TBW ($p<0.01$), PI ($p<0.05$) against women. In Madiga women, significantly higher averages of skin folds of biceps, triceps and calf ($p<0.01$), RFPI, AMA, TSF6 ($p<0.01$) and %BF ($p<0.05$) were observed when compared to the men (Table 17.1).

Significantly higher averages of weight, height, sitting height, diameters of biacromial, wrist, elbow and ankle and knee ($p<0.01$), circumferences of upper arm ($p<0.05$) and forearm, WHR ($p<0.01$), RFPI ($p<0.05$), AMC, AMA, PI, body density, FFW, BMC and TBW ($p<0.01$) were observed in rural Madiga men against women. In contrast to men, rural Madiga women showed significantly higher averages of skin folds of biceps, triceps, subscapular, suprailiac, abdominal and calf ($p<0.01$), hip circumference, BMI, height index, TSF3, TSF6, %BF and BF ($p<0.01$) (Table 17.1).

Residence

Significantly higher averages of skinfolds of biceps, triceps, calf ($p<0.01$) and suprailiac ($p<0.05$), diameters of biacromial, biilliac and ankle, TSF6, %BF ($p<0.01$), and body fat ($p<0.05$) were observed in urban against rural Reddy men whereas in rural Reddy men, averages of diameters of wrist, elbow, ankle, forearm circumference, TE, AMC, AMA ($p<0.01$), RFPI, BMC ($p<0.05$) were found to be significantly higher when compared to the urban Reddy men.

In urban Reddy women, averages of weight, skin folds of biceps, triceps, subscapular, suprailliac and abdominal, diameter of biilliac and knee, circumferences of hip and calf, BMI, TSF3, TSF6, AMC, HWR, %BF, body fat ($p<0.01$), elbow diameter, TE ratio, FFW, TBW ($p<0.05$) were significantly higher than rural Reddy women, in contrast to urban Reddy women, significantly higher averages of WHR and AMA ($p<0.01$) were observed in rural Reddy women.

Urban Golla men showed significantly higher averages of weight, skin folds of calf and biceps, knee diameter, circumferences of hip and calf, BMI, HWR ($p<0.01$), subscapular and suprailiac skinfolds, TSF3,

TSF6, %BF, FFW, TBW and BF ($p<0.05$) against rural Golla men. In rural Golla men significantly higher averages of elbow ($p<0.01$) and ankle diameter ($p<0.05$), forearm circumference, AMC, AMA and PI ($p<0.01$) were observed when compared to the urban Golla men.

In urban Golla women significantly higher averages of weight, skinfolds of suprailiac and abdomen, biilliac diameter, circumference of chest and hip, BMI, TSF3, TSF6, HWR ($p<0.01$), skinfolds of biceps, subscapular, abdominal circumference, TE ratio, %BF, FFW and TBW ($p<0.05$) were observed when compared to the rural Golla women. In contrast, averages of height, sitting height, ankle diameter, RFPI, PI ($p<0.01$), forearm circumference and AMA were significantly, higher in rural against urban Golla women. Significantly, higher averages of weight, sitting height, skinfolds of biceps, triceps, subscapular, suprailiac, abdominal and calf, biacromial diameter, circumferences of hip, waist, upper arm, chest, abdominal, calf ($p<0.01$) and forearm ($p<0.05$), BMI, height index, TSF3, TSF6, HWR, %BF, TE ratio, BF, FFW and TBW ($p<0.01$) were observed in urban against rural Madiga men. In contrast averages of RFPI, AMA, PI and body density ($p<0.01$) were significantly higher in rural when compared to the urban Madiga men.

In urban Madiga women significantly higher averages of skinfolds of biceps, triceps and calf, diameter of elbow ($p<0.01$) and biilliac, TSF6, AMA ($p<0.01$), %BF and BF ($p<0.05$) were observed when compared to the rural Madiga women. Significantly, higher mean of TE ratio was observed in rural against urban Madiga women ($p<0.01$).

Ethnicity

One way analyses of variance (one way ANOVA) was performed between men and women of urban and rural areas in three ethnic groups to investigate significant differences in the mean values.

In urban male, significant difference in the mean values of weight, BMI, TBW, HWR, FFW, AMC, upper arm and hip circumference, knee and biilliac diameter ($p<0.01$), sitting height, elbow diameter, forearm, waist and abdominal circumferences, TE ratio and RFPI ($p<0.05$), was observed between three ethnic groups.

Significant difference in averages of weight, sitting height, skinfolds of biceps, triceps, subscapular, suprailiac and abdominal, diameters of biacromial, billiac, elbow, ankle and knee, circumferences of hip, upper arm, chest, waist, abdominal and calf, BMI, TE ratio AMC, AMA, HWR, PI, FFW, BMC, TBW, BF, body density, TSF3, TSF6, height index and

%BF ($p<0.001$), was found in urban women between three endogamous populations.

In rural males, significant difference in the average values of weight, height, sitting height, skinfolds of biceps, triceps, subscapular, suprailiac, abdominal and calf, diameters of biacromial, billiac, elbow and ankle, circumferences of hip, upper arm, forearm, chest, waist, abdominal and calf, BMI, height index, TE ratio AMC, AMA, HWR, PI, body density, FFW, BMC, TBW, BF, %BF, RFPI, TSF3 andTSF6 ($p<0.001$), was noticed between three endogamous populations.

Statistically significant difference in the mean values was observed in rural women between three caste populations in the following anthropometric variables. Weight, sitting height, diameters of knee and elbow, skinfold of calf, circumferences of upper, forearm, calf, hip, waist and chest, BMI, TBW, FFW, HWR, TE ratio, AMC, PI, RFPI, BMC, height index ($p<0.01$), diameter of biilliac, BF and abdominal circumference ($p<0.05$).

Effect of Gender, Ethnicity and Residence on Anthropometric Variables

Effect of gender was observed on all anthropometric parameters except calf circumference and body fat and demonstrated that gender is a significant variable that influences most of the anthropometric variables/indices. The effect of gender was higher on height (65.9)` followed by sitting height (55.8%), bone mineral content (52%), diameters of biacromial (49.4%), wrist (42.1%) and ankle (41.8%), FFW (32.4%), TBW (30.1%), forearm circumference (26.6%), AMC (27.2%), WHR (22.8%) and AMA (22.4%). The effect of gender on anthropometric variables/indices ranges from 1.2-65.9 per cent. Except RFPI and WHR, ethnicity showed significant effect on all anthropometric parameters/indices in the investigated populations and ranged from 1.8-14.3 per cent, the highest on knee diameter and lowest on biceps skin fold was observed. Compared to gender, effect of ethnicity was found to be lesser on anthropometric parameters/indices. Residence showed no effect on sitting height, elbow diameter, TE ratio and BMC. Effect of residence on anthropometric variables/indices ranged from 1-11.5 per cent the highest effect on AMA (11.5%) and least effect on sitting height (1%). Among the studied variables of gender, ethnicity and residence, the effect of gender was found to be highest followed by ethnicity and residence (Table 17.2).

Table 17.2: Influence of gender, residence and ethnicity on anthropometric parameters analysed by two-way multivariate analysis of variance

Variable	*Gender*			*Ethnicity*			*Residence*		
	F value	*P Value*	*Partial Eta²*	*F value*	*P Value*	*Partial Eta²*	*F value*	*P Value*	*Partial Eta²*
Weight (kg)	180.117	0.000	0.169	52.142	0.000	0.105	37.124	0.000	0.040
Height (cm)	171.93	0.000	0.659	4.179	0.016	0.009	3.641	0.057	0.004
Sitting Height	112.13	0.000	0.558	22.128	0.000	0.000	0.606	0.437	0.001
Biceps SFT (mm)	166.161	0.000	0.158	9.883	0.000	0.022	84.144	0.000	0.087
Triceps SFT (mm)	208.929	0.000	0.190	8.366	0.000	0.018	102.145	0.000	0.103
Subscapular SFT (mm)	78.709	0.000	0.081	12.604	0.000	0.026	55.708	0.000	0.059
Suprailiac SFT (mm)	19.619	0.000	0.022	11.315	0.000	0.025	94.610	0.000	0.096
Abdominal SFT (mm)	10.817	0.001	0.012	12.580	0.000	0.028	71.611	0.000	0.075
Calf SFT (mm)	78.612	0.000	0.081	5.774	0.003	0.013	62.855	0.000	0.066
Biacromial Dia (cm)	866.487	0.000	0.494	14.646	0.000	0.032	20.863	0.000	0.023
Biiliac Dia (cm)	7.004	0.008	0.008	41.996	0.000	0.086	61.541	0.000	0.065
Wrist Dia (cm)	646.778	0.000	0.421	3.866	0.021	0.009	11.504	0.001	0.013
Elbow Dia (cm).	573.663	0.000	0.392	20.221	0.000	0.044	1.194	0.275	0.001
Knee Dia (cm)	31.282	0.000	0.034	74.120	0.000	0.143	12.307	0.000	0.014
Ankle Dia (cm)	638.240	0.000	0.418	3.886	0.021	0.009	10.396	0.001	0.012
Waist Cir (cm)	34.698	0.000	0.038	38.339	0.000	0.079	9.220	0.002	0.010
Hip Cir (cm)	38.871	0.000	0.042	48.064	0.000	0.098	42.499	0.000	0.046
Upperarm Cir (cm)	41.851	0.000	0.045	37.676	0.000	0.078	4.596	0.032	0.005
Forearm Cir (cm)	322.024	0.000	0.266	23.242	0.000	0.050	7.195	0.007	0.008
Chest Cir (cm)	11.051	0.001	0.012	29.375	0.000	0.062	21.009	0.000	0.023
Abdominal Cir (cm)	25.585	0.000	0.028	29.752	0.000	0.063	13.374	0.000	0.015
Calf Cir (cm)	0.012	0.913	0.000	52.045	0.000	0.105	31.431	0.000	0.034
BMI (Kg/m²)	14.293	0.000	0.016	53.881	0.000	0.108	57.265	0.000	0.061

(Contd.)

Contd.

WHR	262.025	0.000	0.228	1.695	0.184	0.004	8.924	0.003	0.010
Height Index	8.005	0.005	0.009	18.845	0.000	0.041	10.174	0.001	0.011
TSF3	31.714	0.000	0.034	13.242	0.000	0.029	81.678	0.000	0.084
TSF6	82.012	0.000	0.085	12.736	0.000	0.028	100.850	0.000	0.102
TE Ratio	129.580	0.000	0.127	4.828	0.008	0.011	1.399	0.237	0.002
RFPI	25.311	0.000	0.028	0.064	0.938	0.000	23.419	0.000	0.026
AMC	332.045	0.000	0.272	39.125	0.000	0.081	21.443	0.000	0.024
AMA	256.250	0.000	0.224	10.039	0.000	0.022	115.041	0.000	0.115
HW Ratio	27.946	0.000	0.031	55.082	0.000	0.110	48.103	0.000	0.051
Ponderal Index	150.301	0.000	0.145	57.948	0.000	0.115	53.870	0.000	0.057
Body Density	107.345	0.000	0.108	14.618	0.000	0.032	87.709	0.000	0.090
%BF	108.103	0.000	0.109	14.551	0.000	0.032	89.029	0.000	0.091
FFW	425.280	0.000	0.324	59.134	0.000	0.118	13.718	0.000	0.015
Bone Mineral content	963.303	0.000	0.520	25.573	0.000	0.054	0.555	0.456	0.001
TBW	382.186	0.000	0.301	59.305	0.000	0.118	15.065	0.000	0.017
Body Fat	0.081	0.776	0.000	29.987	0.000	0.063	79.677	0.000	0.082

Discussion

While attempting to find predictors of disease or clinical outcomes in studies in which anthropometric parameters are included, the role of gender, residence and ethnicity are suspected as confounding variables. Till now the role of these variables on only few anthropometric variables or indices, is known. Ever increasing studies are bringing the information on the role of new anthropometric variables in various disease conditions. To know the effect of gender, ethnicity and residence on the new emerging anthropometric variables, researchers have to perform further analysis. If the information on the effect of gender, residence and ethnicity on anthropometric variables or indices if known on most of these variables it will be handy information to the researchers and can be used to control their effects. In this direction, the present investigation attempts to provide the information on the effect of gender, ethnicity and residence on 38 anthropometric variables/indices.

Irrespective of caste and residence, significantly higher averages of height, weight, sitting height, diameters of biacromial, elbow, wrist and ankle, circumferences of waist, forearm, upper arm and abdominal, WHR, PI, FFW, BMC, TBW, HWR, AMC, AMA were observed against women (Table 17.1). In women significantly higher averages of skinfolds of biceps, triceps, subscapular, abdominal and calf, hip circumference, TSF3, TSF6, RFPI and %BF were observed when compared to the men (Table 17.1).

Without regard to ethnic group, significantly higher averages of skinfolds of biceps, triceps, calf ($p<0.01$) subscapular and supraillIiac ($p<0.05$), biacromial diameter, circumferences of hip and calf, TSF3, TSF6, BMI, %BF, FFW, HWR, TBW ($p<0.01$) and BF ($p<0.05$) in urban when compared to the rural men. In contrast averages of elbow and knee diameter, fore arm circumference, AMC, AMA, RFPI and PI ($p<0.01$) were significantly higher in rural against urban men. Significantly higher averages of weight, skin folds of biceps, triceps, subscapular, suprailliac and abdominal, hip circumference, billiac diameter, BMI, TSF3, TSF6, HWR,%BF ($p<0.01$), TE ratio, FFW, BF and TBW ($p<0.05$) were observed in urban against rural women. In contrast averages of height, sitting height, RFPI, PI, ankle diameter ($p<0.01$), AMA and forearm circumference ($p<0.05$) were significantly higher in rural when compared to the urban women.

In men irrespective of urban or rural residence, significant average differences across the endogamous groups were observed in variables of weight, HWR, TBW, AMC, upper arm and hip circumferences, diameters of billiac and elbow, FFW, RFPI, TE ratio ($p<0.01$), sitting height, waist and abdominal circumferences ($p<0.05$). Only in rural men significant difference in the averages of skinfolds of biceps, triceps, subscapular, suprailliac and calf and %BF was observed across the Caste groups.

In women without regard to the residence, significant difference in averages of weight, sitting height, diameters of elbow and knee, circumferences of hip, chest and upper arm, BMI, TBW, TBW, FFW, HWR, PI, height index, TE ratio, BMC, AMC ($p<0.01$), BF and abdominal circumference ($p<0.05$) was observed across the endogamous populations. With regard to the differences, only in urban women, significant average difference was observed in skinfolds of biceps, triceps, subscapular, suprailiac and abdominal, diameters of biacromial, ankle and knee, TSF3, TSF6 and %BF ($p<0.001$) across the Caste populations, whereas only in rural women across the endogamous populations significant average difference was observed in calf skinfold, circumferences of forearm and calf ($p<0.001$) and billiac diameter ($p<0.005$).

Gender was shown to influence anthropometric variables and indices to the extent of 1.2 per cent-65.9, residence and ethnicity to the tune of 1 per cent-11.5 per cent and 1.8 per cent-14.3 per cent respectively suggesting that gender has a larger effect when compared to residence and ethnicity on anthropometric variables/indices. Researchers have to take gender in account for controlling its effect while attempting to find predictors of various clinical conditions.

To know whether the gender, ethnicity and residence act alone or in combination influences the anthropometric variables/indices, we performed two way MANOVA and the results are presented in Table 17.3. In this table, we have given only the variable in which interactants interacted significantly. A total of 29 anthropometric variables/indices on which either two or three of the gender or ethnicity or residence variables were found to be interacting significantly. These observations suggest that either alone or in combination these variables are interacting and influencing the anthropometric variables/indices. Interaction of variables such as gender, ethnicity and residence has been shown to contribute 0.9 per cent to 5.7 per cent variation in anthropometric variables/indices.

Table 17.3: Interactions of gender, ethnicity and residence on anthropometric variables and indices

Interacting variables	*F value*	*P Value*	*Partial Eta^2*
Height			
Gender*residence	4.049	0.018	0.009
Sitting height			
Residence*ethnicity	7.391	0.001	0.016
Weight			
Gender*residence*ethnicity	4.499	0.011	0.010
Biceps			
Residence*ethnicity	6.775	0.001	0.015
Gender*ethnicity	6.122	0.002	0.014
Triceps skinfold			
Gender*ethnicity	11.215	0.000	0.025
Residence*ethnicity	11.123	0.000	0.024
Gender*residence*ethnicity	3.564	0.029	0.008
Subscapular skin fold			
Gender*ethnicity	3.063	0.047	0.007
Residence*ethnicity	2.445	0.087	0.005
Gender*residence*ethnicity	6.990	0.001	0.015
Suprailiac skin fold			
Residence*ethnicity	3.913	0.020	0.009
Gender*residence*ethnicity	14.133	0.000	0.031
Abdominal skin fold			
Residence*ethnicity	3.093	0.046	0.007
Gender*residence*ethnicity	16.796	0.000	0.036
Calf skin fold			
Gender*residence	14.726	0.000	0.016
Gender*ethnicity	7.303	0.001	0.016
Residence*ethnicity	10.458	0.000	0.023
Biacromial diameter			
Gender*residence	23.283	0.000	0.026
Gender*residence*ethnicity	6.766	0.001	0.015
Biilliac diameter			
Gender*ethnicity	5.575	0.004	0.012
Ethnicity*residence	7.165	0.001	0.016
Elbow diameter			
Gender*ethnicity	3.735	0.024	0.008
Gender*residence	25.789	0.000	0.028
Ethnicity*residence	12.059	0.000	0.026
Knee diameter			
Gender*ethnicity	4.433	0.012	0.010
Gender*ethnicity*residence	3.317	0.037	0.007
Ankle diameter			
Gender*ethnicity	7.514	0.001	0.017
Ethnicity*residence	6.048	0.002	0.013
Gender*ethnicity*residence	7.550	0.001	0.017

Hip circumference			
Gender*ethnicity*residence	3.951	0.020	0.009
Upper arm circumference			
Gender*ethnicity	11.463	0.000	0.025
Gender*residence	4.226	0.040	0.005
Ethnicity*residence	3.144	0.044	0.007
Forearm circumference			
Gender*ethnicity	4.808	0.008	0.011
Ethnicity*residence	10.120	0.000	0.022
Chest circumference			
Ethnicity*residence	3.200	0.041	0.007
Calf circumference			
Gender*ethnicity	3.641	0.027	0.008
Gender*ethnicity*residence	17.253	0.000	0.037
Body mass index			
Gender*ethnicity*residence	5.721	0.003	0.013
Height index			
Gender*ethnicity	7.041	0.001	0.016
Gender*residence	22.890	0.000	0.025
Ethnicity*residence	6.078	0.002	0.014
Sum of three trunk skinfolds			
Ethnicity*residence	3.463	0.032	0.008
Gender*ethnicity*residence	13.665	0.000	0.030
Sum of the six skinfolds			
Gender*ethnicity	3.569	0.029	0.008
Ethnicity*residence	6.203	0.002	0.014
Gender*ethnicity*residence	7.882	0.000	0.017
The trunk extremity ratio			
Gender*ethnicity	16.809	0.000	0.036
Ethnicity*residence	4.637	0.010	0.010
Gender*ethnicity*residence	26.921	0.000	0.057
Relative fat pattern index			
Gender*ethnicity	5.941	0.003	0.013
Gender*residence	5.135	0.024	0.006
Gender*ethnicity*residence	7.218	0.001	0.016
Arm muscle circumference			
Gender*ethnicity	3.257	0.039	0.007
Gender*residence	3.201	0.041	0.007
Arm muscle area			
Gender*ethnicity	9.356	0.000	0.021
Gender*residence	17.461	0.000	0.019
Ethnicity*residence	10.011	0.000	0.022
Gender*ethnicity*residence	5.714	0.003	0.013
Height to weight Ratio			
Gender*ethnicity*residence	5.168	0.006	0.012
Ponderal index			
Gender*ethnicity*residence	5.827	0.003	0.013

Body density			
Gender*ethnicity	5.196	0.006	0.012
Gender*residence	5.198	0.023	0.006
Ethnicity*residence	8.333	0.000	0.018
Gender*ethnicity*residence	10.278	0.000	0.023
Per cent of body fat			
Gender*ethnicity	5.121	0.006	0.011
Gender*residence	4.621	0.032	0.005
Ethnicity*residence	8.224	0.000	0.018
Gender*ethnicity*residence	10.205	0.000	0.022
Bone mineral content			
Gender*ethnicity*residence	4.243	0.015	0.009
Body fat			
Ethnicity*residence	3.209	0.001	0.017
Gender*ethnicity*residence	7.490	0.001	0.017

Conclusion

The results of the study suggest that there is a significant influence of gender, ethnicity and residence either alone or in combination on the anthropometric variables and indices. The present study brings important information on the effect of gender, ethnicity and residence on 38 anthropometric variables/indices which may be useful while finding the predictors of clinical conditions in which anthropometric variables and indices are included as independent variables.

REFERENCES

Adediran, O.S., Adebayo, P.B., and Akintunde, A.A. (2013). "Anthropometric differences among natives of Abuja living in urban and rural communities: correlations with other cardiovascular risk factors", *BMC Research Notes, 6*, 123.

Frignani, R.R., Passos, M.A., Ferrari, G.L., Niskier, S.R., Fisberg, M., and Cintra Ide P. (2015). "Reference curves of the body fat index in adolescents and their association with anthropometric variables", *J Pediatr (Rio J), 91*, 248-55.

Goh, L.G.H., Dhaliwal, S.S., Welborn, T.A., Lee, H., and Della, P.R. (2014). "Ethnicity and the association between anthropometric indices of obesity and cardiovascular risk in women: A cross sectional study", *BMJ Open*, 4, e004702.

Mohan, I., Gupta, R., Misra, A., Sharma, K.K., Agrawal, A., Vikram, N.K. Sharma, V., Usha, S., and Pandey, R.M. (2016). "Disparities in Prevalence of Cardio-metabolic Risk Factors in Rural, Urban-Poor, and Urban-Middle Class Women in India", *PloS one, 11*, e0149437.

Mohan Reddy, B., Latheef, S.A.A., and Pranavchand, R. (2019). "The burden of non-communicable disease risk factors and haematological indicators of infections among the rural, semiurban and urban inhabitants of the Yanadi tribal Population of south India", *J Indian Anthrop Soc*, 54, 137-169.

National Health and Nutrition Examination Survey III.1988. Body Measurements (Anthropometry), West at Inc., Maryland NCD Risk Factor Collaboration (NCD-Risk). (2017). Worldwide trends in blood pressure from 1975 to 2015: a pooled analysis of 1479 population-based measurement studies with 19.1 million participants. *Lancet (London, England), 389*, 37-55.

Latheef, S.A.A., Subramanyam, G., and Reddy, B.M. (2018). "Utility of anthropometric traits and indices in predicting the risk of coronary artery disease in the adult men of southern Andhra Pradesh", *Indian Heart J,* 70 Suppl 3, S133-S139.

Lutoslawska, G., Malara, M., Tomaszewski P, Mazurek, K., Czajkwoska, A., Keska, A., and Tkaczyk, J. (2014). "Relationship between the percentage of body fat and surrogate indices of fatness in male and female Polish active and sedentary students", *J Physiol Anthropol*, 33, 10.

Reddy, N. (1998). "Blood pressure and adiposity: A comparative study of socio-economically diverse groups of Andhra Pradesh, India", *Am J Hum Biol, 10*, 5-21.

Shaik, S., Das, R., Saha, R., Das, S., and Dasgupta, P. (2020). "Age and sex specific variations in body composition in Indian urban Bengali Hindu children, adolescents and young adults aged 7–21 years", *Anthropological Review*, *83*, 1-17.

Venkatramana, P. and Reddy, P.C. (2002). "Association of overall and abdominal obesity with coronary heart disease risk factors: Comparison between urban and rural Indian men", *Asia Pac J Clin Nutr, 11*, 66-71.

PART IV

Psychological Health and Wellbeing

18

Adolescent Mental Health in Conflict Settings

Anthropological Insights

Urfat Anjem Mir, Shwetha Gopalakrishnan and *Anushka Singh*

Introduction

The term 'adolescence' has come to be used to refer to the age-group between 10 and 19 years of age (WHO, 2014). Throughout this chapter, the standard meaning of the terms 'children' and 'adolescents' will be used interchangeably while referring to children ranging between the age of 13 and 18. Adolescence has been known to be a critical and vulnerable period of life as an individual's growth is impacted by development of their physical and psychological abilities during this period (Patton *et al.*, 2016). Exposure to any adverse or negative experience during this stage in life has been noted to hamper the life-long functioning of an individual (Soleimanpour, Geierstanger, & Brindis, 2017). Traumatic episodes of violence have been linked to detrimental effects on the emotional and cognitive development of an individual.

Recent findings on adolescent health however, have raised concerns about their mental health conditions. Self-harm, interpersonal violence and depressive disorders have been found to be common causes of distress among adolescents (Ameratunga & Denny, 2016). Further exposure to an array of traumatic experiences in an already vulnerable state increases the risk of developing mental health concerns among adolescents (Dekovik, Koning, Stams & Buist, 2008). These traumatic events can include a range of personal experiences like bereavement and accidents to more community-based experiences like political and ethnic conflict (Obermeyer, Bott, & Sassine, 2015). The contemporary times have witnessed increasing episodes of political strife all over the world. Political conflict and violence has been recurring in countries like Israel,

Palestine, India, Sri Lanka, Afghanistan, Nepal and many other parts of the world. A growing body of literature has investigated the adverse psychological impact as a consequence of such trauma on the people living in these conflict zones (Franzese, Vovey, Tucker, McCoy & Menard, 2014). Much research work has been carried out to investigate the impact of these experiences on children (Varela & Hensley-Maloney, 2009), adolescents (Lubit, Rovine, Defreancisci & Eth, 2003), and adults (Sousa, Kemp & El-Zuhairi, 2014) in these regions. Most researches conducted on adolescent mental health in these areas have either been aimed at assessing the prevalence of mental health disorders (Williams, Alexander, Bolsover & Bakke, 2008) or towards identification of risk/and protective factors which mediate the relationship between exposure to trauma and the development of mental disorders (Dubow *et al.*, 2012). However, the subjective meaning ascribed by adolescents to traumatic experiences and the social-psychological impact on them has been largely neglected by previous research. Hence, a key step in understanding adolescent mental health and their psychological distress is to know how adolescents perceive and make sense of adverse experiences. This in-depth understanding of psychological distress and mental health would facilitate the development of nuanced and efficient psycho-social interventions for the adolescent population in the years to come.

This chapter aims at emphasizing the importance of studying adolescent mental health with a special focus on regions affected by political conflict. It illustrates the various findings in the area of adolescent mental health especially in the context of trauma experiences due to exposure to political conflict. Furthermore, the study by presenting research based evidence, highlights the need for an individual-centric, socially mediated and culturally applicable approach to the study of trauma and mental health among adolescents.

Adolescent Mental Health

Research conducted on adolescents provides abundant evidence to highlight their precarious state by indicating that the onset of most psychological disorders is between the ages of 12 and 24 years (Patel, Fisher, Hetrick & McGorry, 2007). A longitudinal study which looked at the trajectory of development of mental health issues revealed that individuals are at a high risk of developing mental health problems between the ages 7 and 12 years and after 19 years (Ravens-Siebere, Otto, Kriston, Rothenberger, Dopfner, Herpertz-Dahlmann *et al.*, 2015). Furthermore, in the past fifty years, there has been a rapid upsurge in the prevalence of mental health concerns in adolescents. Researches have noted an escalation in episodes of self-harm among young females and suicide rates in young men (Maughan, Iervolino & Collishaw, 2005). Currently, an estimate of 10-20 per cent of the world's adolescents are enduring mental disorders (Kieling, Baker-Henningham, Belfer, Conti, Ertem, Omigbodun *et al.*, 2011). Most of past researches have been conducted on high-income American (Maughan, Lervolino & Collishaw, 2005; Gutterman, Hahm & Cameron, 2002) and European (Ravens-Siebere *et al.*, 2008) nations. However, recent researches have started to explore adolescent mental health in low and middle-income countries (Obermeyer, Bott & Sassine, 2015). Research in the Asian continent demonstrated that the prevalence rate of mental health disorders was equitable to the global rates with Asperger's syndrome Attention deficit hyperactivity disorder (ADHD) and Post-Traumatic Stress Disorder (PTSD) (Srinath, Kandasamy & Golhar, 2010). A recent review of literature conducted in Iran found that the prevalence rate of mental health disorders to be ranging between 16.7 per cent to 36.4 per cent. Moreover, mental health concerns like suicide, depression, drug Abuse, autism, Attention deficit hyperactivity disorder (ADHD) were the most prevalent disorders (Sharifi, Mojtabai, Shahrivar, Alaghband-Rad, Zarafshan *et al.*, 2016). A study that examined high school adolescents in Iran found that an estimated 19.5 per cent of them obtained scores that were above the threshold for that mental health disorder (Emami, Ghazinour, Rezaeishiraz & Richter, 2007). Indian studies also have shown concerning figures with respect to the prevalence rates of mental health disorders in adolescents with a range of prevalence between 1.81 to 24.7 per cent (Aggarwal & Berk, 2015). A research conducted in Assam found 31.6 per cent of the children to be symptomatic of mental health disorders (Harikrishnan, Arif & Sobhana, 2017). With such high prevalence rates of disorders, it becomes imperative to engage in the elaborate study of the mental health of adolescents to gain a more comprehensive knowledge about it.

Adolescence, as has been previously discussed is a period of vulnerability (Danielson *et al.*, 2006) and being exposed to a traumatic event during this period can significantly increase an adolescent's risk of developing mental disorders (Cavanaugh & Huston, 2008; Lubit, Rovine, Defreancisci & Eth, 2003). Therefore, exposure to trauma acts as a significant mediator in the process of development of mental health disorders. Many adolescents are exposed to various traumatic situations in their life. 70 per cent of females and 85 per cent of males were found to be exposed to at least one traumatic event in their lives according to an Indian study (Rasmussen, Karsberg, Karsoft & Elklit, 2013). Exposure to traumatic experiences like family violence, bereavement, natural disasters, abuse, conflict and violent situations have been linked with high prevalence of mental health disorders (Soleimanpour, Geierstanger, & Brindis, 2017; Stikkelbroek, Bodden, Reitz, Vollebergh & Baar, 2015; Franzese, Covey, Tucker, McCoy & Menard, 2014; Kieling *et al.,* 2011; Varela & Hensley-Maloney, 2009). Being exposed to traumatic events like these has been associated with the development of an array of mental health concerns including PTSD-Post Traumatic Stress Disorder (Wang, Chan & Ho, 2013; Williams, Alexander, Bolsover & Bakke, 2008; Seethalakshmi, Dhavale, Gawande & Dewan, 2006), depressive disorders (Paul, Felton, Adams, Welsh, Miller & Ruggiero, 2015), anxiety disorders (Wang, Chan & Ho, 2013; Slone & Shechner, 2009), behavioural problems (Foltz, Dang, Daniels, Doyle, McFee & Quisenberry, 2013; Lubit, Rovine, Defreancisci & Eth, 2003), and substance abuse (Danielson *et al.*, 2006).

These findings add to the previously discussed literature on adolescent mental health. Hence, it can be argued that exposure to trauma has a significant impact on adolescent mental health and wellbeing and may be one of the most important variables which needs to be studied in the context of adolescent mental health. Furthermore, the relationship between trauma and mental health is not unidirectional and is mediated by many variables such as gender, traumatic event etc. Research shows that young men are at a higher risk of being exposed to traumatic events, however, it is young women who are at a greater risk of developing mental distress with such an exposure (Yazdani, Zainab & Shafi, 2015). These findings call for a more comprehensive assessment of mental health in adolescents to gain an in depth understanding of the socio-cultural dynamics of trauma and mental health experiences.

Conflict Settings and Mental Health of Adolescents

Political conflict and violence has become a common cause of trauma across the globe. Research findings across the world found an escalation in the development of mental health concerns following political violence in many countries like Israel (Schmid & Muldoon, 2013), Palestine (Al-Krenaxi, Graham & Sehwail, 2004), Afghanistan (Panter-brick, Grimon, Kalin & Eggerman, 2015); Nepal (Luitel *et al.*, 2013), and India (Jong *et al.*, 2008) to name a few. Individuals living in regions afflicted by political conflict often find themselves unprotected to multiple traumatic events such as arrests, forced labour, crossfire, kidnappings, torture, rapes, round up raids, and sexual violence (Jong *et al.*, 2008). These events can impact the psychological and social functioning of individuals who are either (1) directly exposed to such instances as a victim or (2) are bystanders or (3) have been indirectly exposed through stories of others. Exposure to political violence not only affects adults (Luitel *et al.*, 2013), but also children (Willian, Alexander, Bolsover & Bakke, 2008) and adolescents (Punter-Brick, Eggerman, Gonzalvez & Safdar, 2009) living in these areas.

Exposure to armed conflict at a tender age is also another factor that exacerbates the risk of developing mental disorders (Kieling *et al.*, 2011). Exposure to political violence has been reported to have an adverse impact on the social (Al-Krenawi & Graham, 2012) and psychological (Shaw, 2000) functioning of children and adolescents and has led to increased risks of developing Post-traumatic stress disorder (PTSD) (Moussa, Kholy, Enaba, Ali, Nasreldin, Gabal *et al.*, 2015; Rabaia, Saleh & Giacaman, 2014; Dubow, Boxer, Huesmann, Landau, Dvir, Shikaki *et al.*, 2012; De Jong, Komproe, Ommeren, El Masri, Araya, Kaled *et al.*, 2001; Rosenthal, 2000), depressive and anxiety symptoms (Obermeyer, Bott & Sassine, 2015; Rabaia, Saleh & Giacaman, 2014; Dimitry *et al.*, 2011; Slone & Shechner, 2009; Lubit, Rovine, Defreancisci & Eth, 2003), substance abuse (Schiff *et al.*, 2007; Reijneveld, Crone, Schuller, Verhulst & Verloove-Vanhorick, 2005; Spooner, 1999), and somatic disorders (Slone & Mayer, 2015), among children and adolescents. Moreover, these traumatic experiences do not occur as one-off instances but are recurrent and rampant in areas suffering from political conflict. Exposure to such recurrent traumatic instances further escalates the risk of developing mental disorders among adolescents and is also linked with the development of more debilitating symptoms (Rabaia, Saleh & Giacaman, 2014). Even in cases of one-off instances of exposure to traumatic episodes, the psychological impact of these traumatic experiences (natural and man-made) may last over a long period (Bal & Jensen, 2007) and may persist well into adulthood (Franzese, Vovey, Tucker, McCoy & Menard, 2014). Research on adolescents exposed to trauma has recognized Post-Traumatic Stress Disorder (PTSD) and related symptoms to be the most commonly occurring form of mental distress (Dubow *et al.*, 2012; Ai, Rana & Ali, 2011). The prevalence of PTSD may range from 8.6 per cent in children exposed to natural disasters (Ali, Rana & Ali, 2011) to 10 per cent in Indian adolescents exposed to traumatic events like accidents, death of a closed one, coming close to being injured or killed, witnessing someone get injured or killed. (Rasmussen, Karberg, Karstoft & Elklie, 2013). Furthermore, research shows that 50-70 per cent children exposed to political violence and war-like situations in the Middle East end up developing the symptoms of this disorder (Dimitry, 2011). A study done on high school students also showed similar results, with increased symptoms of PTSD and somatization disorder after exposure to political violence. Research also emphasized how being exposed to political violence post the age of 12 can put an individual at a significant risk of developing PTSD (de Jong, Komproe, Ommeren, El Masri, Araya, Kaled *et al.*, 2001). As discussed earlier, the prevalence of mental disorders in general and PTSD in specific is higher among children who experience recurrent violence (Dubow *et al.*, 2012; Harder, Mutiso, Khasakhala, Burke & Ndetei, 2012). Hence, there is an evident need to study adolescent mental health in the context of political conflict as it is a ubiquitous and recurrent form of trauma which adversely affects adolescents.

Why Anthropological Approach?

As illustrated in the previous section, most of the research that has investigated the impact of trauma on adolescent mental health has aimed at providing epidemiological summaries of mental disorders (Wang, Chan & Ho, 2013; Caffo, Forresi & Lievers, 2006). Others have aimed at engaging in quantitative analysis of various factors which mediate the relationship between the life circumstance of an adolescent and their risk of developing mental disorders (Yazdani, Zainab & Shafi, 2015; Shaw, 2000). Similarly, in the context of political conflict and its impact on mental health and wellbeing of adolescents, similar approaches have been applied (Moussa, Kholy, Enaba, Ali, Nasreldin, Gabal *et al.*, 2015; de Jong *et al.*, 2001). However, these researches fall short at exploring the phenomenon of political conflict and adolescent mental health in its entirety (Tol, Rees & Silove, 2013). While research in this area has identified many variables which mediate the relationship between exposure to political conflict and mental health (Rosenthal, 2000) they have failed at providing any in-depth understanding of these variables and their impact on this relationship. On the other hand, other research initiatives have been aimed at identifying the various pathological conditions associated with exposure to political conflict (Rabaia, Saleh & Giacaman, 2014) but the understanding of the experience of trauma and the meanings that adolescents assign to this experience has not been studied in so much detail.

The study of trauma and mental illness lacks a thorough investigation of the meaning and significance of the experience of trauma and mental illness for the individuals going through it on an everyday level. Kleinman (2012) argued that the understanding of pathology is insufficient without incorporating the social and cultural context of an individual. These aspects of an individual's life are significant indicators to illustrate the difference between social suffering that a person experiences because of the prevailing social conditions in which they live in and the development of pathological symptoms. This distinction is especially important to make in the case of adolescents experiencing trauma because what is usually seen as a pathological pattern of behaviours and emotions in adolescents may be a natural and acceptable reaction to the prevailing trauma and conflict in their environment. It is important to note that psychological distress is never experienced in a vacuum and it is invariably the result of social and community based stressors (Drake, 2015). Anthropological scholarship emphasizes on the notion of suffering being determined by social and cultural realities and various other determinants of collective suffering (Lim, Stock, Oo, Joote, 2013). Hence, understanding the meaning that the context holds for an individual is crucial to holistically understand the distress experienced by individuals in such social and cultural contexts. The perception of mental suffering and healing differ from place to place and are complicated in their nature. A limitation with research discussed in the previous section has been that the psychiatric understanding of distress has been a restricted way of defining this very distress that the individual experiences (Nichter, 1981).

The meanings of diagnosis and medical epidemiology change and the scientific knowledge of/around a medical condition is subject to use by the various actors involved in a conflict in various ways during a socio-political conflict. These processes are associated with the idea of the state imposed citizenship and entitlement and hence lead to a unique form of health care economy (Young and Rees, 2011). Imposing a rigid diagnostic model of psychiatric healing in conflict zones, has also been perceived as appropriating the suffering of people at multiple levels. Some mental health interventions in post conflict regions have attempted to create job opportunities for psychosocial practitioners, clinicians and social workers who especially help people with "coping" with mental health issues like depression and trauma (Baingana, Bannon & Thomas, 2005). However, one cannot justify use of political conflicts and violence. Another interesting dimension to explore would be whether psychiatric diagnosis and treatment are used as an institutional or state means to silence the voice of resistance by turning structural violence into stigma and misfortune of individuals and reduce the traumatic reactions to pathological conditions which may be delinked from structural violence. Structural violence has also selectively erased people's histories by de-socializing its context and by building a new narrative around it (Farmer, 2004). Psychiatry and Psychobiology have given birth to a new form of suffering which is rooted in the rule of science and is affirmed in the phenomenon referred as "Psychogenic trauma" (Young, 1996). The anthropological perspective towards trauma, however, holistically covers both the social and biological elements, which helps to gain a wider understanding of the local social and cultural context. In order to be able to deal better with the limitations of the psychiatric approach, anthropologists have urged for an understanding of the bio-social history of the disease itself (Farmer, 2004).

Often times, the tools used to diagnose mental health disorders are the ones that are the result of Western contributions and also appropriately applicable to a western population. It is, thus, important that Psychiatry develops ways of diagnosing individuals that are not rooted in assumptions of the "normal" according to a western notion (Baingana, Bannon, Thomas, 2005). Questionnaires like The Harvard Trauma Questionnaires have been adapted several times according to the different cultural requirements and the General Health Questionnaire (GHQ) has also been modified to suit the Burundi Population and more such efforts need to be done to measure the cultural and subjective meanings and metaphors. There are ideas and beliefs related to the mind-body relationship that are locally embedded in the cultural repertoire of the people, which are expressed in the forms of "idioms of distress" (Hinton, Fernandez, 2010). Even in the case of political conflict and violence, the mind-body relationship has cultural connotations. Insecurity, feelings of powerlessness and violence that is often a normal/new normal in protracted conflict situations and can find expression in these "idioms of distress". In some communities in Rwanda and Kosovo, the impact of trauma has infiltrated in the everyday lives of the people, and so societal healing is recognized by people and is used to process this social suffering by making deliberate attempts to turn down psychiatric diagnosis for the purpose of cure (Drake, 2015). This is evidence to the fact that sometimes psychiatric medication can be far from the everyday lives of people and might not be able to comprehend the cultural values, beliefs and personal experiences of the trauma narrative of a collective.

Posttraumatic Stress Disorder (PTSD) through Anthropological Lens

Thc critique of diagnostic model of Post-Traumatic Stress Disorder in anthropological perspective is primarily due to the importance of social and cultural factors in construction of suffering and mental health. When it comes to the study of psychological health and illness and the specific case of studying mental disorders, the prevalent psychiatric methodology uses diagnostic criteria and tools to give clinical labels to the experience of individuals. However, in this process, the individual's experience and understanding of their condition gets ignored. The diagnosis—treatment model of cure has been critiqued by researchers for having a confined perspective and has also been perceived as inadequate for tranquilizing a population with pain related medications and antidepressants (Drake, 2015). The anthropological lens on the other hand, helps in understanding and locating agency in the social beings who face the trauma and political violence and seek refuge in the local community systems to cope with the traumatic situations. The anthropological perspective draws our attention towards the link of mental health with the problem of social injustice.

An important question that emerges out of existing research on trauma work around PTSD is that how does this diagnosis-treatment model cater to those families who do not seek treatment in the first place. There is an existing critique of PTSD which argues that the diagnosis itself emerges from structural power play, profit making and conspiracy that goes against the community related meanings of distress (Weiner, Chafe, 2008). Trauma is built, adjusted and manipulated through diagnostic narratives in this diagnostic trauma paradigm. PTSD and trauma cannot be perceived and construed as wholly psychiatric problems as the link between trauma and history cannot be overlooked. The history of trauma can often include components of structural violence where the trauma is not only an occurrence of inhumanity but a living evidence of humanity. (Young and Rees, 2011).

Hence, an approach which studies the 'Idioms of Distress' used by an individual is more appropriate (Kohrt, Mendenhall and Brown, 2016) for a holistic comprehension of mental health in regions of political conflict. These are language based notions derived from the cultural and social context of an individual and highlight the lived experience of the person undergoing the psychological ordeal and the associated distress. This approach to pathological conditions associated with traumatic violence can help give insights into the language of the said distress as used and understood by these adolescents. Moreover, it helps to understand the interconnections between human rights violations and mental health issues through the lens of ethno-psychology. Present scholarship in the arena of adolescent mental health (in the context of trauma) is critiqued for the lack of focus on these very 'Idioms of Distress' (Tol, Rees & Silove, 2013).

Anthropology, which aims at studying an individual embedded in their social and cultural context comes as a ready means of rescuing mental health research from these shortcomings (Kohrt, Mendenhall and Brown, 2016; Drake, 2015). An anthropological approach will help understand the experience of not just pathology but also the register of social suffering as is experienced by people embedded in the specific context of political conflict. Moreover, such an approach will fulfil the need to understand trauma in terms of the individual and society which is something that research on political violence lacks at present (Pederson, 2002).

The Need for Alternatives and Acceptance

A comprehensive understanding of local ideas of mental health and health care is imperative to ensure efficient mental health interventions at a public level (Ventevogel, Jordans, Reis, Jong, 2013). The mental health professionals ought to be more accepting of the local, regional alternative processes of cultural healing (Thirthalli *et al.*, 2016). Such collaborations between professionals from the biomedical sector, alternative medicine sector; traditional, religious healers have proven to be successful. Often, the local understanding of mental health is different from universal categories of psychiatric model such as DSM. For instance, Kwajana in South Sudan have various categories of madness such as *Moul, Wehie Arir, Nger Yec* which would be classified similar to psychotic disorders in DSM-V but the five symptoms of psychotic disorders according to DSM-V are not necessarily present in the local understanding of this mental illness. (Ventevogel, Jordans, Reis, Jong, 2013). Such complications and nuances cannot be overlooked and need to be better addressed in the psychiatric approach to mental health not specifically in conflict settings across the globe but in general approach as well.

Conclusion

A review of literature on adolescent mental health illustrates that adolescents are at a significant risk of developing multiple mental health concerns including anxiety disorders, depressive disorders, post-traumatic stress disorder, substance abuse, self-harm behaviour and suicidal ideation.

The risk associated with the development of these and other disorders increases manifolds if the adolescent is exposed to traumatic events such as bereavement, abuse, accidents, community, and political conflict. Furthermore, the frequency of adolescents who are exposed to these traumas is very high across the world. In terms of specific traumas, the contemporary times have seen an increase in the prevalence of political conflict across the world. Exposure to political conflict is also seen as a major risk factor when it comes to the development of mental disorders. Hence, the study of mental illness and health in the context of adolescents living in areas of political conflict becomes a very important area of study. Over the years, much work has been done on mental health of adolescents exposed to political trauma but most of this work has been limited to quantifying the effects of trauma, identifying prevailing rates of mental disorders or identifying risk and protective factors. However, these research initiatives have neither been able to study the meaning attached to this trauma nor understand the language used by adolescents to describe these meanings and experiences. Psychiatric approach has been criticized for appropriating people's collective political pain and for its lack of engagement with structural concerns related to political violence. Hence, there is a need to study the 'Idioms of Distress' employed by individuals exposed to political trauma as they describe the experience of trauma and the associated psychological distress. Anthropology, which is an approach embedded in the study of culture can come as a saviour in the light of these methodological constraints. An anthropological approach to the study of adolescent mental health in areas of political conflict will help researchers and mental health practitioners understand the lived experience of trauma and mental illness embedded with the social and cultural context.

Acknowledgments:

The authors would like to acknowledge the financial support of Indian Council of Social Sciences Research (ICSSR) under MRP scheme for the year 2017-2019. This chapter is based on the research carried out as part of that study.

REFERENCES

Aggarwal, S. and Berk, M., (2015). "Evolution of Adolescent Mental Health in a Rapidly Changing Socioeconomic Environment: A Review of Mental Health Studies in Adolescents in India over Last Ten Years", *Asian Journal of Psychiatry*, *13*, 3-12.https://doi.org/10.1016/j.ajp.2014.11.007

Al-Krenawi, A., Graham, J.R., and Sehwail, M. (2004). "Mental health and violence/trauma in Palestine: Implications for helping professional practice", *Journal of Contemporary Family Studies, 35*(2), 185–209.https://doi.org/10.3138/jcfs.35.2.185

Al-Krenawi, A., and R. Graham, J. (2012). "The impact of political violence on psychosocial functioning of individuals and families: The case of Palestinian adolescents", *Child and Adolescent Mental health, 17*(1), 14-22. https://doi.org/10.1111/j.1475-3588.2011.00600.x

Ali, M.W., Rana, M.H., and Ali, S. (2011). "Psychosocial Impact of October 2005 Earthquake on Children and Adolescents Aged 9 to 18 Years, Assessed after One Year in Kashmir, Pakistan", *Pakistan Journal of Medical Research, 50*(4), 123-129.

Ameratunga, S., and Denny, S. (2016). "GBD 2013: A window into the world of young people", *The Lancet, 387*(10036), 2353-2354.https://doi.org/10.1016/s0140-6736(16)30296-3

Baingana, F.K., Bannon, I., and Thomas, R. (2005). *Mental health and conflicts: Conceptual framework and approaches*. Washington, DC: World Bank.

Bal, A., and Jensen, B. (2007). "Post-traumatic stress disorder symptom clusters in Turkish child and adolescent trauma survivors", *European Child and Adolescent Psychiatry, 16*(7), 449-457. https://doi.org/10.1007/s00787-007-0618-z

Black, J.J., and Rofey, D.L. (2018). "An overview of common psychiatric problems among adolescent and young adult females: Focus on mood and anxiety", *Best Practice and Research Clinical Obstetrics and Gynaecology, 48*, 165-173. https://doi.org/10.1016/j.bpobgyn.2017.08.007

Caffo, E., Forresi, B., and Lievers, L.S. (2005). "Impact, psychological sequelae and management of trauma affecting children and adolescents", *Current Opinion in Psychiatry, 18*(4), 422-428. https://doi.org/10.1097/01.yco.0000172062.01520.

Cavanagh, S.E., and Huston, A.C. (2008). "The timing of family instability and children's social adjustment", *Journal of Marriage and Family, 70*(5), 1258–1270. https://doi.org/10.1111/j.1741-3737.2008.00564.x

Danielson, C.K., De Arellano, M.A., Ehrenreich, J.T., Suárez, L.M., Bennett, S.M., Cheron, D.M., Goldstein, C.R., Jakle, K.R., Landon, T.M., and Trosper, S.E. (2006). "Identification of high-risk behaviours among victimized adolescents and implications for empirically supported psychosocial treatment", *Journal of Psychiatric Practice, 12*(6), 364-383. https://doi.org/10.1097/00131746-200611000-00004

David, S., Gazi, R., Mirzazada, M.S., Siriwardhana, C., Soofi, S., and Roy, N. (2017). "Conflict in South Asia and its impact on health", *BMJ, 357*(j1537), 1-5 https://doi.org/10.1136/bmj.j1537

Deković, M., Koning, I.M., Jan Stams, G., and Buist, K.L. (2008). "Factors associated with traumatic symptoms and internalizing problems among adolescents who experienced a traumatic event", *Anxiety, Stress and Coping, 21*(4), 377-386. https://doi.org/10.1080/10615800701791161

Dimitry, L. (2011). "A systematic review on the mental health of children and adolescents in areas of armed conflict in the Middle East", *Child: Care, Health and Development, 38*(2), 153-161. https://doi.org/10.1111/j.1365-2214.2011.01246.x

Drake, R.E. (2015). "Anthropology and mental health care", *Epidemiology and psychiatric sciences, 24*(4), 283-284.https://doi.org/10.1017/S2045796015000402

Dubow, E.F., Boxer, P., Huesmann, I.R., Landau, S., Dvir, S., Shikaki, K., and Ginges, J. (2012). "Cumulative Effects of Exposure to Violence on Posttraumatic Stress in Palestinian and Israeli Youth", *Journal of Clinical Child and Adolescent Psychology, 41*(6), 837-844. https://doi.org/10.1080/15374416.2012.675571

Dubow, E.F., Huesmann, L.R., Boxer, P., Landau, S., Dvir, S., Shikaki, K., and Ginges, J. (2012). "Exposure to Political Conflict and Violence and Posttraumatic Stress in Middle East Youth: Protective Factors", *Journal of Clinical Child and Adolescent Psychology, 41*(4), 402-416.https://doi.org/10.1080/15374416.2012.684274

Emami, H., Ghazinour, M., Rezaeishiraz, H., and Richter. J. (2007). "Mental Health of Adolescents in Tehran, Iran", *Journal of Adolescent Health, 41*(6), 571-576.https://doi.org/10.1016/j.jadohealth.2007.06.005

Farmer, P. (2004). "An Anthropology of Structural Violence", *Current Anthropology, 45*(3), 305-325.https://doi.org/10.1086/382250

Foltz, R., Dang, S., Daniels, B., Doyle, H., McFee, S., and Quisenberry, C. (2013). "When Diagnostic Labels Mask Trauma", *Reclaiming Children and Youth, 22*(2), 12-17.

Franzese, R.J., Covey, H.C., Tucker, A.S., McCoy, L., and Menard, S., (2014). "Adolescent Exposure to Violence and Adult Physical and Mental Health Problems", *Child Abuse Neglect, 38*(12), 1955-1965. https://doi.org/10.1016/j.chiabu.2014.10.017

Guterman, N.B., Hahm, H.C., and Cameron, M, (2002). "Adolescent Victimization and Subsequent use of Mental Health Counselling Services", *Journal of Adolescent Health, 30*(5), 336-345.https://doi.org/10.1016/s1054-139x(01)00406-2

Harder, V.S., Mutiso, V.N., Khasakhala, L.I., Burke, H.M., and Ndetei, D.M. (2012). "Multiple traumas, postelection violence, and posttraumatic stress among impoverished Kenyan youth", *Journal of Traumatic Stress, 25*(1), 64-70. https://doi.org/10.1002/jts.21660

Harikrishnan, U., Arif, A., and Sobhana, H. (2017). "Assessment of Mental Health Status Among School Going Adolescents in North East India: A Cross-Sectional School based Survey", *Asian Journal of Psychiatry, 30*, 114-117. https://doi.org/10.1016/j.ajp.2017.08.021

Hinton, D.E. and Lewis-Fernandez, R. (2010). "Idioms of Distress Among Trauma Survivors: Subtypes and Clinical Utility", *Culture, Medicine and Psychiatry, 34*(2), 209- 218. https://doi.org/10.1007/s11013-010-9175-x

de Jong, J.T.V.M., Komproe, I.H., Van Ommeren, M., El Masri, M., Araya, M., Khaled, N., van de Put, W., and Somasundaram, D. (2001). "Lifetime events and posttraumatic stress disorder in 4 postconflict settings", *JAMA: Journal of the American Medical Association, 286*(5), 555–562. https://doi.org/10.1001/jama.286.5.555

de Jong, K., Ford, N., Kam, S.v., Lokuge, K., Fromm, S., van Galen, R., Reilley, B., and Kleber, R. (2008). "Conflict in the Indian Kashmir Valley I: exposure to violence", *Conflict and Health, 2*, 10. https://doi.org/10.1186/1752-1505-2-10

Kieling, C., Baker-Henningham, H., Belfer, M., Conti, G., Ertem, I., Omigbodun, O., Rohde, L.A., Srinath, S., Ulkuer, N., and Rahman, A. (2011). "Child and adolescent mental health worldwide: Evidence for action", *The Lancet, 378*(9801), 1515–1525. https://doi.org/10.1016/S0140-6736(11)60827-1

Kleinman, A. (2012). "Medical Anthropology and Mental Health: Five Questions for the Next Fifty Years", In M.C. Inhorn and E.A. Wentzell (Ed.), *Medical Anthropology at the Intersections: Histories, Activisms, and Futures* (pp. 116-129). Durham, USA: Duke University Press.

Kohrt, B.A., Mendenhall, E., and Brown, P.J. (2016). "How anthropological theory and methods can advance global mental health", *The Lancet Psychiatry, 3*(5), 396-398. https://doi.org/10.1016/s2215-0366(16)00046-8

Lim, A.G., Stock, L., ShweOo, E.K., and Jutte, D.P. (2013). "Trauma and mental health of medics in eastern Myanmar's conflict zones: A cross-sectional and mixed methods investigation", *Conflict and Health, 7*(1). https://doi.org/10.1186/1752-1505-7-15

Lubit, R., Rovine, D., Defrancisci, L., and Eth, S. (2003). "Impact of trauma on children", *Journal of Psychiatric Practice, 9*(2), 128–138. https://doi.org/10.1097/00131746-200303000-00004

Luitel, N.P., Jordans, M.J., Sapkota, R.P., Tol, W.A., Kohrt, B.A., Thapa, S.B., Komproe, I.H., and Sharma, B. (2012). "Conflict and mental health: A cross-sectional epidemiological study in Nepal", *Social Psychiatry and Psychiatric Epidemiology, 48*(2), 183-193. https://doi.org/10.1007/s00127-012-0539-0

Maughan, B., Iervolino, A.C., and Collishaw, S. (2005). "Time trends in child and adolescent mental disorders", *Current Opinions in Psychiatry, 18*(4), 381-385. https://doi.org/10.1097/01.yco.0000172055.25284.f2

Moussa, S., Kholy, M.E., Enaba, D., Salem, K., Ali, A., Nasreldin, M., Gabal, M., Emadeldin, M., and Moselhy, H.F. (2015). "Impact of political violence on the mental health of school children in Egypt", *Journal of Mental Health, 24*(5), 289-293. https://doi.org/10.3109/09638237.2015.1019047

Nichter, M. (1981). "Idioms of distress: Alternatives in the expression of psychosocial distress: A case study from South India", *Culture, Medicine and Psychiatry, 5*(4), 379-408. https://doi.org/10.1007/bf00054782

Obermeyer, C.M., Bott, S., and Sassine, A.J. (2015). "Arab Adolescents: Health, Gender, Social Context", *Journal of Adolescent Health*, *57*(3), 252-262. https://doi.org/10.1016/j.jadohealth.2015.01.002

Panter-Brick, C., Eggerman, M., Gonzalez, V., and Safdar, S. (2009). "Violence, suffering, and mental health in Afghanistan: A school-based survey", *The Lancet*, *374*(9692), 807-816. https://doi.org/10.1016/s0140-6736(09)61080-1

Panter-Brick, C., Grimon, M., Kalin, M., and Eggerman, M. (2014). "Trauma memories, mental health, and resilience: A prospective study of Afghan youth", *Journal of Child Psychology and Psychiatry, 56*(7), 814-825. https://doi.org/10.1111/jcpp.12350

Patel, V., Flisher, A.J., Hetrick, S., and McGorry, P. (2007). "Mental health of young people: a global public-health challenge", *The Lancet*, *369*(9569), 1302-1313. https://doi.org/10.1016/s0140-6736(07)60368-7

Patton, G.C., Sawyer, S.M., Santelli, J.S., Ross, D.A., Afifi, R., Allen, N.B., Arora, M., Azzopardi, P., Baldwin, W., Bonell, C., Kakuma, R., Kennedy, E., Mahon, J., McGovern, T., Mokdad, A.H., Patel, V., Petroni, S., Reavley, N., Taiwo, K., Waldfogel, J., … Viner, R.M. (2016). "Our future: a Lancet commission on adolescent health and wellbeing", *Lancet (London, England)*, *387*(10036), 2423–2478. https://doi.org/10.1016/S0140-6736(16)00579-1

Paul, L.A., Felton, J.W., Adams, Z.W., Welsh, K., Miller, S., and Ruggiero, K.J. (2015). "Mental Health Among Adolescents Exposed to a Tornado: The Influence of Social Support and its Interactions with Sociodemographic Characteristics and Disaster Exposure", *Journal of Trauma Stress, 28*(3), 232-239. https://doi.org/10.1002/jts.22012

Pedersen, D. (2002). "Political violence, ethnic conflict, and contemporary wars: broad implications for health and social well-being", *Social Science and Medicine, 55*(2), 175-190. https://doi.org/10.1016/s0277-9536(01)00261-1

Rabaia, Y., Saleh, M.F., and Giacaman, R. (2014). "Sick or Sad? Supporting Palestinian Children Living in Conditions of Chronic Political Violence", *Children and Society, 28*(3), 172-181. https://doi.org/10.1111/chso.12061

Rasmussen, D.J., Karsberg, S., Karstoft, K.-I., and Elklit, A. (2013). "Victimization and PTSD in an Indian youth sample from Pune City", *Open Journal of Epidemiology, 3*(1), 12-19. https://doi.org/10.4236/ojepi.2013.31003

Ravens-Sieberer, U., Wille, N., Erhart, M., Bettge, S., Wittchen, H., Rothenberger, A., Herpertz-Dahlmann, B., Resch, F., Hölling, H., Bullinger, M., Barkmann, C., Schulte-Markwort, M., Döpfner, M., and BELLA study group. (2008). "Prevalence of mental health problems among children and adolescents in Germany: Results of the BELLA study within the national health interview and examination survey", *European Child and Adolescent Psychiatry*, *17*(S1), 22-33. https://doi.org/10.1007/s00787-008-1003-2

Ravens-Sieberer, U., Otto, C., Kriston, L., Rothenberger, A., Döpfner, M., Herpertz-Dahlmann, B., Barkmann, C., Schön, G., Hölling, H., Schulte-Markwort, M., Klasen, F., and BELLA Study Group. (2014). "The longitudinal BELLA study: Design, methods and first results on the course of mental health problems", *European Child and Adolescent Psychiatry, 24*(6), 651-663. https://doi.org/10.1007/s00787-014-0638-4

Reijneveld, S.A., Crone, M.R., Schuller, A.A., Verhulst, F.C., and Verloove-Vanhorick, S.P. (2004). "The changing impact of a severe disaster on the mental health and substance misuse of adolescents: Follow-up of a controlled study", *Psychological Medicine, 35*(3), 367-376. https://doi.org/10.1017/s0033291704003575

Rosenthal, B.S. (2000). "Exposure to community violence in adolescence: Trauma symptoms", *Adolescence, 35*(138), 271-284.

Schiff, M., Zweig, H.H., Benbenishty, R., and Hasin, D.S. (2007). "Exposure to Terrorism and Israeli Youth's Cigarette, Alcohol, and Cannabis Use", *American Journal of Public Health, 97*(10), 1852-1858.https://doi.org/10.2105/ajph.2006.090514

Schmid, K., and Muldoon, O.T. (2013). "Perceived Threat, Social Identification, and Psychological Well-Being: The Effects of Political Conflict Exposure", *Political Psychology, 36*(1), 75-92. https://doi.org/10.1111/pops.12073

Seethalakshmi, R., Dhavale, H.S., Gawande, S., and Dewan, M. (2006). "Psychiatric morbidity following motor vehicle crashes: A pilot study from India", *Journal of Psychiatric Practice, 12*(6), 415-418. https://doi.org/10.1097/00131746-200611000-00012

Sharifi, V., Mojtabai, R., Shahrivar, Z., Alaghband-Rad, J., Zarafshan, H., and Wissow, L. (2016). "Child and adolescent mental health care in Iran: Current status and future direction", *Archives of Iranian Medicine, 19*(11), 797-804.

Shaw, J.A. (2000). "Children, adolescents and trauma", *Psychiatric Quarterly, 71*(3), 227–243. https://doi.org/10.1023/A:1004630127000

Slone, M., and Mayer, Y. (2015). "Gender differences in mental health consequences of exposure to political violence among Israeli adolescents", *Children and Youth Services Review, 58*, 170-178. https://doi.org/10.1016/j.childyouth.2015.09.013

Slone, M., and Shechner, T. (2009). "Psychiatric consequences for Israeli adolescents of protracted political violence: 1998–2004", *Journal of Child Psychology and Psychiatry, 50*(3), 280-289. https://doi.org/10.1111/j.1469-7610.2008.01940.x

Soleimanpour, S., Geierstanger, S., and Brindis, C.D. (2017). "Adverse childhood experiences and resilience: Addressing the unique needs of adolescents", *Academic Pediatrics, 17*(7S), S108-S114. https://doi.org/10.1016/j.acap.2017.01.008

Sousa, C.A., Kemp, S., and El-Zuhairi, M. (2014). "Dwelling Within Political Violence: Palestinian women's narratives of home, mental health, and resilience", *Health Place, 30,* 205-214. https://doi.org/10.1016/j.healthplace.2014.09.005

Spooner, C. (1999). "Causes and correlates of adolescent drug abuse and implications for treatment", *Drug and Alcohol Review, 18*(4), 453-475. https://doi.org/10.1080/09595239996329

Srinath, S., Kandasamy, P., and Golhar, T.S. (2010). "Epidemiology of child and adolescent mental health disorders", *Current Opinion in Psychiatry, 23*(4), 330-336. https://doi.org/10.1097/YCO.0b013e32833aa0c1

Stikkelbroek, Y., Bodden, D.H., Reitz, E., Vollebergh, W.A., and van Baar, A.L. (2016). "Mental health of adolescents before and after the death of a parent or sibling", *European child and adolescent psychiatry, 25*(1), 49–59. https://doi.org/10.1007/s00787-015-0695-3

Thirthalli, J., Zhou, L., Kumar, K., Gao, J., Vaid, H., Liu, H., Hankey, A., Wang, G., Gangadhar, B.N., Nie, J., and Nichter, M. (2016). "Traditional, complementary, and alternative medicine approaches to mental health care and psychological wellbeing in India and China", *The Lancet Psychiatry, 3*(7), 660-672. https://doi.org/10.1016/s2215-0366(16)30025-6

Tol, W.A., Rees, S.J., and Silove, D.M. (2013). "Broadening the scope of epidemiology in conflict-affected settings: Opportunities for mental health prevention and promotion", *Epidemiology and Psychiatric Sciences, 22*(3), 197-203. https://doi.org/10.1017/s2045796013000188

Varela, R.E. and Hensley, M.L. (2009). "The Influence of Culture on Anxiety in Latino Youth: A review", *Clinical Child Family Psychology Review, 12*(3), 217-23. https://doi.org/10.1007/s10567-009-0044-5

Ventevogel, P., Jordans, M., Reis, R., and De Jong, J. (2013). "Madness or sadness? Local concepts of mental illness in four conflict-affected African communities", *Conflict and Health, 7*(1). https://doi.org/10.1186/1752-1505-7-3

Wang, C., Chan, C.L., and Ho, R.T. (2013). "Prevalence and trajectory of psychopathology among child and adolescent survivors of disasters: A systematic review of epidemiological studies across 1987–2011", *Social Psychiatry and Psychiatric Epidemiology, 48*(11), 1697-1720. https://doi.org/10.1007/s00127-013-0731-x

Weine. S.M. and Chae. S.R. (2008). "Trauma, disputed knowledge, and storying resilience", University of Illinois, Chicago. *Incore.* 1-47.

World Health Organization. (2014). Adolescents: Health risks and solutions. Fact sheet 345; Available at: http://www.who.int/mediacentre/factsheets/fs345/en/

William, R., Alexander, D.A., Bolsover, D., and Bakke, F.K. (2008). "Children, resilience and disasters: Recent evidence that should influence a model of psychosocial care", *Current Opinion in Psychiatry, 21*(4), 338-344. https://doi.org/10.1097/yco.0b013e328305b6e4

Yazdani, A., Zadeh, Z.F., and Shafi, K. (2015). "Gender differences in adolescents experiencing vicarious trauma", *Pakistan Journal of Clinical Psychology, 14*(1), 27-39.

Young, A. (1996). "Suffering and the Origins of Traumatic Memory", *Daedalus, 125*(1), 245-260.

Young, A. (2012). "The Social Brain and the Myth of Empathy", *Science in Context, 25*(3), 401-424. https://doi.org/10.1017/s0269889712000129

Young, A., and Rees, T. (2011). "Medical Anthropology Enters the 21st Century", *The Journal of Nervous and Mental Disease, 199*(8), 592-596. https://doi.org/10.1097/nmd.0b013e318225f344

19

Psychological Health and Wellbeing among Infertile Women

A Hospital-based Case-Control Study from North India

Chakraverti Mahajan, Apoorva Sharma, Manju Puri, Nandita Babu and *Kallur Nava Saraswathy*

Introduction

Infertility is defined as the state of failure to conceive after one year of unprotected sexual intercourse. Infertility affects millions of individuals and couples, and the estimates vary from 48.5 million couples to 120 million women worldwide (Njagi, 2020). The prevalence of infertility ranges between 8 per cent and 12 per cent worldwide, with high infertility prevalence in South Asia, sub-Saharan Africa, the Middle East and North Africa, Central and Eastern Europe and Central Asia (Inhorn and Patrizio, 2015). In low-income countries, such as India, the burden of infertility is considered to be even higher. The total number of infertile people in India stands close to 13.9 million (Ganguly and Unisa, 2010). The Indian Society for Assisted Reproduction (ISAR) has stated that in India, 'up to one in six couples have difficulties in conceiving and many seek medical advice and treatment' (ISAR, 2017).

Infertility, apart from being a medical condition, also has a social dimension. As biological and social beings, humans bear an inherent desire to reproduce. Procreation is seen as a critical endeavour in human society, and it is strongly related to the ultimate goals of completeness, happiness and family integration. Failure to procreate can have social and psychological consequences on the individual. These may range from overt ostracism or divorce to more subtle forms of social stigma leading to isolation and mental distress (World Health Organization, 2003; Rutstein and Shah, 2014). Thus, infertility serves as a poorly-controlled, chronic stressor with severe, long-lasting negative social and psychological consequences on the couples. Studies reveal that infertility driven stress has 'direct and indirect effect on infertile couples that decreases their evaluations of life-as-a-whole, self-efficacy, marriage, intimacy, and health' (Andrews *et al.*, 2020). Both infertile women and men tend to have more psychiatric morbidity than women and men not experiencing infertility. In highly pro-natalist and patriarchal societies like India, women suffer from the brunt of childlessness's social, psychological and physical consequences. Infertility also leads to abuse, marital instability, social isolation, and loss of self-esteem (Behboodi-Moghadam *et al.*, 2010).

The present chapter is based on an ongoing study that seeks to understand the relationship between infertility and psychological health and wellbeing. Funded by the National Commission of Women (NCW), the study is being conducted by the Department of Anthropology, University of Delhi, in collaboration with the Department of Obstetrics and Gynaecology at Lady Hardinge Medical College (LHMC), New Delhi and the Department of Psychology, University of Delhi. The study aims to understand the impact of infertility on the psychological health and wellbeing of women who have primary infertility. The study attempts to answer whether infertility is associated with the psychological health and wellbeing of women. What are the factors that determine psychological health and wellbeing in infertile women? How is their life affected by the experience of infertility and its treatment? Can there be a social intervention tool that can help clinicians provide better treatment and care to infertile women? This chapter shares some of the preliminary findings of the more extensive study on these research questions.

Research Settings and Methods

The present case-control study is being carried out at the Department of Obstetrics and Gynaecology at the Lady Hardinge Medical College (LMHC), New Delhi. A total of 500 women were included; out of which 250 are women with primary infertility (cases) and another 250 age-matched fertile women (controls). Sample size is calculated using the formula: n = (Z2 × P (1 / P)) /e2 (Daniel, 1999)

P = 0.20; e = 0.05; Z = 1.96;
n = 3.84 × 0.20 × (1-0.20) / (0.05)2
n = 0.6144 / 0.0025
n = 245.76 ~ 246

Where:

Z is value from standard normal distribution corresponding to desired confidence level (Z = 1.96 for 95% CI)

P is expected true proportion

e is desired preciseness (half desired CI width).

The inclusion criteria for age of cases were married women with primary infertility and their age ranging from twenty years to thirty-five years. The exclusion criterion for cases was women with successful pregnancy outcomes. Inclusion Criteria for the age of controls was similar to cases, i.e. twenty to thirty-five years. The women with successful pregnancy and having at least one child who was older than one year were considered fertile.

The data were collected from August 2020 to February 2021. The non-probability consecutive sampling method was used for collecting data from the infertile women and fertile women. Non-probability consecutive sampling means the information was collected from one infertile woman or fertile women after another until the number of cases and controls had been reached. We interviewed the infertile women in the Out Patient Department (OPD) of the Department of Gynaecology and Obstetrics of the LMHC. Within the Department of Gynaecology and Obstetrics, every Tuesday, between 1:00 pm to 3:00 pm, the doctors provide consultation and treatment services to infertile women. Therefore, the field team visited the department on Tuesdays to interview infertile women.

Initially, the concerned doctor referred the women (who consented to participate) with primary infertility for the interview. Later, the team began to identify women with primary infertility from the waiting room in the OPD. Also, word spread from one interviewed woman to another, and women seemed interested in being interviewed. The field team was provided with a separate room at the department to interview the women in private. For every infertile woman the team interviewed at the department, a fertile woman of the same age who came from a similar socio-economic background and area was interviewed. Interviewing the control group women were less challenging than interviewing the infertile women as the latter group was more reserved about divulging details of their private lives.

For interviewing women, a pretested quantitative interview schedule was used. The first part of the schedule included demographic variables such as name, age, household composition, educational status, occupational status, social-economic status, family structure and reproductive profile.

The second part of the schedule consisted of psychological tools for stress, anxiety, depression, psychological and emotional wellbeing. For each variable, Psychological tools related were administered in English and Hindi version to all the participants, i.e. both the cases and the controls.

During these interviews, women opened up about the challenges they faced in their personal lives regarding infertility. There were numerous occasions where women broke out in tears while narrating the ordeals they faced because of failing to bear children. Stories of domestic abuse, financial constraints and disgrace in everyday life surfaced up during the interview sessions.

The Ethical Committee at Lady Hardinge Medical College granted ethical approval for the study. The study participants were fully informed about the aim of the study. Before data collection, written informed consent was obtained from each participant. After reaching an adequate sample size, data were analyzed using statistical tools.

Statistical Analysis

Pearson's chi-square test or Fisher's exact test was carried out for comparing categorical data. For all statistical tests, $p<0.05$ was considered to be statistically significant. Odds Ratio of having poor wellbeing was calculated using logistic regression analysis in which infertility and fertility are independent variables and wellbeing is the dependent variable. The known confounding factors available in the data set: age, education, occupation of husband, family income, family structure reproductive age, age at marriage and married for how long were selected for the model. All statistical analyses were carried out using SPSS, IBM version 21, with a significance level of 0.05. Descriptive statistics were used for quantitative variables and were expressed as mean, standard deviation or frequencies and percentage.

Psychological Tools used for Psychological Variables

Stress: Perceived Stress Scale (PSS) was used to measure the perception of stress. It is a measure of the degree to which situations in one's life are estimated as stressful. The questions in the PSS ask about feelings and thoughts experienced by the participants during the previous month.

Anxiety: The participants were screened for anxiety through the generalized anxiety disorder seven-item (GAD-7) psychological parameter or tool for anxiety (Spitzer *et al.*, 2006). GAD-7 has seven items, which measure the severity of various signs of GAD according to reported response categories with assigned points (Lowe *et al.*, 2008). The questionnaire includes questions on (i) nervousness; (ii) inability to stop worrying; (iii) excessive worry; (iv) restlessness; (v) difficulty in relaxing; (vi) easy irritation; and (vii) fear of something awful happening.

Depression: To assess the severity of depression and response to treatment, we used the Patient Health Questionnaire 9-Items (PHQ-9) in the study. It scores each of the 9 DSM-IV criteria as "0" (not at all) to "3" (nearly everyday).

Psychological Tools for Wellbeing Variables

Psychological Wellbeing: WHO 5 perceived wellbeing scale for measuring psychological wellbeing among the participants. The WHO-5 is a five-item questionnaire assessing general functional and psychological wellbeing (Topp *et al.*, 2015). It was derived from the WHO (Ten) Well Being Index (Bech, Gudex, & Johansen, 1996) and is used to measure psychological wellbeing. In the questionnaire, respondents rate the five positively worded items on WHO-5 on a six-point Likert scale, from 0 representing 'a total absence of wellbeing' to 5 representing 'a strong feeling of wellbeing'.

Emotional Wellbeing: Positive and Negative Affect Schedule-Short Form (PANAS SF) is a tool that comprises twenty items relating to a 'positive affect' domain—containing ten items and a 'negative affect' domain—containing ten items. A five-point Likert scale is used for scoring in the PANAS where a score of 1 represents 'very slightly or not at all, and a score of 5 represents 'extremely'. For both PANAS domains, scores can range from 10 to 50. A higher score in the positive affect domain indicates a more significant positive effect (e.g. reflecting happiness), whereas a higher score in the negative affect domain indicates a significant adverse effect (e.g. reflecting a depressed or dysphoric state)(Watson, D. 1988). Scores less than the mean positive score describe less positive emotional wellbeing, and more than the mean positive score describes better positive wellbeing.

Results and Conclusions

The cases (n = 250) interviewed in the study included 44 per cent of women between the reproductive ages of 26-30. A total of 39 per cent of women belonged to up to 25 years of age. Women with more than 30 years of ages were less in number. It was probably because, by the age of 30, women either had successful pregnancies resulting in childbirth or had developed better coping mechanisms with their increasing age. Among various psychological or mental health factors, infertile women were at a higher risk to be anxious than fertile women, and they also were more prone to stress than fertile women. The infertile women showed a higher risk of being depressed, and their day-to-day functioning was severely affected. We found that the emotional wellbeing of infertile women had fewer scores of positive wellbeing and more scores for negative wellbeing. The poor wellbeing resulted in reduced work efficiency for the couples, tumultuous relationship between the couple which threatened their marriage and poor social interaction with friends and family.

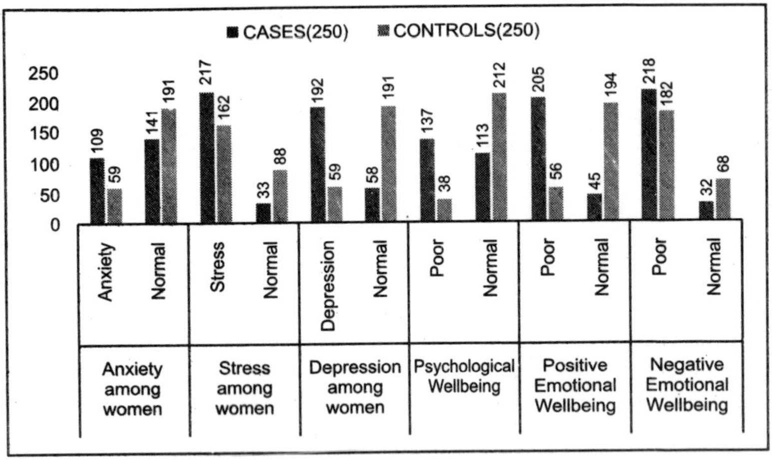

Fig. 19.1: Psychological and emotional wellbeing among cases and controls

Psychological Health and Infertility

Psychological factors of infertile women were diagnosed with the help of three variables, i.e. stress, anxiety and depression.

Stress: According to PSS scores in Figure 19.1, 87 per cent of infertile women experienced stress, of which 64 per cent of women experienced moderate stress, and 22 per cent of women experienced severe stress. Among the fertile women, 64 per cent of women were found stressed, of which 60 per cent experienced moderate stress, and 4 per cent of women experienced severe stress.

Stress was higher in infertile women with a significant association (p-value <0.05). According to the regression analysis of various variables with stress, the husband's occupational status was one of the causes of stress among infertile women. The men who were daily wage earners or who did not earn at all caused more stress to infertile women than men in better jobs like government jobs or businesses. Women who slept less than six hours a day tended to be more stressed than women who slept for more than six hours.

Anxiety: According to GAD-7, 44 per cent of infertile women had anxiety, including 27 per cent moderate anxiety and 16 per cent severe anxiety. Among the fertile women, 23 per cent women were found to have anxiety, of which 21 per cent women had moderate anxiety and only 2 per cent women had severe anxiety. The results of the anxiety tool demonstrated significant anxiety among infertile women (p-value <0.05). Among the various demographics, lifestyle and reproductive profile factors, education was the only variable that showed significance among the anxiety levels of infertile women. Women who were more educated, i.e. women who were graduate or had higher qualification than graduation, had higher anxiety levels than the women who were less educated.

Depression: Depression was one of the most common psychiatric disorders found among infertile patients. One of the participants described that she sleeps the entire day and is very lethargic most of the times. She was seeking treatment because her husband and his family pressurize her and fight with her. She also said that she was not sure if she wanted to have children or not. She was further referred for psychiatric help in LHMC. To assess the severity of depression and response to treatment, we used the Patient Health Questionnaire 9-Items (PHQ-9) in the study. According to PHQ-9 responses, 77 per cent of the infertile women had depression, of which 39 per cent women had mild depression, 26 per cent women had moderate depression, 15 per cent women had moderately severe depression and 3 per cent women had severe depression. Among the fertile women, 23 per cent of women were found to have depression, of which 11 per cent women had mild depression, 9 per cent of women had moderate depression and nearly 3 per cent women had moderately severe depression. Depression was higher among infertile women than fertile women with a statistically significant association (p value<0.05). Within infertile women, we evaluated various risk factors which might cause depression. According to the regression analysis, the significant factors that showed its impact on the severity of depression among infertile women were exercise duration, infertility, and bleeding during menstruation. Women who used to exercise more frequently were less depressed as compared to women who did not exercise. Women who suffered from heavy bleeding during menstruation were found to be more depressed. Duration of infertility also had an impact on the severity of depression among infertile women. Infertile women with five to ten years of endurance were more depressed than women who had infertility for less than five years.

Wellbeing and Infertility

Well-being, a prudential value or quality of life, refers to what is intrinsically valuable to someone. Thus, a person's wellbeing is ultimately suitable for this person, in this person's self-interest (Roger, 2017). Wellbeing can also be referred to as both positive and negative wellbeing. In its positive sense, it is sometimes contrasted with ill-being (Heady *et al.*, 1984). In this study, wellbeing was screened based on the psychological and emotional wellbeing of an individual.

Psychological Wellbeing: An individual's emotional health and overall functioning is defined as his psychological wellbeing. Huppert (2009), in his study published in *Applied Psychology: Health and Well-Being*, described psychological wellbeing as the combination of feeling competent and functioning effectively. Infertility was perceived as a stressful life situation and influenced an individual's psychological adjustment. Among infertile women, we found that 55 per cent of respondents had a score indicating flawed psychological wellbeing. There was a prevalence of signs of depression among 17 per cent of infertile women who had scores below seven. Among fertile women, 15 per cent of women indicated poor psychological wellbeing, and 85 per cent indicated average or good psychological wellbeing. There was a significant difference in the psychological wellbeing scores of infertile women and fertile women. These issues were generally related to the duration of infertility, and 'the longer the participants experienced infertility, the more they had poor psychological wellbeing' (Hasanpoor-Azqhdy, 2014). The infertile women for more than five years had more poor psychological wellbeing scores.

Emotional Wellbeing: Emotional wellbeing refers to the emotional quality of an individual's experiences (Kahneman *et al.*, 2010). According to the PANAS SF Positive scores in the study, we found that 82 per cent of the infertile women and 22 per cent fertile women had scored less than the mean positive score for the positive emotional aspects of the PANAS scale. Eighteen per cent of infertile women and 77 per cent of fertile women had scored more than the mean positive score.

We found that positive emotional wellbeing among infertile women was affected by the duration of infertility, physical activity and belief systems. Women who were infertile for less than five years had better wellbeing scores than those infertile for more than five years. Women who were more physically active and more frequent in doing exercise were had positive emotional wellbeing scores. Women who considered themselves highly religious had poorer scores of positive emotional wellbeing. According to PANAS SF Negative scores, 87 per cent of infertile women and 72 per cent of fertile women had scored more than the mean negative score of PANAS. 13 per cent out of total infertile women, and 27 per cent of fertile women had scored less than the mean negative score. Scores more than the mean negative score for PANAS SF negative scale describe more negative emotions, whereas scores below the mean score show normal negative emotions. Occupation of the husband, family structure and educational status of the participants showed significant association with the negative emotional wellbeing scores. Women whose husband's had private jobs and lived in a joint family structure suffered from a more negative emotional state. Women who were highly educated suffered from more negative emotional wellbeing than women who were less educated. There were feelings of loneliness and guilt from items that participants reported. Women with infertility were found to have a poor emotional state as compared to fertile women.

Apart from the physiological problems, women suffered from several preventable problems such as Polycystic Ovarian Syndrome, blocked fallopian tubes, endometriosis, cysts, fibroids, double damage, miscarriages, disturbed menstrual cycles, contraception complications, abortions, and sexually transmitted infections. Despite all the variables, it is evident that infertility is the primary cause affecting women's psychological health and wellbeing.

General Observations

We found that infertile women were more prone to mental health or psychological disorders and poor wellbeing than fertile women. The infertile women often used the expression 'being tensed to express their constant worrying towards childbearing. Infertile women could better understand and respond to the questions asked from the psychological tools as compared to fertile women. The infertile women had experienced a higher degree of psychological duress from their husband, family members and community. They had a constant desire to have a child, and this desire intensified every month, bringing them misery and personal discomfort. This misery and discomfort coupled with failure to achieve a viable pregnancy further affected the sexual life of the infertile couples, which in turn intensified their feeling of hopelessness and reduced their self-worth. Infertile couples who had invested a large sum of money in their treatment with the hopes of attaining parenthood found the prospect of a failed treatment intolerable. Couples felt devastated and bereaved when they found themselves pregnant after the initial treatment, and the pregnancy was interrupted at a later stage. One of the women interviewed at LHMC expressed her anguish in these words, "we expect a lot from this treatment, and when it fails, the disappointment is enormous".

In this section, we have discussed the broader trends observed in the data during the analysis stage. However, a detailed analysis of the data is still ongoing and would be communicated to reputed journals in the coming months.

Discussion

Infertility is becoming a serious concern. Many reasons have been attributed to the increase in infertility rates. Urbanization, family income, husband's occupational status, higher literacy, different contraceptive usages, and nuclear families also play a significant role in infertility. This study attempted to establish this association and assess various psychological or mental health and wellbeing factors about infertility in North Indian women. The study found that infertile women were more prone to psychological disorders and poor wellbeing than fertile women. Our study is supported by Reija Klemetti Jani Raitanen *et al.* (2010), where the author states that infertile women and men report poor psychological symptoms and subjective wellbeing. Mental health factors for infertility were calculated for Stress, Anxiety and Depression. It was found that infertile women were more prone to stress than women with children, and infertility causes stress which is in contrast to a study that states that women and men with infertility report high levels of distress that can impact their quality of life (Rooney, K.L., 2016). Stress in infertile women significantly associated with the husband's occupational status and hours of sleep taken by the women. Infertile women were anxiously trying to conceive, which was very prevalent from the initial interview stage itself. Infertile women were found to be more anxious than fertile women. Because of such pressure, partners may become more anxious to conceive, ironically increasing their sexual dysfunction and social isolation. Women who were more educated, i.e. women who were graduates or had higher qualification than graduation, experienced higher anxiety levels than women who were less educated. Depression being a clinical factor, was also found to be higher among the women who were trying to conceive and were infertile. Lee (2007) shows that the social pressure of non-fulfilment of the wish to have biological children has been associated with depression, anger, anxiety, marital problems and feelings of worthlessness. Significant factors associated with the severity of depression among infertile women were exercise, duration of infertility and bleeding during menstruation. Our study is also supported by research by Lamia Yusuf (2016) where it states that there was a high prevalence of depression, anxiety and stress among females who have infertility compared to females in the control group ($p < 0.05$). Apart from this, the psychological and emotional wellbeing of the respondents was calculated. State of wellness or psychological wellbeing was found to be better among the fertile group of women. Infertility affected couples psychological wellbeing, marital relationships, sexual relationships, and quality of life (Luk and Loke, 2015). Emotional wellbeing was described according to the positive and negative state of mind. Infertile women were found to have poor positive emotional state. Also, the negative emotions were found to be more prevalent among infertile women. More significant observations included a more negative emotional state in women living in joint families than women in nuclear families, demonstrating that instead of providing a healthy coping mechanism, the joint family system negatively impacted infertile women. Women who were highly educated suffered from more negative emotional wellbeing than women who were less educated. Despite the covariants like education, occupational status, family structure, reproductive health having some role, infertility is the significant risk factor affecting mental health and women's wellbeing. During the study, women who were found to be severely depressed, stressed, anxious or experiencing inferior psychological and emotional wellbeing were referred to the psychiatry department at LHMC for further treatment and care. During the interviews, we also found several narratives of alcoholism in the husbands and domestic violence directed at women, alleviating their scores in the assessment and showing their abject suffering in their quest for childhood. In the hospital, women were treated for the disease of their bodies and not the disease of their minds. So psychological and emotional support was provided to most of these women, and the biomedical approach of treating lacked a sensitive approach. Infertility is a highly stigmatized and debilitating experience for couples, and we recommend that the humanization of biomedicine and sensitization of health professionals would go a long way in alleviating the troubles of infertility patients. For this purpose, we also plan to use the data and insight from the present study to develop psychological intervention tools to help clinicians provide a wholesome treatment to infertility patients. We also encourage more qualitative research on infertility and its association with psychological and emotional wellbeing in couples.

Conclusion

Infertile women were more vulnerable to poor psychological health and wellbeing than their fertile counterparts. This study demonstrates that adding professional trained social workers to infertility clinics as a supplemental medical intervention is beneficial. The study found that in the hospital setting, although, women were treated for infertility, their psychological health and wellbeing was not considered. This study records that women struggling with infertility require psychological and emotional support in terms of counseling. Some interventions need to be designed to alleviate the symptoms of stress, depression, anxiety and poor psychological and emotional wellbeing in infertile women. This study suggests that having professional trained social workers as complementary medical interventions in the infertility clinics is central to manage the issue of infertility in all aspects. This professional assistance not only meets the needs on infertile people but also the needs of the social system in which infertile people are living. In this view, social workers can support the rights and needs of infertile people as a means to development planning by policy-makers so that the infertility can be looked upon as a biopsychic social phenomenon.

Acknowledgement : The authors express their gratitude to the research team Rashmi Patel, Navjot Kamboj, Sweta Prasad, Ankita Chandel and Shivani Tyagi. We also thank the National Commission for Women (NCW) of India for funding the project. We are thankful to the staff of Lady Hardinge Medical College, New Delhi, and the participants who cooperated with the research team.

REFERENCES

Andrews, F.M., Abbey, A., and Halman, L.J. (1991). "Stress from infertility, marriage factors, and subjective well-being of wives and husbands", *Journal of health and social behaviour*, *32*(3), 238-253. https://doi.org/10.2307/2136806

Bech, P., Gudex, C., and Johansen, K.S. (1996). "The WHO (Ten) well-being index: validation in diabetes", *Psychotherapy and psychosomatics*, *65*(4), 183-190. https://doi.org/10.1159/000289073

Behboodi-Moghadam, Z., Salsali, M., Eftekhar-Ardabily, H., Vaismoradi, M., and Ramezanzadeh, F. (2013). "Experiences of infertility through the lens of Iranian infertile women: a qualitative study", *Japan Journal of Nursing Science*, *10*(1), 41-46. https://doi.org/10.1111/j.1742-7924.2012.00208.x

Ferreira-Borges, C. (2014). "Mental Health: Strengthening Health and Development Opportunities in the WHO African Region", *International Psychiatry, 11*(1), 3-6. doi:10.1192/S1749367600004161

Hasanpoor, A.S.B., Simbar, M., Vedadhir, A., and AMIRI, F.L. (2016). "Exploring the challenge of adoption from the perspective of Iranian infertile women", *Journal of client centered nursing care, 2*(1), 20-26. https://www.sid.ir/en/journal/ViewPaper.aspx?id=523508

Huppert, F.A. (2009). "Psychological well-being: Evidence regarding its causes and consequences", *Applied Psychology: Health and Well-Being*, *1*(2), 137-164. https://doi.org/10.1111/j.1758-0854.2009.01008.x

Inhorn, M.C., and Patrizio, P. (2015). "Infertility around the globe: New thinking on gender, reproductive technologies and global movements in the 21st century". *Human reproduction update*, *21*(4), 411-426. https://doi.org/10.1093/humupd/dmv016

Indian Society for Assisted Reproduction. (2017). Retrieved on 18th April, 2021, from https://www.isarindia.net/general_info.php.

Kahneman, D., and Deaton, A. (2010). "High income improves evaluation of life but not emotional well-being", *Proceedings of the National Academy of Sciences, 107*, 16489-16493. https://doi.org/10.1073/pnas.1011492107

Kazandi, M., Gunday, O., Mermer, T.K., Erturk, N., and Ozkınay, E. (2011). "The status of depression and anxiety in infertile Turkish couples", *Iranian journal of reproductive medicine*, *9*(2), 99-104. https://www.ncbi.nlm.nih.gov/pmc/articles/PMC4216443/#__ffn_sectitle

Klemetti, R., Raitanen, J., Shiva, S., Saarni, S., and Koponen, P. (2010). "Infertility, mental disorders and well-being—A nationwide survey", *Acta obstetricia et gynecologica Scandinavica*, *89*(5), 677-682.https://doi.org/10.3109/00016341003623746

Lee, M. (2017). "Don't give up! A cyber-ethnography and discourse analysis of an online infertility patient forum", *Culture, Medicine, and Psychiatry*, *41*(3), 341-367. https://doi.org/10.1007/s11013-016-9515-6

Löwe, B., Decker, O., Müller, S., Brähler, E., Schellberg, D., Herzog, W., and Herzberg, P.Y. (2008). "Validation and standardization of the Generalized Anxiety Disorder Screener (GAD-7) in the general population", *Medical care*, 266-274. https://www.jstor.org/stable/40221654

Luk, B.H.K. and Loke, A.Y. (2015). "The impact of infertility on the psychological well-being, marital relationships, sexual relationships, and quality of life of couples: A systematic review", *Journal of sex and marital therapy, 41*(6), 610-625. https://doi.org/10.1080/0092623X.2014.958789

Manimekalai, K., Poulpunitha, S., and Veeramani, P. (2020). "Infertility: An Alarming Situation in India", *International Journal of Scientific and Technology Research, 9*(2), 2606-2609.

Njagi, P., Groot, W., Arsenijevic, J., Dyer, S., Mburu, G., and Kiarie, J. (2020)."Economic costs of infertility care for patients in low-income and middle-income countries: A systematic review protocol", *BMJ open, 10*(11), e042951.doi: 10.1136/bmjopen-2020-042951

Oberhelman, D.D. (2001), "Stanford Encyclopedia of Philosophy", *Reference Reviews, 15* (6), 9-9. https://doi.org/10.1108/rr.2001.15.6.9.311

Onat, G., and Beji, N.K. (2012). "Marital relationship and quality of life among couples with infertility", *Sexuality and Disability, 30*(1), 39-52. https://doi.org/10.1007/s11195-011-9233-5

Ramezanzadeh, F., Aghssa, M.M., Abedinia, N., Zayeri, F., Khanafshar, N., Shariat, M., and Jafarabadi, M. (2004). "A survey of relationship between anxiety, depression and duration of infertility", *BMC women's health, 4*(1), 1-7. https://doi.org/10.1186/1472-6874-4-9

Rooney, K.L., and Domar, A.D. (2016). "The impact of stress on fertility treatment", *Current Opinion in Obstetrics and Gynecology, 28*(3), 198-201. doi: 10.1097/GCO.0000000000000261

Max Roser (2014). "Fertility Rate". Published online at *Our World In Data*. Retrieved from: https://ourworldindata.org/fertility-rate

Rutstein, S.O. and Shah, I.H. (2004). *Infecundity, Infertility, and Childlessness in Developing Countries* (No. 9). ORC Macro, MEASURE DHS.

Skakkebaek, N.E., and Giwercman, A. (1994). Pathogenesis and Management of Male Infertility. *The Lancet, 343*(8911), 1473-1479.

Topp, C.W., Østergaard, S.D., Søndergaard, S., and Bech, P. (2015). *The WHO-5 Well-Being Index: A Systematic Review of the Literature. Psychotherapy and Psychosomatics, 84*(3), 167-176. doi:10.1159/000376585

Ganguly, S., and Unisa, S. (2010). "Trends of infertility and childlessness in India: Findings from NFHS data", *Facts, views and vision in ObGyn, 2*(2), 131-138.

Watson, D. (1988). "Intraindividual and interindividual analyses of positive and negative affect: their relation to health complaints, perceived stress, and daily activities", *Journal of personality and social psychology, 54*(6), 1020-1030. https://psycnet.apa.org/doi/10.1037/0022-3514.54.6.1020

World Health Organization. (2003). "Towards adulthood: exploring the sexual and reproductive health of adolescents in South Asia", *World Health Organization.*

Yusuf, L. (2016). "Depression, anxiety and stress among female patients of infertility: A case control study", *Pakistan journal of medical sciences, 32*(6), 1340-1343. https://www.ncbi.nlm.nih.gov/pmc/articles/PMC5216278/

20

Disability and Adoption

Anthropological Reflections on Mental Health and Well-Being of Children with 'Special Needs' in India

Mitashree Srivastava and *Tajinder Kaur*

Introduction and Overview

Disability and Health is a major area of concern for anthropologists now a days. Ablon (1995) explained that people with disabilities are often labelled as "the Other," that separated them to those who does not have any kind of disability. According to Reid-Cunningham (2009), anthropologist's sincere interests with 'the Other' can logically inform the field of disability studies, but not been fully utilized. Therefore, this article attempts to explore the multidimensional nature of the problem of disability by linking it to the problem of adoption of children with disabilities and their mental and social well-being.

The multidimensional nature of the anthropological contribution to disability studies and adoption can be grasped through the perspective of kinship studies and can be viewed through the following interpretations; adoption solely for acquiring a legal and spiritual heir or son rather than training and caring for a child especially in the context of Indian culture, belongingness of a particular person or an infant in a family according to parents expectation, birth being not the only thing which can incorporate an infant into a family, religious ceremonies matter; adoption being "social kinship or nothing" and a debate among anthropologists about the treatment of adoption as equivalent or dissimilar to kinship as both take in account related to variability of biogenetic substance (Bhardwaj, 2016; Modell, 1994; Durkheim, 1896; Schneider, 1980). According to Jessica (2018), there is a difference between the 'social kinship' and 'biological kinship' in the case of the adoption and disability, which deviates from the norms formulated by the society. Although, very little adoption literature addresses the often unspoken needs of families who want to adopt or have adopted children with disabilities (Gretchen, 2016). Therefore, in this study, as one of the objectives; we are trying to examine the role of prospective adoptive parents, who want to adopt and bring a child with 'special' needs into their family; irrespective of the norms fabricated by the society. On the contrary, it also spoke about the challenges and struggles faced by them in the time-consuming process of adoption.

Rationale: Considering that both disability and adoption are regarded as social problems in India and are both attached to notion of stigma that adds up to their vulnerability zones, the problem of disability and adoption deserves to be explored disability and adoption in India. Be it lesser opportunities of adoption of children with 'special needs' or be it the PAPs (Prospective Adaptive Parents) disabled PAP's who are denied rights of adoption of children, the cases seem gloomy. An anthropological investigation may highlight the mental health challenges at both fronts and look into the issues of their marginalization.

Research Questions

- What are the needs and challenges of children with 'special needs' in India?
- What are the adoption guidelines for children with 'special needs' in India?
- What is the role of a family/home in the mental health and well-being of children with disabilities?
- What are the suitable public policy measures for it?

Aim: The present research study aims to explore the problem of adoption of children with correctable disabilities/'special needs' in India considering their developmental challenges, mental health and social being.

Objectives: The objectives of the study include: firstly, to understand anthropological connotations of two terms—disability and adoption; secondly, to find out various legal rules, regulations or acts for the adoption of disabled children in India; thirdly, to find out mental health challenges of such adopted children, and their PAPs; fourthly, to explore the social mindset of general public towards the process of adoption of disabled children; and fifthly, to suggest policy measure for provisions of better homes to disabled children.

Methodology: The study is anthropological in nature and is based on both primary and secondary sources. The universe of the present study is two non-profit organizations in Delhi; one is in Civil lines, namely Palna—Delhi Council for Child Welfare and other is in Jangpura, namely, Missionaries of Charity. Palna-DCCW, is a home for abandoned, homeless and destitute children, which operates under Child Adoption Resource Authority (CARA), statutory body of Ministry of Women and Child Development, Government of India and is the biggest non-governmental organization in that particular area. However, Missionaries of Charity is a private and Catholic organization in Delhi, mainly operated on foreign funds in India.

By applying case study method using the technique of interviews, the researcher was able to gather data from the above mentioned organizations about the views and experiences of members and children with 'special needs', to create a broader picture of a child with 'special' needs life using holistic approach. The primary data includes the interviews of authorities like Director of the organization and organization personnel like centre coordinators, children's attendants and volunteers. It was difficult to communicate with the children in the beginning but through volunteer work and participant observation in both the organizations; the researcher was able to collect the experiences and mental health challenges of children with 'special' needs in their natural setting, that is; their orphanage home.

The sampling strategy that the researcher used is the non-probability purposive sampling in which the samples are selected on the researcher's knowledge about the participants and the study, to fulfil the purpose of getting information from the participants and to get the proper understanding about the situations by maintaining the susceptibility of the issue of disability and adoption. The total sample size of present research study is 40; which includes four officials' interviews, two from each organization, and interviews of centre coordinators which was around 11 (six from Missionaries of Charity and five from Palna-DCCW), total 10 volunteers (four from Palna-DCCW and six from Missionaries of Charity) and fifteen children with 'special' needs (both physical and mental disability) which was mostly from Missionaries of Charity, as Palna includes only newborn or slightly elder than that disabled. But, in this study; the researcher tried to provide the cumulative understanding of the topic disability and adoption, by maintaining the anonymity of a particular individual of the organization.

In the beginning, when the researcher became part of the NGO by taking the permission of authorities; the researcher had to struggle to communicate with everyone and it was not easy to ask them direct questions about disability and adoption because of the sensitivity of the topic. Therefore, the researcher had to build some rapport by assisting everyone and step-by-step interaction with children with 'special' needs; after which she was able to conduct interviews with everyone within the period of 2017-2019. It was not possible to get the interviews of different Prospective Adoptive Parents (PAPs), as the authorities were strictly maintaining the anonymity of the parents and did not allow anyone to interact with them. But, to explore the social mindsets of general public and PAPs; the researcher was able to track those five parents who adopted or want to adopt a child from CARA and interviewed them; who was not afraid to present themselves as prospective adoptive parents and wanted to create some awareness about the issue of disability and adoption.

The secondary data was mostly from the CARA website, their guidelines and their online portal, "address your concerns" for PAPs to communicate and interact with the experts. To maintain the authenticity of the information, researcher also explored the websites of Ministry of Social Justice and Empowerment, the Ministry of Women and Child Development and Mental Health foundation.

Findings

I. Meaning of the Two Terms: 'Disability' and 'Adoption'

Disability is the umbrella term for impairments, activity limitations and participation restrictions, referring to the negative aspects of the interaction between an individual (with a health condition) and that individual's contextual factors (environmental and personal factors) (WHO, 2011: 4). Defining disability as an interaction means that "disability" is not an attribute of the person. Progress on improving social participation can be made by addressing the barriers which hinder persons with disabilities in their day-to-day lives. Anthropologists have contributed to the understanding of disability in a social and cultural context, through the use of ethnographic, phenomenological, and cross-cultural methods (McDermott, 1995; Singh's, 2002). So, what can be the anthropological connotations for the term 'adoption'? One way of answering 'what is adoption?' is with another question: 'Well, it depends — what needs and expectations do people have of their families in the cultural context you are wondering about?' (Jessica, 2018). And in India, disability is mostly blamed on misdeeds of person with disability, ancestors, supernatural forces or punishment or individual's destiny. This is often applied to children with disabilities also, as society or family members do not allow prospective parents to adopt a disabled child and prefer 'normal child'.

As per Section 2(2) of the Juvenile Justice (Care and Protection) Act, 2015; adoption is defined as the legal process through which children are permanently separated from their biological parents and become the legitimate children of their adoptive parents with all the rights, privileges and responsibilities that are attached to the relationships. Also, this act has recognized five kinds of adoption, namely (a) an abandoned, surrendered, destitute child/children adopted by unrelated person/s living within the country, (b) an abandoned, surrendered, destitute child/children adopted by unrelated person/s living outside the country, (c) a related child by relatives living within the country, (d) a related child by relatives living outside the country, and (e) adoption of a child by step parents within the country. In India, there are two categories of children fallen under the process of adoption, that is, normal needs and 'special needs'; where 'special needs' encompass a child with minor health issues, correctable disabilities that can be manageable comes under the category of children with 'special needs'.

Recent data suggests that between 93 million and 150 million children live with a disability worldwide (UNICEF, 2013). According to 2011 Census, there are 78,64,636 children with disability in India constituting 1.7 per cent of total child population. According to the data submitted by Child Adoption Resource Authority (CARA), statutory body of Ministry of Women and Child Development, Government of India disclosed that there is a reduction in the adoptions of children with disabilities under the category of 'special needs' with every passing year. Simultaneously, inter-country adoptions increased by 50 per cent last year alone. A total of 355 children with disabilities were inter-country adoptions in 2017-18, and 237 children in the preceding year. But on the contrary, only 46 children were intra-country adoptions in the same year; consecutively 76 in 2015-16 and 49 in 2016-17.

Those children, who suffer from physical or mental ailments and are often surrendered by their guardians at doorsteps of homes and orphanages where after an inquiry by the Child Welfare Committee these children are declared as abandoned, i.e. unaccompanied and deserted. Among these children, those children who have minor and correctable disabilities, that comes under the category of 'special needs' are placed in adoption agencies.

The adoption agencies prime task is to make an effort to restore the abandoned children to their respective families. In case of no clue of their families, the adoption agencies have to look after the best interests of the children by taking appropriate decisions to ensure the physical, emotional, intellectual, social and moral development of the children.

II. Complexity of Legislation and Adoption in India

In India, there exist three major legislations which regulate adoptions. They are the Hindu Adoption and Maintenance Acts of 1956 (HAMA), the Guardians and Wards Act of 1890 (GAWA), and the Juvenile Justice (Care and Protection) Act of 2000, amended in 2006 and 2011 (JJ ACT).

The Hindu Adoption and Maintenance Acts of 1956 (HAMA) covers adoption for the Hindus, Buddhists, Jains and Sikhs. It does not include Muslim and Parsis in its purview because among the Muslims adoption is an act of prohibition and among Parsis an "outsider"' should not enter the Zoroastrian family. Under HAMA, the following guidelines are mentioned with regard to adoption: married couples or singles both can adopt, legally only the man adopts with the consent of the wife, a single man or woman can also adopt, if a biological child already exists in the family a child of the opposite sex can only be adopted, children adopted under this act should get the same rights as that of the biological children, children under the age of 15 years can be adopted, a single man adopting a girl should be at least 21 years elder to the child.

The Guardian and Wards ACT, 1890 (GAWA) states that even the non-Hindus could adopt. Prior to the Juvenile Justice Act, this Act was the only Act which gave relief to the non-Hindu PAPs. Under this Act, the parents adopting a child is a "guardian" and the child is a "ward". The guardianship can be revoked by the courts or by the guardian; a will is required for any property or good to be bequeathed the child. This shall be legally contested by the blood relatives also. Here both the PAPs can be guardians in contrast to HAMA where only the man adopts with consent of the wife. Under GAWA single person can also adopt without any age difference in restriction.

The Juvenile Justice (Care and Protection) Act which is mainly for care and rehabilitation of children in conflict with the law. It states that there is a need for children having the same law or themselves whether they are biological or adopted. It also states that there is also a need for a law which delinks adoption of children from their religious backgrounds. Juvenile Justice Act added small but significant sub-section in adoption laws. Under this Act any Indian citizen can adopt a child who is legally free for adoption, the adoptee gets the same rights as that of the biological child might get, the religion of the adoptee is irrelevant, single people can adopt, the adoption is irrevocable, sometime limits have to be set to ensure that the child is legally free for adoption, the thrust is on the best interest of the child. While the Act covers the whole of India, it is possible to adopt children *via* this Act only at places where the juvenile justice boards have been constituted. Further the Act states no clarity over the fact that if adoptions for Muslims may also be included in its purview. The Juvenile Justice Act can be treated as a general law for adoption but how will it override the other personal laws is a matter of question.

The Government of India looks after the safety, security and development of the disabled children and instructs adoption agencies to follow certain guidelines for adoption and make their best efforts to place such children in suitable families *via* a safe and secured process of adoption. But in India, due to social stigma being attached to the parenting of disabled children, adoption of disabled children becomes a taboo. Reservations towards adoption of children and specifically the disabled children result in children waiting in long queue for their adoption.

Overall it can be said that though we have several adoption laws in our country yet no common general adoption law exists which addresses both adoption issues as well as rights issue of the children and it is because successive governments seem reluctant to enact such a law in view of opposition from certain sections of society belonging to different religious groups.

Procedures and Guidelines Related to Inter- and Intra-Country Adoptions

Adoption is a sensitive issue, be it inter-country adoptions or intra-country adoptions. In case of special needs children inter-country adoptions occur more commonly but with it is also associated certain risks for children. The disabled children may become victims of child trafficking, prostitution etc. For this reason, Ministry of Social Justice and Empowerment and the Ministry of Women and Child Development works together to look after the sensitive issue of disability rights and adoption of the disabled.

For the purpose of adoption, Central Adoption Resource Authority (CARA) takes care that the prospective parents should be informed about all the Acts of adoption and the ramifications of provisions of each Act. CARA has listed certain general guidelines of adoption which have to be followed by homes and adoption agencies before the actual petition for adoption is to be filed under any chosen Act for adoption. CARA's guidelines ensure that adoptions are in best interest of the child and all adoptions are legally processed through licensed homes and institutions only and not any fraudulent agencies.

CARA's Categorization for 'Special Needs' Children

CARA has categorized 'special needs' children into four categories, children having visible or serious medical or physical conditions, the older children, the siblings, and extremely low birth weight children. It has further listed thirty different sorts of ailments or disabilities or serious medical conditions which may be considered as disabilities. A child suffering from a disease or deformity which does not have a long term residual effect and which may be corrected shall not be categorized as a special needs child. Children above five years shall also be considered as special needs children as placement of such children in adoption agencies is difficult as the prospective adoptive parent usually come to adopt the younger children and the infants and ignore the elder ones. Siblings are also considered as special needs children as their placement in the same family is also a difficult task. A child having specially delayed milestone may also be considered as a special needs child for adoption.

CARA lists down adoption procedures of these children and criterion for the prospective adoptive parents also known as PAPs. Prospective adoptive parents in general have to ensure atleast two years of stable marital relationship before going for adoption. Couples in live-in relationship are not allowed to adopt a child. To adopt a child in the age group of 0-3 years the couple must have a composite age of below 90 wherein the individual age of the prospective adoptive parents should not exceed 25 years and should not be more than 50 years. To adopt children of over three years the composite age of the prospective adoptive parent should not be more than 105 years where the individual age of the PAPs should not be less than 25 and more than 55. In case a single prospective adoptive parents wish to adopt, he or she should not be less than 30 years of age and shall not be more than 50 years of age. The maximum age shall be 45 years to adoption of a child for 0-3 years and 50 years for adopting children above three years. An unmarried or single male person is not allowed to adopt a girl child. The prospective adoptive parents should have adequate financial resources for adoption to provide a good upbringing of the child. The PAPs should maintain good health and should not be suffering from any contagious disease or terminal disease or any other mental or physical condition which may prevent them from taking care of the child. Adoption of a second child by the PAPs is permissible only when the legal adoption of the first child is finalized but this is not applicable in case of siblings.

For Foreign prospective adoptive parents (FPAP) the criterion of marital stable relationship is of five years at least, with the composite age of the prospective parents being 90 years. This composite age is relaxed for children of special needs, single persons never married widowed or divorced can adopt. The age difference of single adoptive parent from child may be a minimum of 21 years else, the FPAP should not be less than 30 years and more than 55 years. Same Sex couples not allowed cost of adopting a special needs child is low. In India no special law for inter country adoption is present. All the procedures are expensive, time consuming and uncertain in the foreign nationals are given the last priority in the list of adoptions. Foreigners interested in child adoption in India believe that if challenges involved in inter country adoption are taken care of many homeless children can get joy.

In case of adoption of special needs children the prospective adoptive parents are given more priority than the prospective adoptive parents of the other children. Adoption agencies while making a list of such prospective adoptive parents keep many criterions in mind. The PAPs of older age are of more experience tend to be more committed to parent a child with special needs as they are more likely to have the skills, patience and financial means to handle such special needs children. Parents who have some sort of exposure to a particular medical condition are thought to be better equipped to handle parenting of disabled children. Many of the above criterions fixed for the PAPs seem quite subjective in nature as it cannot be assumed that older parents will have the patience and strength to care for a small baby. It could be the other way round also with the younger parents being more energetic to handle overnight waking hours for the baby's care.

In another guideline, CARA lists that it will assess the motivation levels of the PAPs and their level of financial incomes and see if it is enough to handle a special needs child. As far as the income levels are concerned the adoption agencies usually keep Rs. 25000 as the minimum monthly income limit for a private employee and a decent amount of salary for a government employee. The adoption agency should clearly list down the present medical condition of the child as per current medical reports and should inform the PAPs about the future medical interventions that may be required for the child. This helps the PAPs to be aware of all realities of the child and prevents all sorts of ambiguities and future conflicts within the PAPs and the adoption agencies. The PAPs of special needs children are to be given top priority in the waiting list. The adoption of special needs children should be carried as expeditiously as possible by the concerned authorities and time lines lay down for adoption of special needs children in these guidelines is strictly adhered to. Special care must be taken while processing the cases for adoption of special needs children so that the PAPs is aware and ready to provide extra care and attention that the child needs.

III. Mental Health Challenges and Psychosocial Needs of Children with Disabilities and Prospective Adoptive Parents, Concerns

According to WHO, health is a state of complete physical, mental and social well-being and not merely the absence of disease or infirmity; and one of the important point of this definition is that mental health is more than just the absence of mental disorders or disabilities. And out of many, one specific way to upgrade mental health initiatives is to make early childhood interventions; in which they receive a desirable environment of a home and a proper parental guardianship, without any threats or harm to child's mental health and developmental growth; and include psychosocial support and encouragement. Different policies and legislations related to a child adoption process should comprise these issues to promote mental health and well-being of a child with disabilities in India.

But, on the contrary, according to Rosenthal and Groza (1991), children with 'special needs' adoption process often affects their behaviour and mental health like soiling, stealing and hoarding in a group of children whose adoption had disrupted; and child can react with extreme verbal abuse or with physical aggression, provocative deviant behaviour such as running away and threats. Therefore, when one is adopting a child with disability; then one should keep in mind that they need an entire family not just parents and your decision can change or disrupt a child's future and mental well being. According to Berry and Barth (1989), both management training and intensive family preservation services should be utilized with the adoptive families in order to maintain the mental well-being of a child with 'special needs'. Also, family preparedness, financial stability and good relationships with adoption agencies can give sufficient results which can ease the adoption process of children with disabilities.

Little literature is available on the mental health challenges and needs of children with disabilities and PAPs; and no authorized support is available for the parents who want to adopt a child with 'special needs'.

The fatigue of pre- and post-adoption processes can give anxiety and stress to PAPs, which can often lead to discontinuation of the adoption and put the mental health of both child with disability and prospective parents in question.

Both the child welfare and the legal systems often lack the capacities to track and monitor the progress of cases through the adoption processes, making it difficult to identify the source of delays and develop strategies to overcome them (Dodson, 1998). This delayed capacity of tracking and monitoring the progress of adoption process often impedes the psychosocial needs and mental wellbeing of a child. Therefore, the role of policies and acts should formulate to consider the mental wellbeing of both of them; that can smooth the lengthy process of adoption and does not disrupt the relation of PAPs and adoption agencies; which will ultimately not allow anyone to play with the future of a child.

IV. Perspectives/'Social Mindset' of Society Towards Adoption of Disabled Children

In spite of clear-cut guidelines by Child Adoption Resource Authority (CARA), adoption of special needs children with suitable Prospective Adoptive Parents (PAPs) is a difficult task. PAPs complain of the long exhaustive procedures to be followed for adoption. Case studies report that couples have been waiting for more than two years waiting for their chance in spite of the fact that infants are present in the adoption centres. PAPs often complain of CARA closing their online registration process at random notice. PAPs also complain of difficulty in adopting child from interstate adoption agencies though it is clearly mentioned in CARA guidelines that such interstate adoptions can be made. There are many PAPs who complain about the strictness of these guidelines, their subjective nature which constitutes the major loopholes in the whole process of adoption. PAPs opine that they have to be in a long waiting queue in spite of their strong motivational will to adopt a child. Due to this long waiting queue many PAPs are willing to adopt children with minor correctable disabilities because such adoptions are more speedily done.

One of the young couple in the reputed adoption centre of Delhi said to the authorities that, "*thodi si aankh kharab haina, par hum adopt kar lenge*" (Only minor issue in the eye, but we will adopt).

Adoption centre share contrary view to what has been discussed. The adoption agencies find interstate adoptions as a big problem as it reduces the chances of intra-state adoptions of children and also encourages growth of social stigma attached to the whole concept of adoption. PAPs prefer to adopt from interstate placement agencies rather than intra-state agencies in order to minimize the chances of relatives knowing or inquiring about the adopted child is minimum and in many cases the PAPs want to conceal the fact they are going to adopt a child. For this reason, it is only after ascertaining the motivational levels of the PAPs and conducting a home study report which ascertains the social economic status, family status and background description of standard of living, relationship with any other spouse, relationship with any other, family member's health and hygiene status, educational levels of the PAPs. After matching the qualities of the child with the qualities of the PAPs, a suitability criterion is made, PAPs are decided, petition under a particular adoption act is filed and the child is handed to the PAP. Before that, a counselling of both the PAPs and the adopted child is done. After handling of the child a two year follow-up is also mandatory to track the development of the child in the family. This follow-up may happen after every six months or so.

Some of the other problems which adoption agencies usually meet in placing a special needs child with suitable PAPs are the choice of the special needs child to be adopted. The PAPs ask weird questions before deciding for a child to be adopted. They assess if the child to be adopted would grow up to resemble their caste people and can easily camouflage in their society.

In a case study it was revealed that the PAPs were looking for a child who resembled the Aggarwal caste. In their words, "*agarwal jaisa dikhta haikya..?*" (Does the child look like Aggarwal..?). And the placement in charge answering "*dikhta nahi to banadena*" (If not, then make him/her). Such narrow mindedness is often discouraged by the adoption agencies as they have seen the hardships the children have to undergo to even survive up to a few years. For this reason the adoption agencies many a times lose their patience and often give straightforward answers while satisfying the queries of the PAPs. They may, therefore, appear rude to the PAPs but they are not wrong in a way. In many instances, a disagreement between the wife and husband leads to a delay in the process of deciding which child to adopt. In one instance PAPs expressed their guilt to the placement agency after spending months of decision making and not coming up with any conclusion. The placement in charges do not blame on to the PAPs as they feel that after all it is their life decision.

Guidelines are indeed strict but all are devised keeping in mind the sensitivity of an adoption of disabled children. The majority of cases of adoption of special needs children are inter-country rather than intra-country as governments of many foreign countries provide subsidies for caring the disabled children and have proper infrastructural arrangements for the disabled children like ramps at public places etc. In majority countries there exists no fear of any social stigma attached with parenting of disabled children. They are in fact even eager to adopt children with HIV. Adoption agencies also face problems in placing elder, i.e. above five age group children to suitable homes in India whereas abroad they are easily adopted. As told by one adoption centre coordinators, one reason behind differences in this attitude is that in India a lot of emphasis is laid on the intellectual potential and sense of achievement of that child and the child's academic achievements. In countries abroad each sort of labour is recognized and credited whereas in India it is more related to position held and status of work. Even if one child turns to be a farmer and the other a director, not many comparisons are being made. Children above five usually land up to the orphanages and homes at that age because perhaps their parents abandon them only after visible manifestations of uncorrectable disabilities. By the time these children reach adoption centres they have already wasted three to four years of their lifetime which could be utilized in providing them with basic school education say pre-nursery etc. which could help them to get admission in a good school. PAPs are worried to adopt such children as they are unsure of their admissions in school and their development in comparison to other children of the same age. Moreover, if they already have an elder child they have to see that a match is their between the two children.

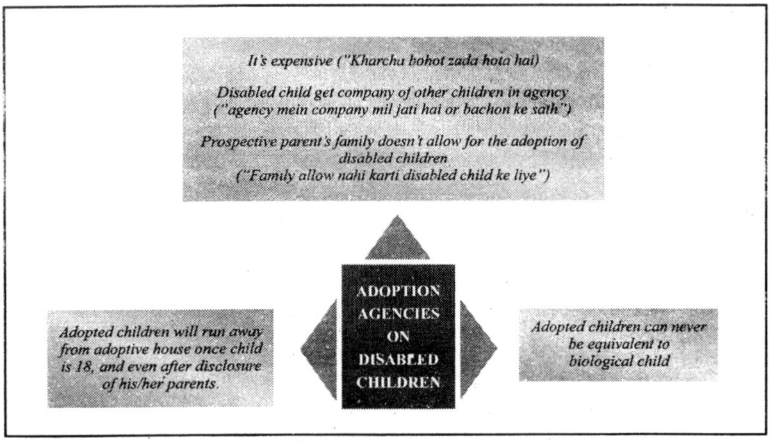

In spite of strict and time-bound guidelines for adoption of children, the process of adoption of disabled children occurs at a very slow pace in India. At one of the leading adoption centres of Delhi, it was found that there have been just three to four cases of adoption of disabled children in past decade. Prospective adaptive parents in India rarely opted for adopting a disabled child. The trend seems to be changing now with certain prospective adoptive parents volunteering for adoption of the disabled children. Over the period of time, meanings of disability have been changing. These changing interpretations of the term 'disability' is a reflection of the mindset of the society ranging from conservative to liberal and the government's concern for the disabled.

V. Role of Policy Reformation for the Welfare of Children with 'Special Needs' and Adoption Agencies in India

According to Adoption agencies, the government guidelines should give proper worth and respect to adoption procedures but some lacunae definitely lie in the implementation aspects. For instance, there is a scarcity of homes and orphanages for the children where the abandoned children can be kept and trained. Usually infants are abandoned in front of such adoption agencies, so adoption agencies are forced to pick them up and care for them with the resources available for few children of their centre. Reason instruction from Ministry of Women & Child Development on distributing *Adhaar* card to all the children of the adoption agencies is not a very logical idea as such children would be soon adopted and get a different *Adhaar* card in their respective PAPs family and even if they do not get adopted they would spend most of their time in the particular homes as they arc physically and mentally challenged. Government should also provide for adoption subsidies to encourage the PAPs to at least think for once of adopting children of special needs. If one sort of child care support system is provided by the government in form of more number of subsidized crèches etc. more number of childless couples can think for adopting a child with special needs.

With many PAPs complaining of long procedures of CARA and the adoption agencies finding the PAPs as unsuitable, the government is now trying to make the adoption procedure simplified by making the adoption procedures online and minimal. In fact, eliminating the role of adoption agencies in such a system that by logging onto the site of photographs and other biodata details and medical history, five children at once will be presented to the PAPs who can choose one and block the rest they may further contact the particular placement agency and claim for the child. In such a case it will become very difficult for an adoption agency to say no to the PAPs. Adoption agencies in the normal course prefer first assessing the motivational levels, intellectual levels, moral levels etc. of PAPs before placing a particular child to them. For example, a bright child if placed in compromised family settings may land up achieving just a moderate life due to his capabilities being unrecognized and undernourished.

However, Adoption agencies does not seem to be comfortable with the new guideline changes because they feel that the ultimate decisions of placing the children should depend on the PAPs as they are the ones who know the child and they are the ones who care for them. After all adoption is an issue where in a case some problem occurs, they will be the first people to be contacted and held responsible. At that time the government would perhaps not come to share the responsibility. Many instances have been reported where disabled children are picked up by middlemen and forced into illicit child trafficking, begging etc. For this reason, the first task of an adoption agency should be restoring an abandoned child to his or her original home. In order to prevent such illegal activities, the government has to bring in awareness towards the safety, security and dignity of the disabled children.

Discussions

The article rests on the belief that the human potential especially that of children can be discovered and nurtured only when they receive a desirable environment of a home and a proper parental guardianship, which can affect their mental health and developmental changes. But in India, with growing trend of nuclear families and working couples in Delhi chances of adoption of 'special needs' children by childless couples even reduces. With those who are in a joint family, it is difficult to present their children proudly in front of all because of the attached social stigma and unawareness of rights. Adopted child has equal rights on property as one biological child rights so many a times in Indian society parents hesitate to adopt children with 'special needs' who can own and look after the property after their death.

Along with changes in government policies, the mindset of the people have to be changed and more adoptive parents support group should be created in the country like India. Parent resource materials should be prepared. But first of all, the primary task should be to restore the child to the biological parents, so that their growth and development will not get affected by the frequent change of foster homes or undesirable environment. If they do not know the concept of family or relative, how can they identify themselves without any proper parental guardianship?

Conclusion

There is a need of proper implementation of policies and measures for the welfare of both children with 'special needs' and Prospective Adoptive Parents (PAPs). The multidimensional nature of this issue often stigmatized and marginalized them that affect their mental and social wellbeing, and also restrict their integration in the society through the process of adoption. With decrease in intra-country adoptions as compared to inter-country, one can see the complexity of different policies and legislations in India, with their strict guidelines and lengthy adoption process often put PAPs in the waiting line that can take three-four years of their life which can easily resonate on the lives of children with 'special needs'. On the contrary, issue of abandonment and disruption of adoption process in between fatigued and frustrate both adoption agencies and a child with disability. Proper implementation of rules given by government can ease out the struggle of adoption agencies to handle the increasing amount of abandonment cases in scarcity of resources. Different selection criterion for the adoption of a disabled child like online portals can shorten the adoption process for both agency and prospective parents. Therefore, a family/home provides financial, emotional and social security to an adopted child, which encourages their mental wellbeing and ensures acceptance. Also, if the adoption's guidelines and policies, given by both government and reputed adoption agencies like CARA loosens its grip; and social mindsets of the society does not stigmatize and abandoned a child with 'special needs'; we can be successful in safeguarding the future of a child and will prevent children from becoming a puppet to the system.

Acknowledgements: The first author, Dr. Mitashree Srivastava contributed to conceptualization of the theme of research, preparing its methodology of investigation, and collecting narratives on adoption, and the second author, Ms. Tajinder Kaur contributed to the paper by analyzing the narratives in light of mental health challenges of children with 'special needs' in India. The research is personally funded and sponsored.

REFERENCES

Ablon, J. (1995). "The elephanlt man" as "self" and "other": The psychosocial costs of a misdiagnosis", *Social Science and Medicine*, *40*: 1481-1489.

Barth, R.P., and Berry, M. (1988). *Modern applications of social work. Adoption and disruption: Rates, risks, and responses.* Aldine de Gruyter.

Bharadwaj, A. (2016). *Conceptions: infertility and procreative technologies in India.* New York: Berghahn Books.

Census of India (2011). *Data on Disability.* Office of the Registrar General & Census Commissioner, New Delhi, 27-12-2013.
Available at: http://www.disabilityaffairs.gov.in/upload/uploadfiles/files/disabilityinindia2011data.pdf

Dodson, D. (1998). Finding Families for Waiting Kids: The Challenge of Special Needs Adoption in the 90s and Beyond, presented at the Policy Institute for Family Impact Seminar, Washington, DC, 1998. Washington, DC: Family Impact Seminar. Available at https://www.purdue.edu/hhs/hdfs/fii/wp-content/uploads/2015/06/pf_fis42report.pdf

Durkheim, E. 1896. Review of Kohler, *J. ZurUrgeschichte der Ehe. Totemismus, Gruppenehe, Mutterrecht (Contribution à l'histoire primitive du mariage. Totémisme, mariage collectif, droit maternel). L'Année sociologique* 1, 306-319.

Gretchen A. Good (2016). Adoption of children with disabilities: an exploration of the issues for adoptive families, *Early Child Development and Care, 186*:4, 642-661, DOI: 10.1080/03004430.2015.1040786

Leinaweaver, J. (2018). "Adoption", In *The Cambridge Encyclopedia of Anthropology* (eds.) F. Stein, S. Lazar, M. Candea, H. Diemberger, J. Robbins, A. Sanchez & R. Stasch. http://doi.org/10.29164/18adopt.

McKenzie, J. (1993). "Adoption of Children with Special Needs", *The Future of Children, 3*(1), 62-76. DOI: 10.2307/1602402

Modell, J.S. (1994). *Kinship with strangers: adoption and interpretations of kinship in American culture.* Berkeley: University of California Press.

Reid-Cunningham, A.R. (2009). "Anthropological Theories of Disability", *Journal of Human Behaviour in the Social Environment, 19*:99-111. DOI: 10.1080/10911350802631644.

Rosenthal, James & Groza, Victor. (1991). "Behavioural problems of special needs adopted children", *Children and Youth Services Review. 13*: 343-361. https://doi.org/10.1016/0190-7409(91)90025-D

Schneider, D.M. 1980 [1968]. *American kinship: a cultural account.* Chicago: University Press.

The Gazette of India (2016, January 1). Juvenile Justice (Care and Protection of Children) Act, 2015. Available at http://wcd.nic.in/sites/default/files/JJ%20Act,%202015%20_0.pdf

The Guardian and Wards Act of 1890 (GAWA), 21 March, 1890. Accessed on: 11.03.2021.
Available at: http://www.ijtr.nic.in/family%20matters/Guardians%20and%20Wards%20Act,%201890.pdf

The Hindu Adoption and Maintenance Act of 1956 (HAMA), 21 December, 1956. Accessed on: 11.03.2021.

Available at: https://tcw.nic.in/Acts/Hindu%20adoption%20and%20Maintenance%20Act.pdf

United Nations Children's Fund (UNICEF), *The State of World's Children 2013: Children with Disabilities,* May 2013.
Available at: https://www.unicef.org/sowc2013/files/SWCR2013_ENG_Lo_res_24_Apr_2013.pdf

World Health Organization, & World Bank. (2011). *World report on Disability.* Geneva, Switzerland: World Health Organization.
Available at: http://www.who.int/disabilities/world_report/2011/report.pdf

PART V

Women's Health and Wellbeing

21

Folic Acid Supplementation in Pregnancy

An Anthropological Insight

Kallur Nava Saraswathy, Imnameren Longkumer and *Jyoti Mishra*

"Babies are not simply born; they are being shaped for their future health and subsequent generations through intra-uterine programming; which depends on the mother's health status preconceptionally and throughout gestations of pregnancy".

(Mishra *et al.*, 2020).

Pregnancy is a biological phenomenon which is important in women's life in different dimensions. Giving birth to a child gives emotional, psychological and social support to women. This is a very vital stage and is an important interphase between biology and social aspects of a women's life. Social environment in terms of economic status primarily decides the nutrition or quality and quantity of food intake, and thus the outcome of pregnancy (Kim *et al.*, 2018). Emotional environment in terms of family ties, human relations and social networking in turn lead to correction in hormonal imbalances. As pregnancy is a dynamic state involving a myriad of biological mechanisms during different trimesters, this immuno-compromised state demands for social and emotional support to enable a successful pregnancy.

Pregnancy and One Carbon Metabolic Pathway

One Carbon Metabolic Pathway (OCMP), also referred to as Homocysteine Metabolic Pathway is driven by folate and methionine cycles and plays an important role in the synthesis of thymidylate, purines and methyl transferase reactions (Guéant *et al.*, 2013). It participates in key metabolic reactions, like in DNA synthesis which mediates cell division and production of methyl groups for methylation reaction, which is one of the most stable epigenetic mechanisms (Crider *et al.*, 2012). This pathway is mediated by B vitamins such as folate (Vitamin B_9), cobalamin (Vitamin B_{12}), pyridoxine (Vitamin B_6) etc. which act as critical co-factors and play a crucial role in the maintenance of one-carbon metabolism (Lyon *et al.*, 2020). During pregnancy, maternal bioavailability of folate plays a central role to embryonic and fetal development as well as for maternal health (Waterland and Jirtle, 2003; Reynolds, 2006). It also plays a major role in the fetal epigenetic programming *via* OCMP (Crider *et al.*, 2012). Additionally, both genetic mutations and also epigenetic alteration are likely to affect gene expression (over- or under-expression) which can aiter the fetal viability and development. Mutations in the genes involved in the pathway such as Methylenetetrahydrofolate Reductase (MTHFR), Cystathione Beta Synthase (CBS), Methionine Synthase (MTR), Methionine Synthase Reductase (MTRR) etc. impact the availability of methyl groups, both for the mother and fetus (Guéant *et al.*, 2013; Del Gobbo *et al.*, 2018). Hence, the effect of maternal nutrition (first generation) *via* folate bioavailability not just lies in the fetal viability (second generation) but it also impacts the embryonic germ cell lining of the fetus during its development (third generation). Therefore, supplementation with folic acid during pregnancy has an impact not just on mother but also on subsequent generations, i.e. the mother's nutrition is affecting not only her health but her child's and grandchild's health as well (Padmanabhan *et al.*, 2016). Thus, a successful pregnancy and subsequent child and maternal health depends crucially on OCMP.

Folate/Folic Acid and Neural Tube Defects

Neural Tube Defects (NTDs) refer to congenital malformations of the spine, spinal cord or cranium resulting from failure of normal neural tube closure during early pregnancy. It has long been estimated that approximately 300,000 neonates are born with NTDs each year worldwide (Botto *et al.*, 1999). Several studies have indicated the role of folate in association with NTDs and clinical trials during 1980s and 1990s have conclusively showed that periconceptional folic acid intake resulted in decreased prevalence of NTDs (De-Regil *et al.*, 2015). As a consequence, pre-and peri-conceptional folic acid supplementation is recommended in many countries. Thus, folic acid, which is a synthetic form of folate, is supplemented either through fortified foods or nutritional supplements (Berry *et al.*, 2010; Crider *et al.*, 2011) and studies indicated reduced risk of the occurrence of NTDs by as much as 62 per cent to 70 per cent (Blencowe *et al.,* 2010). Folate, which is a key co-factor in OCMP involving synthesis of DNA and certain amino acids, it is suggested that higher amount of folate is required during pregnancy due to rapid rate of cellular and tissue growth for the development of fetus; thus, maternal folate deficiency during this period may have detrimental and irreversible effects on the growing fetus (Dolin *et al.,* 2018).

The burden of NTDs in India is reported to be significant given the 27 million annual births (Bhide *et al.,* 2013) and is associated with maternal folate deficiency (Smithells *et al.,* 1976). This significant association and results from clinical trials lead to the most cost effective public health intervention (Yi *et al.,* 2011), of periconceptional Iron Folic Acid (IFA) supplementation to pregnant women. A prophylactic dose of 300 µg (0.3 mg) per day throughout pregnancy was suggested in 1968 by the World Health Organization (WHO, 2012). This supplemental dose was increased to 400 µg (0.4 mg) of folic acid per day in 1998 following publication of several studies supporting the periconceptional use of folic acid in the prevention of NTDs (WHO, 2012). In India, the guidelines of Maternal Health Division under the Ministry of Health and Family Welfare advises daily IFA tablet consumption (100 mg elemental iron and 0.5 mg folic acid) for at least 100 days among pregnant women (Maternal Health Division Guidelines, 2005).

The Presumed Safety of Folic Acid Supplementation

Folic acid supplementation during pregnancy is considered safe due to its water soluble characteristic (Butterworth and Tamura, 1989) and hence motivated some countries to opt for folic acid fortification in cereal products. The first country to achieve national-scale fortification of flour with folic acid to prevent NTDs was Oman and in 1998 wheat fortification programmes were established in United States and Canada (Wang *et al.,* 2016). By 2008, an estimated 22,000 birth defects were prevented due to this intervention (Bell and Oakley, 2009). Since then, flour fortification is mandatory in more than 70 countries worldwide. These countries have reported 31 per cent to 58 per cent reductions in NTDs (Berry *et al.,* 2010).

Folic acid has been successfully supplemented for more than 40 years, however, recent evidence raises concerns about its safety. Indiscriminate supplementation of folic acid (despite the benefits) was found to be posing risk (US population) for other serious diseases and nutritional deficiencies (Smith *et al.,* 2008). Many studies worldwide have concluded that folic acid supplementation has little or no effect upon birth outcomes (Chiaffarino *et al.,* 2010) or even to prevent Cardiovascular Diseases (Yang *et al.,* 2012). In some animal studies, folate deficiency was found to be protective as compared to supplementation, which was found to increase experimental carcinogenesis (Kim, 2004). Another Randomised Clinical trial conducted at 9 clinical centres between July 6, 1994 and October 1, 2004 (10 years) has found an association of folic acid with higher risk of having three or more adenomas and non-colorectal cancers (Cole *et al.,* 2007). A study by Collin *et al.* (2010a) constituting a case-control study, systematic review and meta-analysis reported that high levels of blood folate were found to be associated with increased prostate cancer risk. Other studies have shown the adverse effects of high intakes of folic acid on health in the form of tumorigenesis (Collin *et al.,* 2010b; Stevens *et al.,* 2010; Ly *et al.,* 2011) which indicates future health risk both for the mother and the child. The mechanism through which excess folic acid promotes cancer is unclear till date, however, animal experiments indicate that these compounds induce a cancer causing reaction, i.e. hypermethylation in the DNA of cancer cells (Ly *et al.,* 2011). In a study of 70,656 postmenopausal women who were followed from 1992 until 2005 (14 years), dietary folate intake (from both folic acid and folate) was positively associated with breast cancer risk (Stevens *et al.,* 2010).

Years after implementing folic acid fortification and maternal folic acid supplementation during pregnancy, there is evidence that the number of reported spontaneous abortions is increasing (Windham *et al.,* 2000; Czeizel, 2001). Voluntary fortification has been practiced for several years in various countries like U.K., Ireland, Spain, Portugal, Austria and Switzerland (Fletcher *et al.,* 2004). However, in other member states, i.e. Denmark, Finland and Sweden, voluntary fortification is restricted and not allowed. This is because the increase in folic acid intake was larger than predicted and could have resulted from a number of enriched products containing higher concentration of folic acid than required by law (Rader, 2002; Choumenkovitch *et al.,* 2002). Evidences are on accumulation on how folic acid supplementation are raising red flags about its potential risks of therapy, possibly as a result of excessive consumption. Both genetic and epigenetic mechanisms are likely to be influenced by high unmetabolized folic acid because naturally occurring and artificially synthesized folic acid have different metabolizable routes. Both are bound to influence OCMP and alter genetic and epigenetic mechanisms leading to adverse health adversities both at maternal and fetal fronts (embryonic development). All these effects depend on the maternal folate status before supplementation and also their genetic makeup.

Although folic acid supplementation is deemed necessary and safe for pregnant women and it reduces pregnancy complications, the untold story of indiscriminate folic acid supplementation is now raising concern over its safety. Especially, in counties like India where folate sufficiency is assumed to be common due to their predominantly vegetarian diet, an indiscriminate folic acid supplementation irrespective of actual folate levels in pregnant women may have detrimental effect on the mother and fetus. In view of this, a study by Katre *et al.* (2010) among Indian pregnant women demonstrated that almost all recruited women who had folate replete at baseline and supplemented with folic acid during their pregnancy progression was not associated with reduction of total homocysteine, which is a metabolite known for causing pregnancy complications. In another study, a high dose maternal folic acid supplementation was associated with an increased risk for infant asthma (Yang *et al.,* 2015). However, despite the impending ill effects of folic acid supplementation, most obstetricians and medical practitioner still have an impression that folic acid is harmless even in high doses as it is water soluble, and are unaware of the growing concern about high dose folic acid supplementation and fortification. Thus, the history and success of folic acid as a nutritional supplement seemed to be enterprising and encouraging till recently but it is increasingly becoming a matter of concern.

High Intakes of Folic Acid: Is It Safe?

The tolerable upper intake level (UL) of folic acid is 1000µg/day (1mg/day) as established by the Institute of Medicine in 1998 as one fifth of the lowest observed adverse effect level (5000µg/day or 5mg/day) associated with a potential adverse outcome in early case reports (Institute of Medicine, 1998). Despite the beneficial effects known of folic acid fortification on folate status and NTDs in countries that implemented in addition to the promotion of supplement use, concern continues that folic acid might also have adverse effects (Cornel *et al.,* 2005). Although folate is safe and almost toxicity free, concerns that folic acid fortification could mask symptoms of vitamin B12 deficiency and precipitate neurological complications have been raised (Cornel *et al.,* 2005). Other examples of potential safety issues are interactions with drugs, hypersensitivity reactions and cancer promotion rate (Campbell, 1996).

Experimental and population based evidence shows that folate influences the epigenetic mechanisms that underlie intrauterine growth retardation (IUGR), fetal programming, and embryo-fetal brain development (Forges *et al.,* 2007; Stover, 2011). One of the key genes in the folate pathway, i.e. *MTHFR* and its mutation *C677T* is the most studied polymorphism and causes a 70 per cent reduction in MTHFR activity in *TT* mutant homozygotes as compared to the *CC* homozygotes and hence affects folate distribution (Stover *et al.,* 2011). A study on mouse models by Pickell *et al.* (2011) revealed adverse fetal outcomes, i.e. fetal anomalies as a result of extra intake of folic acid. Moreover, NTD occurrence can be attributed to specific folate-gene interactions. The *MTHFR 677C>T* polymorphism and other variations can increase the folate requirement and susceptibility for an NTD-affected pregnancy. Prior to the fortification era, a case-control study showed that both red blood cell and serum folate concentrations were significantly lower in pregnant women with the *TT* and *CT* variants compared to the wild-type *CC* genotype (Guenther *et al.,* 1999). Insufficient production of 5-Methyltetrahydrofolate (5-MTHF) leads to an increase in homocysteine levels, as the methyl group of 5-MTHF is no longer available to a sufficient extent for the re-methylation of homocysteine into methionine. Thereby, participants with the *MTHFR 677 C>T* mutation need more dietary folate to achieve an adequate plasma folate levels (de Bree *et al.* 2003). However, when the folic acid supplementation is in excessive form, accumulation of unmetabolized folic acid in the serum can be observed. In a small randomized trial in women of reproductive age (N = 38) receiving 30 weeks of daily supplementation with either 1.1 mg or 5 mg of folic acid resulted in the transient appearance of unmetabolized folic acid in blood over the first 12 weeks of supplementation (Tam *et al.,* 2010). In addition, a study conducted on postmenopausal women also raised concerns about the effect of exposure to unmetabolized folic acid on immune function (Troen *et al.,* 2006). These studies have highlighted the deleterious effects of high serum folic acid levels in women which make them more prone to complex diseases. The proposed mechanism could be epigenetic changes occurring *in utero* in women during pregnancy because of unmetabolized folic acid and critically, folic acid supplementation is the first external exposure affecting both mother and the fetus. In this regard, a study by Plumptre *et al.,* (2015) showed that a daily high folic acid dose resulted in detectable level of unmetabolized folic acid both in maternal and fetal blood.

Research Output from Laboratory of Biochemical and Molecular Anthropology, University of Delhi

Studies by the authors, in collaboration with Lady Hardinge Medical College and Smt. Sucheta Kriplani Hospital, New Delhi, observed folate deficiency to be almost negligible among the pregnant women and also among the women in their reproductive ages. Surprisingly, one of the metabolite of OCMP, i.e. homocysteine, is found to be significantly high among women with pregnancy complications such as preeclampsia (PE), recurrent miscarriages (RM) and preterm premature rupture of membranes (PPROM) as compared to respective controls. The deficiency of another important cofactor, i.e. vitamin B_{12} was found to be a significant risk factor for RM (Puri *et al.,* 2013; Mishra *et al.,* 2018). Most importantly, despite the folate repletion among cases, hyperhomocysteinemia was found to be significantly associated with preeclampsia, recurrent miscarriages (Puri *et al.,* 2013) and preterm premature rupture of membranes cases (Mishra *et al.,* 2018) posing significant 3.2, 2.1 and 8.16 fold increased risk for the cases, respectively. All these results obtained, question the role of folic acid supplementation in the reduction of homocysteine levels, a significant marker associated with pregnancy complications. This is suggestive of the fact that folate repletion is in no way preventing adverse pregnancies (PE, RM) and outcomes such as Intrauterine Growth Restriction and Preterm Birth, neither independently nor by reducing homocysteine levels, which is found to be a major risk factor for all the pregnancy complications. Further, at epigenetic level there seems to be transgenerational alterations at fetal front among the women with pregnancy complications (Mishra *et al.,* 2019). The effect of folate on this phenomenon could not be evaluated because almost all women whether it is a case or control were found to be folate replete. In fact, not just replete but most of them possess extra physiological levels, which can conveniently be attributed to folic acid supplementation.

In one of the pilot study conducted by the authors, the trends of folate and vitamin B_{12} in pregnancy progression and its outcomes were assessed (Mishra *et al.,* 2020). In this follow up study, all the recruited pregnant women were found to be mostly replete (97%) with folate even prior to folic acid supplementation as compared to insufficient vitamin B_{12} stores. More than half of the pregnant women (60%) were found to be vitamin B_{12} deficient in the 1st trimester at their booking visit irrespective of their pregnancy outcomes. The levels of folate among the recruited pregnant women were found to be increased in the 2nd trimester as a result of folate supplementation and declining in the 3rd trimester consequent to maximum utilization of folate by the growing fetus. There is evidence that suggests high folate status could exaggerate or increase the level of serum homocysteine in Vitamin B_{12} deficient individuals (Selhub *et al.*, 2007). However, with the notion of preventing NTDs, several pregnant women are getting exposed to high intake of folic acid rendering the individual susceptible to complex disorders. Moreover, this intervention is expected to reduce pregnancy complications but women with pregnancy complications are found to have excess circulating unmetabolized folic acid levels.

Folic Acid Supplementation: Through an Anthropological Lens

In India, as a part of routine antenatal care a dose of 5mg (5000µg) folic acid (folvite) once a day is given to all the pregnant women during first trimester (Mishra *et al.,* 2018) as against 0.4mg (400 µg) recommended by WHO. This supraphysiological dose (5mg) of folic acid given to Indian pregnant women is 12.5 times the recommended dose, which makes it a matter of concern as folate is the first external exposure for the fetus. Another point of concern is the timing of giving the folic acid because most of the pregnant women in India attend the antenatal care unit only after the first month post-conception when the neural tube is already been closed, hence the purpose of supplementing with folic acid, i.e. to prevent Neural Tube Defects is not met. In addition, recent literature has highlighted the ill effects of high intake of folic acid both on mother's and child's future health. Giving folic acid seems to be justifiable in Western context as majority of them practice non-vegetarianism as against in India, where majority are vegetarians; hence are expected to be folate replete and vitamin B_{12} deficient (Pawlak *et al.*, 2014). Thus folic acid supplementation to folate replete pregnant women is debatable in India where this programme is being implemented since early 1970s. In Indian context, food restrictions and food taboos are practiced during pregnancy in some regions and also in some communities. Some foods are more preferred for others depending on the flora and fauna available in that area. Going by the food habits, Western societies are predominantly non-vegetarian (Vitamin B_{12} rich) as compared to Indian societies where majority of people practise vegetarianism (Folate rich) for various reasons like religion, or economic status and so on. Even those who claim to be non-vegetarians in Indian context consume it with negligible frequency because of many factors. These different dietary habits may widely affect OCMP where folate is one of the important cofactor along with vitamin B_{12} (micronutrients). Vegetarians are expected to be deplete in vitamin B_{12} and non-vegetarians to be deplete in folate. Folic acid supplementation is justifiable in the Western context (non-vegetarianism) as compared to India, where they are expected to be replete in folic acid. Thus, indiscriminate supplementation of folic acid in Indian context is debatable and in this case, controversy arises when the folic acid dose of supplementation (5 mg) exceeds the upper intake level (1 mg) or recommended level (0.4 mg).

Suggestions and Future Directions

Folic acid supplementation in the absence of its deficiency has not demonstrated health benefits, and there are worrying signals that it may raise cancer risks, possibly by "feeding" existing cancers. The relative paucity of data indicates that there is an urgent need to develop further (future) studies focusing on health outcomes of folic acid supplementation after the first trimester. More well-designed, prospective cohort studies are needed to find the association of folic acid supplementation and adverse health outcomes both at the maternal and fetal front, so that the indiscriminate supplementation of folic acid to pregnant women can be challenged. Moreover, the role of *in utero* exposure of folic acid through maternal intake is emerging as a major question. Screening of folate and vitamin B_{12} levels prior to supplementation is suggested during pregnancy to prevent indiscriminate supplementation to all. Such information is critical for making appropriate dietary and supplement recommendations throughout pregnancy to insure healthy birth outcomes. Though this chapter is exclusively dealing with folic acid supplementation, the authors believe that any indiscriminate consumption of vitamins without knowing the status should be discouraged. Any supplement that enters human body in artificial form has a different route of metabolism and is likely to disturb the cycle or pathway in which it is involved.

REFERENCES

Bell, K.N., and Oakley Jr, G.P. (2009). "Update on prevention of folic acid-preventable spina bifida and anencephaly", *Birth Defects Research Part A: Clinical and Molecular Teratology*, *85*(1), 102-107.

Berry, R.J., Bailey, L., Mulinare, J., Bower, C., and Dary, O. (2010). "Fortification of flour with folic acid", *Food and nutrition bulletin*, *31*(1_suppl 1), S22-S35.

Bhide, P., Sagoo, G.S., Moorthie, S., Burton, H., and Kar, A. (2013). "Systematic review of birth prevalence of neural tube defects in India", *Birth Defects Research Part A: Clinical and Molecular Teratology*, *97*(7), 437-443.

Blencowe, H., Cousens, S., Modell, B., and Lawn, J. (2010). "Folic acid to reduce neonatal mortality from neural tube disorders", *International journal of epidemiology*, 39(suppl_1), i110-i121.

Botto, L.D., Moore, C.A., Khoury, M.J., and Erickson, J.D. (1999). "Neural-tube defects", *New England journal of medicine*, *341*(20), 1509-1519.

Butterworth Jr, C.E., and Tamura, T. (1989). "Folic acid safety and toxicity: A brief review". *The American journal of clinical nutrition*, *50*(2), 353-358.

Campbell, N.R. (1996). "How safe are folic acid supplements?". *Archives of Internal Medicine*, *156*(15), 1638-1644.

Chiaffarino, F., Ascone, G.B., Bortolus, R., Mastroia-Covo, P., Ricci, E., Cipriani, S., and Parazzini, F. (2010). "Effects of folic acid supplementation on pregnancy outcomes: A review of randomized clinical trials", *Minerva ginecologica*, *62*(4), 293-301.

Choumenkovitch, S.F., Selhub, J., Wilson, P.W., Rader, J.I., Rosenberg, I.H., and Jacques, P.F. (2002). "Folic acid intake from fortification in United States exceeds predictions", *The Journal of nutrition*, *132*(9), 2792-2798.

Cole, B.F., Baron, J.A., Sandler, R.S., Haile, R.W., Ahnen, D.J., Bresalier, R.S.,... and Polyp Prevention Study Group. (2007). "Folic acid for the prevention of colorectal adenomas: a randomized clinical trial", *Jama*, *297*(21), 2351-2359.

Collin, S.M., Metcalfe, C., Refsum, H., Lewis, S.J., Smith, G.D., Cox, A.,... and Martin, R.M. (2010b). "Associations of folate, vitamin B_{12}, homocysteine, and folate-pathway polymorphisms with prostate-specific antigen velocity in men with localized prostate cancer", *Cancer Epidemiology and Prevention Biomarkers*, *19*(11), 2833-2838.

Collin, S.M., Metcalfe, C., Refsum, H., Lewis, S.J., Zuccolo, L., Smith, G.D.,... and Martin, R.M. (2010a). "Circulating folate, vitamin B_{12}, homocysteine, vitamin B_{12} transport proteins, and risk of prostate cancer: a case-control study, systematic review, and meta-analysis", *Cancer Epidemiology and Prevention Biomarkers*, *19*(6), 1632-1642.

Cornel, M.C., De Smit, D.J., and De Jong-van den Berg, L.T.W. (2005). "Folic acid—The scientific debate as a base for public health policy", *Reproductive Toxicology*, *20*(3), 411-415.

Crider, K.S., Bailey, L.B., and Berry, R.J. (2011). "Folic acid food fortification—its history, effect, concerns, and future directions", *Nutrients*, *3*(3), 370-384.

Crider, K.S., Yang, T.P., Berry, R.J., and Bailey, L.B. (2012). "Folate and DNA methylation: A review of molecular mechanisms and the evidence for folate's role", *Advances in nutrition*, *3*(1), 21-38.

Czeizel, A.E. (2001). "Miscarriage and use of multivitamins or folic acid", *American journal of medical genetics*, *104*(2), 179-180.

de Bree, A., Verschuren, W.M., Bjørke-Monsen, A.L., Van der Put, N.M., Heil, S.G., Trijbels, F.J., and Blom, H.J. (2003). "Effect of the methylenetetrahydrofolate reductase 677C→ T mutation on the relations among folate intake and plasma folate and homocysteine concentrations in a general population sample". *The American journal of clinical nutrition, 77*(3), 687-693.

Del Gobbo, G.F., Price, E.M., Hanna, C.W., and Robinson, W.P. (2018). No evidence for association of MTHFR 677C> T and 1298A> C variants with placental DNA methylation. *Clinical epigenetics, 10*(1), 1-16.

De-Regil, L.M., Peña-Rosas, J.P., Fernández-Gaxiola, A.C., and Rayco-Solon, P. (2015). "Effects and safety of periconceptional oral folate supplementation for preventing birth defects", *Cochrane database of systematic reviews*, (12).

Dolin, C.D., Deierlein, A.L., and Evans, M.I. (2018). "Folic acid supplementation to prevent recurrent neural tube defects: 4 milligrams is too much", *Fetal diagnosis and therapy*, 44(3), 161-165.

Fletcher, R.J., Bell, I.P., and Lambert, J.P. (2004). "Public health aspects of food fortification: a question of balance", *Proceedings of the Nutrition Society, 63*(4), 605-614.

Forges, T., Monnier-Barbarino, P., Alberto, J.M., Gueant-Rodriguez, R.M., Daval, J.L., and Gueant, J.L. (2007). "Impact of folate and homocysteine metabolism on human reproductive health", *Human reproduction update, 13*(3), 225-238.

Guéant, J.L., Namour, F., Guéant-Rodriguez, R.M., and Daval, J.L. (2013). "Folate and fetal programming: A play in epigenomics?", *Trends in Endocrinology and Metabolism*, 24(6), 279-289.

Guenther, B.D., Sheppard, C.A., Tran, P., Rozen, R., Matthews, R.G., and Ludwig, M.L. (1999). "The structure and properties of methylenetetrahydrofolate reductase from Escherichia coli suggest how folate ameliorates human hyperhomocysteinemia", *Nature structural biology, 6*(4), 359-365.

Institute of Medicine. (1998). "Dietary Reference Intakes for Thiamin, Riboflavin, Niacin, Vitamin B6, Folate, Vitamin B12, Pantothenic Acid, Biotin, and Choline", National Academy Press; Washington, DC, USA.

Katre, P., Bhat, D., Lubree, H., Otiv, S., Joshi, S., Joglekar, C.,... and Yajnik, C. (2010). "Vitamin B12 and folic acid supplementation and plasma total homocysteine concentrations in pregnant Indian women with low B12 and high folate status", *Asia Pacific journal of clinical nutrition, 19*(3), 335-343.

Kim, M.K., Lee, S.M., Bae, S.H., Kim, H.J., Lim, N.G., Yoon, S.J.,... and Jo, M.W. (2018). "Socioeconomic status can affect pregnancy outcomes and complications, even with a universal healthcare system", *International journal for equity in health, 17*(1), 1-8.

Kim, Y.I. (2004). "Folate, colorectal carcinogenesis, and DNA methylation: lessons from animal studies", *Environmental and molecular mutagenesis, 44*(1), 10-25.

Ly, A., Lee, H., Chen, J., Sie, K.K., Renlund, R., Medline, A.,... and Kim, Y.I. (2011). "Effect of maternal and postweaning folic acid supplementation on mammary tumor risk in the offspring", *Cancer research, 71*(3), 988-997.

Lyon, P., Strippoli, V., Fang, B., and Cimmino, L. (2020). "B Vitamins and One-Carbon Metabolism: Implications in Human Health and Disease", *Nutrients, 12*(9), 2867.

Maternal Health Division, Ministry of Health and Family Welfare. Guidelines for Pregnancy Care and Management of Common Obstetric Complications by Medical Officers. New Delhi: Government of India; 2005.

Mishra, J., Puri, M., Sachdeva, M.P., Kaur, L., and Saraswathy, K.N. (2018). "Hyperhomocysteinemia and Folate deficiency in preterm premature rupture of membranes: A hospital based case control study (India)". *J Womens Health, Issues Care* 7, 4, 2.

Mishra, J., Talwar, S., Kaur, L., Chandiok, K., Yadav, S., Puri, M.,... and Saraswathy, K.N. (2019). "Differential global and MTHFR gene specific methylation patterns in preeclampsia and recurrent miscarriages: A case-control study from North India", *Gene, 704*, 68-73.

Mishra, J., Tomar, A., Puri, M., Jain, A., and Saraswathy, K.N. (2020). "Trends of folate, vitamin B12, and homocysteine levels in different trimesters of pregnancy and pregnancy outcomes", *American Journal of Human Biology, 32*(5), e23388.

Padmanabhan, V., Cardoso, R.C., and Puttabyatappa, M. (2016). "Developmental programming, a pathway to disease", *Endocrinology, 157*(4), 1328-1340.

Pawlak, R., Lester, S.E., and Babatunde, T. (2014). "The prevalence of cobalamin deficiency among vegetarians assessed by serum vitamin B12: A review of literature", *European Journal of Clinical Nutrition, 68*(5), 541-548.

Pickell, L., Brown, K., Li, D., Wang, X.L., Deng, L., Wu, Q.,... and Rozen, R. (2011). "High intake of folic acid disrupts embryonic development in mice". *Birth Defects Research Part A: Clinical and Molecular Teratology, 91*(1), 8-19.

Plumptre, L., Masih, S.P., Ly, A., Aufreiter, S., Sohn, K.J., Croxford, R.,... and Kim, Y.I. (2015). "High concentrations of folate and unmetabolized folic acid in a cohort of pregnant Canadian women and umbilical cord blood", *The American journal of clinical nutrition, 102*(4), 848-857.

Puri, M., Kaur, L., Walia, G.K., Mukhopadhhyay, R., Sachdeva, M.P., Trivedi, S.S.,... and Saraswathy, K.N. (2013). "MTHFR C677T polymorphism, folate, vitamin B12 and homocysteine in recurrent pregnancy losses: A case control study among North Indian women", *Journal of perinatal medicine, 41*(5), 549-554.

Rader, J.I. (2002). "Folic acid fortification, folate status and plasma homocysteine", *The Journal of nutrition, 132*(8), 2466S-2470S.

Reynolds, E. (2006). "Vitamin B12, folic acid, and the nervous system", *The lancet neurology, 5*(11), 949-960.

Selhub, J., Morris, M.S., and Jacques, P.F. (2007). In vitamin B12 deficiency, higher serum folate is associated with increased total homocysteine and methylmalonic acid concentrations. *Proceedings of the National Academy of Sciences, 104*(50), 19995-20000.

Smith, A.D., Kim, Y.I., and Refsum, H. (2008). "Is folic acid good for everyone?" *The American journal of clinical nutrition, 87*(3), 517-533.

Smithells, R.W., Sheppard, S., and Schorah, C.J. (1976). "Vitamin dificiencies and neural tube defects", *Archives of disease in childhood*, *51*(12), 944-950.

Stevens, V.L., McCullough, M.L., Sun, J., and Gapstur, S.M. (2010). "Folate and other one-carbon metabolism-related nutrients and risk of postmenopausal breast cancer in the Cancer Prevention Study II Nutrition Cohort", *The American journal of clinical nutrition*, *91*(6), 1708-1715.

Stover, P.J. (2011). "Polymorphisms in 1-carbon metabolism, epigenetics and folate-related pathologies", *Lifestyle Genomics*, *4*(5), 293-305.

Tam, C., O'Connor, D., and Koren, G. (2010). "Circulating unmetabolized folic acid: relationship to folate status and effect of supplementation", *Obstetrics and gynecology international*, 2012.

Troen, A.M., Mitchell, B., Sorensen, B., Wener, M.H., Johnston, A., Wood, B.,... and Ulrich, C.M. (2006). "Unmetabolized folic acid in plasma is associated with reduced natural killer cell cytotoxicity among postmenopausal women", *The Journal of nutrition*, *136*(1), 189-194.

Wang, H., De Steur, H., Chen, G., Zhang, X., Pei, L., Gellynck, X., and Zheng, X. (2016). "Effectiveness of folic acid fortified flour for prevention of neural tube defects in a high risk region", *Nutrients*, *8*(3), 152.

Waterland, R.A., and Jirtle, R.L. (2003). "Transposable elements: targets for early nutritional effects on epigenetic gene regulation", *Molecular and cellular biology*, *23*(15), 5293-5300.

WHO. Guideline: Daily Iron and Folic Acid Supplementation in Pregnant Women. Geneva: World Health Organization; 2012. [Accessed April 22, 2021]. Available from: https://www.nhp. gov.in/sites/default/files/pdf/9789241501996_eng.pdf

Windham, G.C., Shaw, G.M., Todoroff, K., and Swan, S.H. (2000). "Miscarriage and use of multi-vitamins or folic acid", *American Journal of Medical Genetics*, *90*(3), 261-262.

Yang, H.T., Lee, M., Hong, K.S., Ovbiagele, B., and Saver, J.L. (2012). "Efficacy of folic acid supplementation in cardiovascular disease prevention: an updated meta-analysis of randomized controlled trials", *European journal of internal medicine*, 23(8), 745-754.

Yang, L., Jiang, L., Bi, M., Jia, X., Wang, Y., He, C.,... and Wang, Z. (2015). "High dose of maternal folic acid supplementation is associated to infant asthma", *Food and Chemical Toxicology*, 75, 88-93.

Yi, Y., Lindemann, M., Colligs, A., and Snowball, C. (2011). "Economic burden of neural tube defects and impact of prevention with folic acid: A literature review", *European journal of pediatrics*, *170*(11), 1391-1400.

22

Social Epidemiology of Maternal and Child Health in India

Vipin Gupta and *M.P. Sachdeva*

Introduction

In order to transform the health and wellbeing of the world populations, United Nation's Sustainable Development Goals, namely 3.1 and 3.2 (SDG, 2015), specifically aimed to reduce maternal mortality and to end the preventable newborn deaths and child mortality under 5 years of age, respectively, by 2030 (GBD, 2015, SDG Collaborators). One fifth of the global under-5 deaths occurred in India, highest in the state of Uttar Pradesh (59.7 per 1000 live births) in 2017, with high level of inequality between districts within states (India State-Level Disease Burden Initiative Child Mortality Collaborators, 2020). In 2017, one of the predominant risk factor death in children less than 5 years of age is malnutrition that accounted for 68.2 per cent of total under-5 child deaths (India State-Level Disease Burden Initiative Malnutrition Collaborators, 2019). Focusing only on epidemiological or clinical aspects of health issues pertaining to mother and child health may be grossly insufficient for understanding the "causes of the causes", i.e. intermediary underlying causes of health conditions. The low utilization of health services and neonatal mortality and morbidity are high in India that could be reduced through simple educational interventions (Lassi *et al.,* 2019). The social or anthropological assessment of maternal health issues is the need of the hour for measuring the accumulation of risk and detecting critical time points for understanding health inequalities (Wadsworth, 1997). Several theories of social epidemiology have been proposed, like psycho-social framework or social production of disease or eco-social framework (Krieger, 2001), that had led to some progress in finding the chain of causes underlying health adversities. The present review discussed the primary social factors that directly/indirectly trigger the adverse social pathways for influencing maternal and child health in India.

Race, Ethnicity and Caste

The natural biological sub-divisions of human populations are conceptualized as races which are discrete and permanent units that implies biological homogeneity in somatic traits within the unit to some extent (Keita *et al.,* 2004, Gravlee, 2009). The racial disparity in health outcomes, like maternal and infant mortality, disqualifies the broad agreement on inexistency of race. Whereas ethnicity is a complex socio-cultural construct that describes specific ancestry, structure of relationships among the people, common food habits, language, lifestyle, belief system which regulates the overall behaviour of the community (Dressler *et al.*, 2005; Chaturvedi and Eastwood, 2020). As per WHO and UNICEF (2003) global strategy for infant and young child feeding, breastfeeding up to 2 years of age or beyond is essential for the healthy growth of the child. The partly learned nature of breastfeeding behaviour varies considerably between ethnicities and mostly consequent to the cultural norms and practices. Globally, sub-optimum breastfeeding was estimated to be responsible for 1·4 million child deaths (Black *et al.,* 2008). Choices of food to be cooked in Indian households is influenced by cultural, economic and environmental factors. Under-privileged communities suffer more from gestational malnutrition due to differential dietary energy intakes (Mukhopadhyay and Sarkar, 2009).

In contrast, caste is system of social stratification based on ascribed social status determined (Saroha *et al.,* 2008) at the time of birth among the Hindus and does have biological consequences. An analysis of the National Health Family Survey (NFHS)-3 and NFHS-4 data to measure the explained and unexplained differences in access to Janani Suraksha Yojana (JSY) among different caste groups had found caste-based discrimination in the access and utilization of JSY (Mishra *et al.,* 2021). Saroha *et al.* (2008) had observed that caste influences the utility of maternal health care services in the state of Uttar Pradesh, India, where upper caste women were using health care services, like antenatal care, birth attendant and contraceptives etc. three times more than lower caste women. A study had found that a child belonging to lower castes or tribes has a lower probability of registration compared to the higher castes (Mohanty and Gebremedhin,

2018). Women belong to poor or disadvantaged groups are usually at higher risk due to caste-based discrimination in accessing healthcare services (Baru *et al.,* 2010). Disparity in usage of maternal healthcare facilities in Scheduled Caste and tribal communities of India could be partly explained by availability of water at home and geographical region (Yadav *et al.,* 2020). The socio-biological categories of race, ethnicity and caste generally reflects upon the bio-cultural nature of human presence and must be considered while micro/macro level planning for communities or policy making for maternal and child health in India.

Urban and Rural Differences

The widespread inter- and intra-district inequities in utilization of maternal and child health services exist in India (Prinja *et al.,* 2019). Differential levels of urbanicity, like living in built-up areas, socio-cultural and economic changes, during the process of urbanization, is also associated with various maternal health and child health outcomes. The rapid urbanization has potential to influence cultural practices for example, Andhra Pradesh Children and Parent Study (APCAPS) had found that early stage urbanicity was associated with a shorter duration of breastfeeding (OR-2.4, 95% CI: 1.45-6.05), i.e. discontinuation before the prescribed WHO standard 24 months (Oakley *et al.,* 2017). A study based on household survey had reported that only 79 per cent women in rural areas had institutional deliveries compared to 93 per cent of urban women of Chandigarh (Gupta *et al.,* 2008). Migrant women to urban landscape for employment are poorly informed about the available medical care/services in the urban areas. A study conducted on women labourers working in brick kilns of Haryana have reported that only one-third of them had ever received cash benefits under Janani Suraksha Scheme or hardly used free ambulance service for maternal care (Siddaiah *et al.,* 2018). Highest urban-rural disparity in utilizing institutional delivery was reported in North-Eastern states (Meghalaya—42.3%) and lowest in Southern states (Kerela—0.1%) (Ghosh and Ghosh, 2020). Urban-rural differences in women empowerment has enabled the women of urban communities to be more involved in decision making, selecting their marital partners and more amount of freedom than rural women (Kumar, 1995; Sethuraman *et al.,* 2006).

Maternal Education

Maternal education is associated with range of maternal and child health outcomes like child's nutrition, vaccination, mortality, morbidity etc. (Vikaram and Vanneman, 2020). It is established that educated mothers would be more involved in health seeking behaviour for her child which is contingent upon household's environment (Desai and Alva, 1998). Maternal education is useful only when she is empowered to make decisions about their choices that will enable them to exercise control and power in their regular life (Malhotra and Schuler, 2005; Smith-Greenway, 2013). For example, children of poorly educated mothers experienced greater risk of stunting due to inadequate dietary habits (Krishna *et al.*, 2018). A study had investigated the role of maternal health literacy on child under nutrition in two Indian populations and found that children of mothers with high health literacy had half the likelihood of being severely stunted (Johri *et al.*, 2016). One year rise in mean years of maternal schooling is associated with 1.1-fold rise in the odds of birth registration (Mohanty and Gebremedhin, 2018). Educational interventions for mothers of under-5 children had shown significant improvement in home management of diarrhoea (Mangala, 2001). Thus, education plays a vital role in mother's life with respect to decision making process in order to improve her child's health.

Family Dynamics

Healthy lifestyle during pregnancy is contingent upon family members and neighbouring society. Family as a social unit has deciding role in making multiple arrangements for women health's and related issues (Morrissey, 2008; Allendorf, 2010). The complex decision-making process about sharing of limited food among the family members is critical for maternal health (FAO, 2015). Over 2 million deaths for children younger than 5 years was due to adverse birth outcomes like stunting, severe wasting, and intrauterine growth restriction (Black *et al.*, 2008). Perceived stress during pregnancy is associated with adverse birth outcomes (Staneva *et al.*, 2015), for example, worry of giving birth to a female child against the family expectation of male child in India was associated with stress (Aneja *et al.*, 2018). Mother's social and economic status enhances her bargaining power within the household and determines her mobility for seeking health care services (Mohanty and Gebremedhin, 2018). Similarly, there are several unexplored aspects of family dynamics and its interplay that regulates maternal behaviour and could be crucial in managing child health.

Socio-economic Status (SES)

Poverty is at the core of biosocial mechanisms that cause poor human development, and suggest that strategic investments in child nutrition must be considered as a model of economic development (McGregor, 2007; World Bank, 2008). There is an increased risk of stunting regardless of its social class due to poor socio-economic status (Krishna *et al.,* 2018). Inaccessible health care due to high expenditure is a risk for maternal and neonatal mortality. A Mumbai based study had reported that a high proportion of household spent catastrophically on maternal and neonatal care, and lower SES was associated with more informal spending (Skordis-Worrall *et al.,* 2011). Further, SES inequalities are also associated with child undernutrition which suggest the need of targeted interventions among poor families (Griffiths *et al.,* 2016). Another study on >1000 children from Darjeeling had reported that households with lower income have more prevalence of children with wasting (Tigga *et al.,* 2015). An assessment of a model of clinical social franchising programme in Rajasthan and Uttar Pradesh had found that families of high SES have utilized their antenatal and delivery services (Haemmerli *et al.,* 2018). A carefully designed conditional cash transfer (CCT) schemes can attenuate some of the adverse effects of low SES. A quantitative assessment of conditional cash transfer in *"Mamata"* scheme on household food security in Odisha had found positive impact on food security, registration of the pregnancy, in receiving medicines from health workers (Raghunathan *et al.,* 2017). Health interventions are required to break the structure of poverty for the percolation of health benefits to the lowest economic strata of the society.

Domestic Violence

Domestic violence is prominent cause of social morbidity, which may accelerate during and after gestation, and are associated with poor maternal and child health outcomes. The mother's experience of physical and sexual abuse is associated with high risk of infant and fetal death, and low birth weight (Asling-Monemi, 2003; Jejeebhoy, 1998). The mothers who experience domestic abuse at home are likely to have poor health outcomes and are more prone to suicidal thoughts (Chisholm *et al.,* 2017).

The maternal adverse health outcomes augmented in pregnancy, with an increased risk of preterm birth, likelihood of premature labour, lower infant birth weight, and small for gestational age (Huth-Bocks *et al.*, 2002). The high prevalence of domestic violence in India are due to male centric nature of the patriarchal societies (Kalokhe *et al.*, 2017). A study on women attending antenatal clinics had reported 26.9 per cent physical, 29 per cent mental and 6.2 per cent sexual abuse, irrespective of their age in Delhi (Sarkar, 2013). Moreover, high incidence of post-partum depression in India is partly explained by high frequency of domestic violence in India (Upadhyay *et al.*, 2017). A household based cross-sectional study was conducted in Bihar on mother of 0 to 23 months old children and found association between intimate partner violence and poor maternal outcomes like complications during delivery, miscarriage and labour complications (Dhar *et al.*, 2018). Large-scale societal and household-based studies are required for screening, referral and counselling of the victims of domestic violence (Daley *et al.*, 2020). A study on South Indian population was conducted had found that psychological abuse is associated with mild or greater depressive syndromes (Rao *et al.*, 2016). A study conducted in urban slums of Mumbai had observed that women whose husband consumed alcohol were at significant risk of experiencing domestic violence (Begum *et al.*, 2015) which may continue during pregnancy and after that to influence maternal and child health.

Gender Inequalities

The gender norms, values and expectations are shaped by the culture that determines the roles and opportunities for the people with the communities (Heise *et al.*, 2019). The restrictive gender norms impact the health and wellbeing through inequality in healthcare seeking behaviours (Heise *et al.*, 2019). There are multiple biosocial factors, for instance educational attainment and age at marriage, that usually incorporate gender inequity in assessing its health impacts on maternal and child health. Gender disparities favouring male child is highly common in India, that lead to differences in providing childcare services, like immunization (Gupta *et al.*, 2017). Although, in 2006 mortality rate was higher for girls between age 1 and 5 years than boys and this gap was eliminated due to improvements in survival in 2016 (Alderman *et al.*, 2021). The challenge of making gender neutral health system can only be achieved by balancing the inequities due to gender power relations in the access of health resources. It has been reported that girls usually have lower immunization coverage than boys due to gender inequality in India and also reported late immunization trends and clear-cut gender difference in immunization coverage especially among girls of high birth order (Corsi *et al.,* 2009).

Conclusion

The pattern of health and disease in a community is a reflection of unequal distribution benefits and risks in the societies. The analysis of social inequalities in terms of health is complicated by socio-cultural diversity within and between communities. Social epidemiologists or medical anthropologists can disentangle these complexities in data collection by developing novel research methods and analytical strategies.

REFERENCES

Alderman, H., Nguyen, P.H., Tran, L.M., and Menon, P. (2021). "Trends and geographic variability in gender inequalities in child mortality and stunting in India, 2006–2016", *Maternal and Child Nutrition*, e13179.

Allendorf, K. (2010). "The quality of family relationships and use of maternal healthcare services in India". *Studies in Family Planning, 41*(4), 263-276.

Aneja, J., Chavan, B.S., Huria, A., Goel, P., Kohli, N., and Chhabra, P. (2018). "Perceived stress and its psychological correlates in pregnant women: an Indian study", *International Journal of Culture and Mental Health, 11*(3), 268-279.

Åsling-Monemi, K., Pena, R., Ellsberg, M.C., and Persson, L.Å. (2003). "Violence against women increases the risk of infant and child mortality: A case-referent study in Nicaragua", *Bulletin of the World Health Organization, 81*, 10-16.

Baru, R., Acharya, A., Acharya, S., Kumar, A.S., and Nagaraj, K. (2010). "Inequities in access to health services in India: Caste, class and region", *Economic and political Weekly*, 49-58.

Begum, S., Donta, B., Nair, S., and Prakasam, C.P. (2015). "Socio-demographic factors associated with domestic violence in urban slums, Mumbai, Maharashtra, India", *The Indian journal of medical research, 141*(6), 783.

Black, R.E., Allen, L.H., Bhutta, Z.A., Caulfield, L.E., de Onis, M., Ezzati, M., Mathers, C., Rivera, J.; Maternal and Child Undernutrition Study Group. "Maternal and child undernutrition: global and regional exposures and health consequences", *Lancet*, 2008 January 19; 371(9608):243-60. doi: 10.1016/S0140-6736(07)61690-0.

Chaturvedi, N., and Eastwood, S. (2020). "Prescribing by ethnicity:(im) precision medicine?" *Diabetes Care, 43*(8), 1687-1689.

Chisholm, C.A., Bullock, L., and Ferguson II, J.E. J. (2017). "Intimate partner violence and pregnancy: Epidemiology and impact", *American journal of obstetrics and gynecology, 217*(2), 141-144.

Corsi, D.J., Bassani, D.G., Kumar, R., Awasthi, S., Jotkar, R., Kaur, N., and Jha, P. (2009). "Gender inequity and age-appropriate immunization coverage in India from 1992 to 2006", *BMC international health and human rights*, *9*(1), 1-12.

Daley, D., McCauley, M., and van den Broek, N. (2020). "Interventions for women who report domestic violence during and after pregnancy in low-and middle-income countries: A systematic literature review", *BMC pregnancy and childbirth*, *20*(1), 1-9.

Dandona, R., Kumar, G.A., Henry, N.J., Joshua, V., Ramji, S., Gupta, S.S., Agrawal, D., Kumar, R., Lodha, R., Mathai, M., Kassebaum, N.J., Pandey, A., Wang, H., Sinha, A., Hemalatha, R., Abdulkader, R.S., Agarwal, V., Albert, S., Biswas, A.,... Dandona, L. (2020). "Subnational mapping of under-5 and neonatal mortality trends in India: the Global Burden of Disease Study 2000–17", *The Lancet*, *395*(10237), 1640–1658.

Desai, S., and Alva, S. (1998). "Maternal education and child health: Is there a strong causal relationship?" *Demography*, *35*(1), 71-81.

Dhar, D., McDougal, L., Hay, K., Atmavilas, Y., Silverman, J., Triplett, D., and Raj, A. (2018). "Associations between intimate partner violence and reproductive and maternal health outcomes in Bihar, India: a cross-sectional study", *Reproductive health*, *15*(1), 1-14.

Dressler, W.W., Oths, K.S., and Gravlee, C.C. (2005). "Race and ethnicity in public health research: models to explain health disparities", *Annu. Rev. Anthropol.*, *34*, 231-252.

Dufour, S., Lavergne, C., Larrivée, M.C., and Trocmé, N. (2008). "Who are these parents involved in child neglect? A differential analysis by parent gender and family structure", *Children and Youth Services Review*, *30*(2), 141-156.

Ghosh, A. and Ghosh, R. (2020). "Maternal health care in India: A reflection of 10 years of National Health Mission on the Indian maternal health scenario", *Sexual and Reproductive Healthcare*, *25*, 100530.

Grantham-McGregor, S., Cheung, Y.B., Cueto, S., Glewwe, P., Richter, L., Strupp, B., and International Child Development Steering Group (2007). "Developmental potential in the first 5 years for children in developing countries", *The lancet*, *369*(9555), 60-70.

Gravlee, C.C. (2009). "How race becomes biology: embodiment of social inequality". *American journal of physical anthropology*, *139*(1), 47-57.

Griffiths, P.L., Balakrishna, N., Fernandez Rao, S., and Johnson, W. (2016). "Do socio-economic inequalities in infant growth in rural India operate through maternal size and birth weight?" *Annals of human biology*, *43*(2), 154-163.

Gupta, M., Bosma, H., Angeli, F., Kaur, M., Chakrapani, V., Rana, M., and Van Schayck, O.C. (2017). "Impact of a multi-strategy community intervention to reduce maternal and child health inequalities in India: A qualitative study in Haryana", *PloS one*, *12*(1), e0170175.

Gupta, M., Thakur, J.S., and Kumar, R. (2008). "Reproductive and child health inequities in Chandigarh Union Territory of India", *Journal of Urban Health*, *85*(2), 291-299.

Haemmerli, M., Santos, A., Penn-Kekana, L., Lange, I., Matovu, F., Benova, L., Wong, K.L., and Goodman, C. (2018). "How equitable is social franchising? Case studies of three maternal healthcare franchises in Uganda and India", *Health Policy and Planning*, *33*(3), 411–419.

Heise, L., Greene, M.E., Opper, N., Stavropoulou, M., Harper, C., Nascimento, M., Zewdie, D., Darmstadt, G.L., Greene, M.E., Hawkes, S., Heise, L., Henry, S., Heymann, J., Klugman, J., Levine, R., Raj, A., and Rao Gupta, G. (2019). "Gender inequality and restrictive gender norms: Framing the challenges to health", *The Lancet*, *393*(10189), 2440–2454.

Huth-Bocks, A.C., Levendosky, A.A., and Bogat, G.A. (2002). "The effects of domestic violence during pregnancy on maternal and infant health", *Violence and victims*, *17*(2), 169-185.

Jejeebhoy, S.J. (1998). "Associations between wife-beating and fetal and infant death: impressions from a survey in rural India", *Studies in family planning*, 300-308.

Johri, M., Subramanian, S., Koné, G.K., Dudeja, S., Chandra, D., Minoyan, N., Sylvestre, M.P., and Pahwa, S. (2016). "Maternal Health Literacy is Associated with Early Childhood Nutritional Status in India", *The Journal of Nutrition*, *146*(7), 1402–1410.

Kalokhe, A., Del Rio, C., Dunkle, K., Stephenson, R., Metheny, N., Paranjape, A., and Sahay, S. (2017). "Domestic violence against women in India: A systematic review of a decade of quantitative studies", *Global public health*, *12*(4), 498-513.

Karlsson, O., Kim, R., Joe, W., and Subramanian, S.V. (2019). "Socioeconomic and gender inequalities in neonatal, postneonatal and child mortality in India: a repeated cross-sectional study, 2005–2016", *J Epidemiol Community Health*, *73*(7), 660-667.

Keita, S.O.Y., Kittles, R.A., Royal, C.D., Bonney, G.E., Furbert-Harris, P., Dunston, G.M., and Rotimi, C.N. (2004). "Conceptualizing human variation", *Nature genetics*, *36*(11), S17-S20.

Krieger, N. (2001). "Theories for social epidemiology in the 21st century: an ecosocial perspective", *International journal of epidemiology*, *30*(4), 668-677.

Krishna, A., Mejía-Guevara, I., McGovern, M., Aguayo, V.M., and Subramanian, S.V. (2018). "Trends in inequalities in child stunting in South Asia", *Maternal and child nutrition*, *14*, e12517.

Lassi, Z.S., Kedzior, S.G., and Bhutta, Z.A. (2019). "Community-based maternal and newborn educational care packages for improving neonatal health and survival in low-and middle-income countries", *Cochrane Database of Systematic Reviews*, (11).

Lim, S.S., Allen, K., Bhutta, Z.A., Dandona, L., Forouzanfar, M.H., Fullman, N.,... and Chang, J.C. (2016). "Measuring the health-related Sustainable

Development Goals in 188 countries: A baseline analysis from the Global Burden of Disease Study 2015", *The Lancet*, *388*(10053), 1813-1850.

Malhotra, A. and Schuler, S.R. (2005). "Women's empowerment as a variable in international development", *Measuring empowerment: Cross-disciplinary perspectives*, *1*(1), 71-88.

Mangala, S., Gopinath, D., Narasimhamurthy, N.S., and Shivaram, C. (2001). "Impact of educational intervention on knowledge of mothers regarding home management of diarrhoea", *The Indian Journal of Pediatrics*, *68*(5), 393-397.

Marks, J. (2013). "The nature/culture of genetic facts". *Annual Review of Anthropology*, *42*, 247-267.

McGuire, S. (2015). FAO, IFAD, and WFP. The state of food insecurity in the world 2015: meeting the 2015 international hunger targets: taking stock of uneven progress. Rome: FAO, 2015. *Advances in Nutrition*, *6*(5), 623-624.

Mishra, P.S., Veerapandian, K., and Choudhary, P.K. (2021). "Impact of socio-economic inequity in access to maternal health benefits in India: Evidence from Janani Suraksha Yojana using NFHS data", *Plos one*, *16*(3), e0247935.

Mohanty, I., and Gebremedhin, T.A. (2018). "Maternal autonomy and birth registration in India: Who gets counted?" *PloS one*, *13*(3), e0194095.

Morrissey, T.W. (2008). "Familial factors associated with the use of multiple child-care arrangements", *Journal of Marriage and Family*, *70*(2), 549-563.

Mukhopadhyay, S., and Sarkar, A. (2009). "Pregnancy-related food habits among women of rural Sikkim, India". *Public health nutrition*, *12*(12), 2317-2322.

Oakley, L., Baker, C.P., Addanki, S., Gupta, V., Walia, G.K., Aggarwal, A., Bhogadi, S., Kulkarni, B., Wilson, R.T., Prabhakaran, D., Ben-Shlomo, Y., Davey Smith, G., Radha Krishna, K.V., and Kinra, S. (2017). "Is increasing urbanicity associated with changes in breastfeeding duration in rural India? An analysis of cross-sectional household data from the Andhra Pradesh children and parents study", *BMJ Open*, *7*(9), e016331.

Prinja, S., Balasubramanian, D., Sharma, A., Gupta, R., Rana, S.K., and Kumar, R. (2019). "Geographic inequities in coverage of maternal and child health services in Haryana State of India", *Maternal and child health journal*, *23*(8), 1025-1035.

Raghunathan, K., Chakrabarti, S., Avula, R., and Kim, S.S. (2017). "Can conditional cash transfers improve the uptake of nutrition interventions and household food security? Evidence from Odisha's Mamata scheme", *PLoS One*, *12*(12), e0188952.

Rao, D., Kumar, S., Mohanraj, R., Frey, S., Manhart, L.E., and Kaysen, D.L. (2016). "The impact of domestic violence and depressive symptoms on preterm birth in South India", *Social psychiatry and psychiatric epidemiology*, *51*(2), 225-232.

Sarkar, N.N. (2013). "The cause and consequence of domestic violence on pregnant women in India", *Journal of Obstetrics and Gynaecology*, *33*(3), 250-253.

Saroha, E., Altarac, M., and Sibley, L.M. (2008). "Caste and maternal health care service use among rural Hindu women in Maitha, Uttar Pradesh, India", *Journal of midwifery and women's health*, *53*(5), e41-e47.

Sethuraman, K., Lansdown, R., and Sullivan, K. (2006). "Women's empowerment and domestic violence: The role of sociocultural determinants in maternal and child undernutrition in tribal and rural communities in South India", *Food and nutrition bulletin*, *27*(2), 128-143.

Shiva Kumar, A.K. (1995). "Women's capabilities and infant mortality: Lessons from Manipur", *Women's Health in India,* Oxford University Press, Mumbai.

Siddaiah, A., Kant, S., Haldar, P., Rai, S.K., and Misra, P. (2018). "Maternal health care access among migrant women labourers in the selected brick kilns of district Faridabad, Haryana: mixed method study on equity and access", *International journal for equity in health*, *17*(1), 1-11.

Skordis-Worrall, J., Pace, N., Bapat, U., Das, S., More, N.S., Joshi, W., Pulkki-Brannstrom, A.M., and Osrin, D. (2011). "Maternal and neonatal health expenditure in Mumbai slums (India): A cross-sectional study", *BMC Public Health*, *11*(1), 1–12.

Smith-Greenaway, E. (2013). "Mothers' reading skills and child survival in Nigeria: Examining the relevance of mothers' decision-making power", *Social science and medicine*, *97*, 152-160.

Staneva, A., Bogossian, F., Pritchard, M., and Wittkowski, A. (2015). "The effects of maternal depression, anxiety, and perceived stress during pregnancy on preterm birth: A systematic review", *Women and Birth*, *28*(3), 179-193.

Swaminathan, S., Hemalatha, R., Pandey, A., Kassebaum, N.J., Laxmaiah, A., Longvah, T., Lodha, R., Ramji, S., Kumar, G.A., Afshin, A., Gupta, S.S., Kar, A., Khera, A.K., Mathai, M., Awasthi, S., Rasaily, R., Varghese, C.M., Millear, A.I., Manguerra, H.,... Dandona, L. (2019). "The burden of child and maternal malnutrition and trends in its indicators in the states of India: the Global Burden of Disease Study 1990–2017", *The Lancet Child and Adolescent Health*, *3*(12), 855–870.

The World, B. (2006). "Repositioning Nutrition as Central to Development. A Strategy for Large-Scale Action". *The International Bank for Reconstruction and Development*.

Tigga, P.L., Sen, J., and Mondal, N. (2015). "Association of some socio-economic and socio-demographic variables with wasting among pre-school children of North Bengal, India", *Ethiopian journal of health sciences*, *25*(1), 63-72.

Upadhyay, R.P., Chowdhury, R., Aslyeh Salehi, Sarkar, K., Singh, S.K., Sinha, B., Pawar, A., Rajalakshmi, A.K., and Kumar, A. (2017). "Postpartum depression in India: A systematic review and meta-analysis", *Bulletin of the World Health Organization*, *95*(10), 706–717C.

Victora, C.G., Adair, L., Fall, C., Hallal, P.C., Martorell, R., Richter, L., and Sachdev, H.S. (2008). "Maternal and child undernutrition: consequences for adult health and human capital", *The Lancet*, *371*(9609), 340–357.

Vikram, K. and Vanneman, R. (2020). "Maternal education and the multidimensionality of child health outcomes in India", *Journal of biosocial science*, *52*(1), 57.

Wadsworth, M.E. J. (1997). "Health inequalities in the life course perspective", *Social science and medicine*, *44*(6), 859-869.

World Health Organization. (2003). Global strategy for infant and young child feeding.

Yadav, A.K., and Jena, P.K. (2020). "Maternal health outcomes of socially marginalized groups in India", *International journal of health care quality assurance*.

23
Quality of Life Assessment Among Women in Kosi Flood Affected Areas

Minakshi and *Rahul Kumar*

Introduction

In the post-disaster situation, women's health encompassing their physical, mental and reproductive health has been a major concern and this if taken in its totality has posed a severe risk resulting in the poor quality of life among them. There has been a very important study by Wind, Joshi *et al.,* where in, it has been elucidated that seasonal floods in Northern India have resulted in recurrent disasters leading to severe impact on Mental Health and its functioning (Wind *et al.,* 2013). In another qualitative study conducted in Bahraich, Khattri and colleagues have concluded that floods leading to economic deprivation and increased poverty are related to mental health problems (Khattri *et al.,* 2012). In this chapter also, an attempt has been made to analyze the Quality of life in terms of physical health functioning and mental health functioning among women in Kosi flood affected area of Bihar, India.

Several studies on disaster have tended to focus on the severity of the impact a disaster might have on individual and community mental health status (Green *et al.,* 1985). Further there has been an attempt to examine the mental health impacts in specific disaster situation like flood, earthquake and cyclone (See Kar *et al.*[1], 2004; Irene Van Kamp *et al.,* 2006[2]; Telles, S. *et al.*[3], 2009). Differences between women and men in the nature of psychological impact of disaster have also been reported (Norris *et al.,* 2002, Norris *et al.,* 2004, Carr, V.J. *et al.,*1997). Several studies have found greater proportion of women and girls report suffering from emotional disorders and distress, as compared to men and boys (WHO, 2002).

Anxiety, Depression and PTSD are among the most common mental health problems in the aftermath of disaster (Norris *et al.,* 2004). In post-disaster situation one can also notice the occurrence of increases in alcohol or drug abuse and domestic or interpersonal violence (Norris *et al.,* 2002). With regard to mental health responses to disaster victims, pre-existing condition of hardship due to lower socio-economic and/or gender status can become greatly enhanced throughout the disaster experience from preparation to recovery (Bolin, 1998; Quarentelli, 1985).

Quality of life measures have become a vital and often required part of health outcomes appraisal (Burckhardt *et al.*, 2003). Measurement of Quality of Life especially after disaster situation provides a meaningful way to determine the impact of that catastrophic event on the individuals' overall well-being, including health and health related services. About the natures of Quality of Life, Revicki and colleagues described QoL as idiosyncratic to the individual, but intuitively meaningful and understandable to most people. It implies value based on subjective functioning in comparison with personal expectations and is defined by subjective experiences, states and perceptions (Reviki *et al.*, 2000). So understanding changes in QoL after a disaster may have important implications for managing health related issues in other disaster prone areas. Against this backdrop, purpose or the of the analysis is twofold: to assess quality of life after Kosi flood among women in affected and unaffected areas and to identify factors related with quality of life in the aftermath of flood disaster.

Study design: Cross-Sectional Survey.

Method

Both quantitative and qualitative methods were used for the purpose of the study. For quantitative method, medical outcomes study Short Form -12 (SF-12) and for qualitative methods, FGDs, case-studies and narratives were used, to explore the factors that influence quality of life among both affected and unaffected group. SF-12 is one of the most extensively used assessments of well-being worldwide (Ware *et al.*, 2002). A cross- sectional survey was conducted with the total sample size of 250. 125 from high flood affected areas where population was displaced for longer period of time from its original homeland and the same from the unaffected areas without displacement. It was not possible to conduct random sampling, therefore, purposive sampling was used with those respondents who were willing to be part of the study. Ever-married women aged 17-49 were eligible for the study, which were recruited after informed consent.

Quality of life was studied and examined by using a shortened version of the Medical Outcome Study 36 Item Short-Form Health Survey (SF-36), which is known as the Short Form-12.

Instrument

In the present study, Quality of life was studied and examined by using a shortened version of the Medical Outcome Study 36 Item Short-Form Health Survey (SF-36), which is known as the Short Form-12.

The SF-12 is a multipurpose short form survey with 12 questions, all selected from the SF-36 Health Survey (Ware, Kosinski, and Keller, 1996). Short Form-12 consists of two components that is mental health and Physical Health which includes 12 items altogether. The time period selected for the purpose of study was previous 4 weeks. Mental Health Component and Physical Health Component consist of 4 subscales each. The mental health summary measure includes subscales of: role-emotional functioning, mental health, vitality, and social functioning. The physical health components consist of items focusing on physical functioning, role-physical functioning, pain, and perceived general health (Khattri *et al.*, 2009). The items were further converted into *z*-scores, weighted, and summed to form physical health and mental health summary scales (Ware *et al.*, 2002). This algorithm was designed so that both scales would range from around 0 (worst health) to around 100 (best health), have a mean close to 50, and have a standard deviation close to 10. The internal consistency of both the scales was measured and it was acceptable to be good. In the affected sample the Cronbach's alphas of the mental health component and the physical health component were respectively .56 and .74. In the unaffected sample the Cronbach's alphas of the mental health component and the physical health component were respectively .56 and .73.

Statistical Analysis

At initial level, frequencies, percentage, means and standard deviation were calculated for descriptive data. Further student t-test for independent sample was used to evaluate differences among categorical variables and Pearson correlation coefficient was used to test for significance among continuous variables. Linear regression analysis was done to find the factor associated with quality of life among the affected population. $p<.05$ was considered to be statistically significant. Internal consistency was measured by using cronbach alpha. Data were analyzed with SPSS version 16 for windows.

Results

Overall there are 12 questions in the short form health survey, used to calculate the physical and mental component summary scores for functioning. These 12 items consist of (1) health condition in general (2) Moderate activities such as moving table or sweeping floor, (3) Walking for a few minutes or climbing several flights of stairs, (4) Accomplished less due to physical health, (5) Limited in kind of work due to physical health, (6) Accomplished less due to mental health, (7) Less careful than usual due, to mental problems, (8) Felt calm and peaceful, (9) Felt downhearted and blue, (10) Having lot of energy, (11) Social activities interfered by physical and emotional problems, and (12) Pain interfering normal work.

Less than one-fourth (22.4%) of the respondents among the affected group thought their health status to be 'good', 71.2 per cent as 'fair' and very less (6.4%) as 'poor', whereas in the unaffected areas around half of the respondent (50.4%) stated their health condition to be 'good' or 'very good', 47.2 per cent as 'fair' and only 2.4 per cent as 'poor'. Thus in the affected areas around 78 per cent of the respondents mentioned their health related quality of life as not good. The response for this particular item has 5 scales: excellent, very good, good, fair and poor.

About limitations in doing some moderate activities in daily life, majority of the respondents (79.2%) in the affected areas reported that they have some kind of limitations varying from little to lot, 20.8 per cent have 'no limitations at all'. Contrary to this, 38 per cent of the respondents in unaffected areas had no limitations in performing moderate activities. This item of physical health component has 3 scales: (1) Yes, limited a lot, (2) Yes, limited a little, and (3) No, not limited at all.

Another physical functioning question was asked "Does your health now limit you in doing activities like walking for a few minutes or climbing several flights of stairs, and this also has 3 scales: (1) Yes, limited a lot, (2) Yes, limited a little, and (3) No, not limited at all. Here again majority of the respondents (86.4%) in the affected areas opined that there activities were limited, 13.6 per cent reported no limitations. In unaffected group, 63.2 per cent has some of the limitations and 36.8 per cent has no limitations at all.

Further due to perceived poor physical health, majority of the respondents reported to have physical limitations in performing activities among the affected group. 79.2 per cent accomplished less work than they would like to do. Additionally, 78.4 per cent of the respondents also claimed kinds of work were limited due to physical health.

To delve into the mental health component, limitations in kind of work due to mental health were asked from the respondents. 80 per cent in the affected and only 35 per cent in the unaffected said that they accomplished less due to mental health. Also, 81.6 per cent in the affected and 35.2 per cent in unaffected claimed that they did not do work or activities as careful as usual.

Additionally, emotional wellbeing component of mental health was calculated by asking the respondents firstly, whether they felt calm and peaceful, for which around two-third (68%) of the respondents in the affected group said 'a good bit of time', 8 per cent said 'all or most of the time' and 32 per cent said only 'some of the time', whereas in unaffected group 58.4 per cent said they felt calm and peaceful 'most of the time'. Secondly, they were asked, whether they felt downhearted and blue. 38 per cent of the respondent in the affected areas said a 'good bit of time'. Whereas in unaffected group 47.2 per cent reported to feel downhearted and blue 'a little or none of the time'. Both the items of emotional well-being have six scales: All of the time, Most of the time, A good bit of time, Some of the time, A little of the time and None of the time. While the response for the first one was coded from 100 to 0, second one was from 0 to 100. Another question which was asked was "Did you have a lot of energy during past 4 weeks?", and it has 6 scales: All of the time, Most of the time, A good bit of time, Some of the time, A little of the time and None of the time. Among affected group around half of the respondents (52%) claimed to have a lot of energy only 'some of the time', followed by 38.4 per cent which said 'a good bit of time'. Only 4 per cent said they had lot of energy 'most of the time'. Contrary to this, among unaffected group, 45.6 per cent said most of the time they had a lot of energy, followed by 38.4 per cent which said 'a good bit of time'.

Then, the respondents were asked whether the physical or emotional problems interfered their social activities like visiting friends, relatives etc. and this item has 5 scales: All of the time, Most of the time, Some of the time, A little of the time and None of the time. Around two-third (63.2%) in the affected group and 55.2 per cent in the unaffected group claimed some of the time they had these problems. 18 per cent of the respondents in the unaffected group and none of them from the affected group said that they did not have these problems.

In terms of interruption of work because of pain, respondents were asked how much did pain interfere with their normal work (including both work outside the home and housework), for this only 4 per cent in the affected group stated 'not interrupted at all' and 60.8 per cent said it was interrupted a little bit. In unaffected group 26.4 per cent has no such kind of experience while 59.2 per cent stated that work was interrupted a bit due to pain. This item has 5 scales: Not at all, A little bit, Moderately, Quite a bit and Extremely (Table 23.1).

So, among the affected and unaffected group, differences were found in both physical and mental health domain, thus affecting overall quality of life. Further descriptive analysis by means of mean, standard deviation and p-value will give us differences in functioning between the affected and unaffected groups.

Differences in Functioning Between the Affected and Unaffected Group

The affected group scores significantly lower on the Physical Health Component as an indicator of Functioning (M = 41.14; SD = 17.50) than the unaffected group (M = 61.45; SD = 23.32) (t = –7.78; df = 248; *p* = .000) and Mental Health Component (M = 43.79; SD = 14.83) than the unaffected group (M = 65.86; SD = 20.97) (t = –9.60; df = 248; *p* = .000).

The subscales of the physical health summary scale revealed highly significant differences between the affected and the unaffected group on General Health (M = 29.00; SD = 12.85 for the affected group and M = 40.40; SD = 18.72 for the unaffected group; *t* = –5.61; df = 248; *p* = .000), Physical Functioning (M = 49.60; SD = 26.93 for the affected group and M = 64.40; SD = 28.79 for the unaffected group; *t* = –4.19; df = 248; *p* = .000), Role-Physical (M = 21.20; SD = 39.78 for the affected group and M = 64.80; SD = 47.95 for the unaffected group; *t* = –7.82; df = 248 *p* = .000), and Bodily Pain (M = 64.20; SD = 18.87 for the affected group and M = 75.40; SD = 21.29 for the unaffected group; *t* = –4.40; df = 248; *p* = .000).

Similarly, the subscales of the mental health summary scale also revealed highly significant differences between the affected and the unaffected group on Vitality (M = 48.80; SD = 13.77 for the affected group and M = 65.92; SD = 17.04 for the unaffected group; *t* = –8.73; df = 248; *p* = .000), Social Functioning (M = 54.40; SD = 14.57 for the affected group and M = 64.80; SD = 19.85 for the unaffected group; *t* = –4.72; df = 248; *p* = .000), Role-Emotional (M = 19.20; SD = 38.51 for the affected group and M = 64.80; SD = 46.67 for the unaffected group; *t* = –8.42; df = 248 *p* = .000), and Emotional well-being (M = 52.16; SD = 12.15 for the affected group and M = 67.12; SD = 14.96 for the unaffected group; *t* = –8.67; df = 248; *p* = .000) (See Table 23.2).

Table 23.1: Frequency (%) For Short Form Health Survey-12 (A = Affected, U = Unaffected)

Sl.No.	*Items*		*Excellent*	*Very Good*	*Good*	*Fair*	*Poor*	
1.	General Health	A	–	–	22.4	71.2	6.4	
		U	–	13.6	36.8	47.2	2.4	
			Yes, limited a lot	Yes, limited a little	No, not limited at all			
2.	Moving a table, sweeping floor	A	9.6	69.6	20.8			
		U	5.6	56.8	37.6			
3.	Climbing several flights of stairs	A	26.4	60.0	13.6			
		U	11.2	52.0	36.8			
			Yes	No				
4.	Accomplished less due to physical health	A	79.2	20.8				
		U	35.2	64.8				
5.	Limited in kind of work	A	78.4	21.6				
		U	35.2	64.8				
6.	Accomplished less, due to mental health	A	80.0	20.0				
		U	35.2	64.8				
7.	Less careful than usual, due to mental health	A	81.6	18.4				
		U	35.2	64.8				
			All of the time	Most of the time	A good bit of time	Some of the time	A little of the time	None of the time

(*Contd.*)

(Contd.)

Sl.No.	*Items*		*Excellent*	*Very Good*	*Good*	*Fair*	*Poor*	
8.	Felt calm and peaceful	A	.8	7.2	60.0	32.0	–	–
		U	3.2	55.2	29.6	8.8	3.2	–
9.	Felt downhearted and depressed	A	3.2	8.0	37.6	43.2	8.0	–
		U	–	.80	28.0	24.0	40.0	7.2
10.	Have a lot of energy	A	.80	4.0	38.4	52.0	4.8	–
		U	1.6	45.6	38.4	9.6	4.8	–
			All of the time	Most of the time	Some of the time	Little of the time	None of the time	
11.	Social activities interfered by physical and emotional problems	A	–	9.6	63.2	27.2	–	
		U	–	1.6	55.2	25.6	17.6	
			Not at all	A little bit	Moderately	Quite a bit	Extremely	
12.	Pain interferes normal work	A	4.0	60.8	23.2	12.0	–	
		U	26.4	59.2	4.0	10.4	–	

Table 23.2: Subscales of Functioning in the Affected and Unaffected group (N = 125)

	Flood Affected group Mean (SD)	*Unaffected Group Mean (SD)*	*'t' Value*	*'p' Value*
Physical health component	41.14 ± 17.50	61.45 ± 23.32	-7.78	.000***
General health	29.00 ± 12.85	40.40 ± 18.72	-5.61	.000***
Physical functioning	49.60 ± 26.93	64.40 ± 28.79	-4.19	.000***
Role-physical	21.20 ± 39.78	64.80 ± 47.95	-7.82	.000***
Bodily Pain	64.20 ± 18.87	75.40 ± 21.29	-4.40	.000***
Mental health component	43.79 ± 14.83	65.86 ± 20.97	-9.60	.000***
Vitality	48.80 ± 13.77	65.92 ± 17.04	-8.73	.000***
Social functioning	54.40 ± 14.57	64.80 ± 19.85	-4.72	.000***
Role-emotional	19.20 ± 38.51	64.80 ± 46.67	-8.42	.000***
Emotional well-being	52.16 ± 12.15	67.12 ± 14.96	-8.67	.000***

Note: SD = Standard Deviation. *** '*p*' significant at <0.001.

Further, among the affected group, association of certain socio-economic and demographic variables with that of quality of life was calculated by means of correlation and students t-test. A non-significant relation (p = .132, r = – .135) was found with that of age and quality of life among the respondents (Table 23.3).

Table 23.3: Showing Correlation between Age and QoL using Pearson Correlation Coefficients

Variable	*r value*	*p value*
Age×QoL	-.135	.132

Similarly, non-significant relation was found between respondent's employment status (whether earning money or not) and quality of life, husband consuming alcohol or not and respondent's quality of life, social support (in form of neighbour helping each other) and quality of life (Table 23.4).

Whereas, highly significant relation (p = .001, t = –3.28, df = 123) between quality of life and respondents' literacy status. Among the affected group, those who were literate had better quality of life (mean score = 49.17) than those who were illiterate (mean score = 39.70).

Similarly, the family which has taken loan has lower mean score for quality of life (40.31) than those who has not taken loan (47.39). A significant relation was found (p = .01, t = –2.42, df = 123) in terms of quality of life score between those who have taken loan and those who have not (Table 23.4).

Table 23.4: Showing relationship between Quality of life and categorical variables using Student t-test

Variable	*Mean (±SD)*	*t value*	*p value*
Literacy Status			
Literate	49.17 ± 18.52	-3.28	.001**
Illiterate	39.70 ± 12.59		
Employment Status			
Earning money	43.00 ± 15.75	.264	.792
Not earning money	42.16 ± 14.89		
Husband drink alcohol			
Consuming alcohol	40.77 ± 13.61	-1.13	.259
Never consume alcohol	43.82 ± 16.20		
Social Support			
Neighbour help	43.23 ± 15.63	1.50	.136
Neighbour does not help	37.75 ± 10.51		
Family took loan			
Taken loan	40.31 ± 13.77	-2.42	.01*
Not taken loan	47.39 ± 16.95		

*p is significant at <.05 level, **p is highly significant at <.01 level.

Further, those variables which were found to be significant in bivariate analysis were put to linear regression analysis. For this quality of life was taken as dependent variable and educational status and loan burden as an independent variable. After regression analysis respondents' literacy status (B = 8.98, t = 3.15, p = .002) and financial burden in form of loan respondents' educational status (B = 6.40, t = 2.27, p = .02) was found to be the significant predictor of overall quality of life among the flood affected population (See Table 23.5).

Table 23.5: Predictor for quality of life using linear regression

Dependent Variable	*Predictor*	*Adjusted R Square*	*Beta Coefficient*	*p value*
Quality of Life	Literacy	.103	8.98	.002**
Quality of Life	Loan Burden	.103	6.40	.02*

*p is significant at <.05 level, **p is highly significant at <.01 level.

Correlation of Mental Health Outcomes in Form of Anxiety and Depression and Overall Quality of Life

In addition to certain socio-economic variables relation between mental healths outcomes (anxiety and depression) with that of quality of life was also calculated among both affected and unaffected group. A non-significant relation was found between mental health outcomes and quality of life in the affected group. Whereas, in the unaffected group, highly significant and inverse relation was found between anxiety and quality of life (r = –.400, p = .000) and depression and quality of life (r = –.275, p = .000), using Pearson Correlation Coefficients (See Table 23.6).

Table 23.6: Showing Correlations between Anxiety and QoL and Depression and QoL in the Unaffected Group

Variable	*r value*	*p value*
Anxiety ×QoL	– .400	.000***
Depression ×QoL	– .275	.000***

*** *'p'* significant at <.001.

Discussions

In this section an attempt was made to analyze health related quality of life among flood affected population. For this purpose, quality of life has been viewed from overall perspective, not specifically in terms of physical and mental health. Moreover, the significant and non-significant relation of parameters under test with that of quality of life can be viewed in the light of some definitional aspect, like how social support, economic loss is defined, how literacy is defined and what are the parameters of quality of life. It may be pointed out that quality of life has two important dimensions, i.e. the objective dimensions and the subjective dimensions. While the former referred to the 'reason' or a cognitive part of quality of life, the latter concerns 'emotions' or the affective part, which refers to both the presence of positive affect and the absence of negative affect (Diener, 1994). Further elaborating upon the subjective well-being, Deiner stated that subjective well-being refers to all of the various types of evaluations, both positive and negative, that people make of their lives. It includes reflective cognitive evaluations, such as personal satisfaction and work satisfaction, interest and engagement, and effective reactions to life events such as joy and sadness. Subjective well-being is a cognitive judgmental process that depends on a series of appropriate standards, but on the basis on their own unique set of criteria (Deiner, 2005).

When comparing quality of life, among affected and unaffected group, a highly significant difference was found between the groups, on both the subscales, physical health summary score and mental health summary score. Many studies are conducted to assess the quality of life in the aftermath of disaster (Hurricane Katrina, by Stanley *et al.* in 2011, Chi Chi earthquake, Taiwan by Wu HC *et al.* in 2006, Wenchuan earthquake, by Wen *et al.* in 2012) and found poor quality of life among the survivors due to many factors. But only few studies (Khattri *et al.*, 2009 and Wind *et al.,* 2013) have tried to compare the quality of life among the affected population with that of the unaffected groups and have found significant difference between the groups, same as the present study. The findings are consistent with other studies which accounted that disasters have significant effects on psychological and physical health, especially in those instances in which there was a significant loss of life, extensive property damage and severe economic disruptions of people's lives (Adams *et al.*, 2002; Erikson, 1976; Freedy, Kilpatrick and Resnick, 1993; Green, 1995; Norris *et al.*, 2002). Kosi flood, being unpredictable in nature due to its changing course, also brought huge damage to people's life and property, thereby affecting overall quality of life.

With reference to age, statistically non-significant relation was found between age and the quality of life of the respondents among the affected group while conducting pearson's correlation coefficient ($p = .13$). The findings are not in congruence with other studies as most of them reported higher age with poor quality of life (see Adams *et al.*, 2005; Santos, P.R., 2006; Ardalan *et al.*, 2011). Fran H. Norris, in psychosocial consequences of natural disasters in developing countries summarizes the findings on who is most likely to experience serious and lasting psychological distress in the aftermath of disaster has put older adults at greater risk than were other adults in only a small minority of adult samples where age differences were observed. Findings concerning the effect of age have been inconsistent (Norris *et al.,* 2002). Cross-cultural research suggests that the effects of age may differ across countries according to the social, political, economic, and historical context of the setting involved (Norris, 2005). Findings from this study shows that around 83 per cent of the respondents fall in the age range of 18-38, and only 17 per cent in the age range of 39-48 with mean age of 30 years. It may be possible that respondents age being not falling in much older category; the perceived quality of life does not get affected with age.

Similarly, non-significant relation was found between respondents' occupational status (i.e. working and non-working) and quality of life. Quality of life does not get affected with respondents' earning status may be because those who were earning were more likely to be engaged in part time work or irregular employment, mostly in the form of labour work with less remuneration. This may not contribute towards good material condition or to fill the losses occurred during the flood disaster, thereby having a non-significant role in the overall quality of life of the respondents.

Further, husbands' habit of consuming alcohol also played a non-significant role in the overall quality of life of the respondents. As stated by a lady aged forty nine:

> '*My husband drinks daily, during the evening. He is a rickshaw puller and he needs to drink. Not only has my husband, almost all men in this village consumed alcohol and smoked bidi. But what will happen by telling all these things? Situation is same from last twenty-twenty five years and will remain as such. Moreover he is only feeding me and my family. Others will not come and help me. Therefore, I don't want my husband to get bad name...*'.

As evident from the statement, women are used to of these situations and it does not mark any differences in their day-to-day life. Moreover the act is often legitimized or justified through their socio-cultural and economic condition.

Further, with regard to social support, similar non-significant association was found between quality of life and social support in the form of neighbour's help during the time of crisis. The findings did not cohere with the other studies which assert positive and significant association of quality of life with that of social support. In 'Quality of Life in Hypertensive Clinic Patients Following Hurricane Katrina' Stanley *et al.,* found that increased distance from family and friends, and decreased visits with family and friends were associated with lower quality of life (Stanley *et al.*, 2011).

In the present study, probably, respondents' did not view neighbours support as an important factor that can impinge on their health related quality of life as all of them were in the similar state of suffering in the aftermath of disaster. Presumably, it may also because of the fact that in this study social support were only looked in terms of neighbours help, and not including other parameters as role of family members, friend and other institution within the community.

Whereas, a highly significant association was found between quality of life and respondents' literacy status with p-value .001 by student t-test. Respondents who were literate had better quality of life than those who were illiterate. Recently, scholars have pointed out that literacy has significant advantages in terms of subjective wellbeing (SWB), in addition to its well-known micro-macro-economic and social outcomes (Cornali, 2011). Probable explanation for this association may lie in the fact that literate person has more personal control over their life, as they have more access to economic resources and support from the families. Several authors have shown the importance that education has in increasing the sense of control over life, personal satisfaction and access to stable relationship or in other words on increasing SWB (Cornali, 2011). In the study 'Education and Subjective Quality of life', Ross and Willingen proposes that compared to the poorly educated, well-educated individuals have access to stable social relationship, thereby having better subjective quality of life (Ross and Willingen, 1997). Belief in personal control is a learned, generalized expectation that outcomes are contingent on one's own choices and actions (Mirowsky and Ross, 1989; Rotter, 1966). Education correlates positively with the sense of control, and the sense of control mediates a large part of the negative association between education and distress (Mirowsky and Ross, 1989). High personal control helps people cope actively and flexibly, to avoid problems and to prepare for those that cannot be avoided (Mirowsky and Ross 1989, Turner and Noh, 1983, Wheaton, 1983). In this study also literacy may have provided respondents a kind of personal control, a sense of empowerment which enhanced the problem solving attitude in a situation like disaster. But, this exploratory findings/explanation needs to be better understood and more thoroughly studied and can also be the hypothesis for the further studies. As said by Pearlin, education is rarely the focus of investigation in the sociological study of stress and research has not identified the mechanisms by which education affects psychological well-being (Pearlin, 1989). Further the negative association between education and psychological distress is well documented but the mechanisms by which education affects well-being are not (Ross and Willingen, 1997).

Additionally, literacy was also found as one of the predictor of quality of life among the affected group using the linear regression model.

Similarly, financial crisis in the form of loan burden was found to be highly significant with p-value .01 using student t-tests. Respondents' from those families which have taken loan during last year, in the aftermath of disaster had poor quality of life than those who have not taken loan. The stress caused by the financial burden in form of loan was taking toll on respondents' health and health related quality of life. Similar finding was reported in one study 'Quality of Life in Hypertensive Clinic Patients Following Hurricane Katrina' by Stanley *et al.,* where personal and financial losses were identified as the most common cause of post-disaster stress, reported by 29.6 per cent of participants. In the study, the presence of stress in form of personal and financial loss was a factor associated with poor quality of life (Stanley *et al.*, 2011).

In the present study, loan burden upon family was also found to be the predictor of quality of life in the linear regression analysis, among respondents in the flood affected areas. The finding goes in line with the study 'Survey of quality of life and related risk factors for a Taiwanese village population 3 years post-earthquake' by Wu, H.C. *et al.*, economic problem was identified as one of the predictor for poor quality of life (Wu, H.C. *et al.*, 2006).

Surprisingly, the outcome of the study highlighted that in the affected group, the level of functioning of the individuals was not related with anxiety or depression score. Whereas, in the unaffected group, highly significant and inverse relation was found between anxiety and quality of life and depression and quality of life, which mean higher the anxiety or depression level, lower the quality of life of the respondents. Similar findings were reported by Khattri *et al.* in context of Bahraich flood, India, where they found absence of a relation between functioning and mental health in the affected group. However, among the unaffected group, the mental health problems affected around the one-fourth of the variance of both psychological and physical functioning and anxiety was found to hinder their daily functioning; both psychological and physical (Khattri *et al.*, 2009). Presumably, in the unaffected areas monetary loss was very less as compared to the affected areas, major concern lies within the domain of health, resulting in increased level of anxiety and depression thereby decrease in the quality of life or the subjective well-being of the respondents. Whereas, in the affected areas there were huge loss mainly in terms of property (land, livestock, agricultural produce) resulting in the heavy loan burden on the respondents and her family. The loss was magnified due to the unpredictability of the Kosi flood, denial mode of the villagers (people were not ready to accept that flood will come in their region, since historically this does not happened in the last four decades) and consequentially there was lack of preparedness. All this amounted to heavy monetary loss among the flood affected population. So, it may be said that among the affected group, the material aspects gained precedence over the non-material aspect while describing their overall quality of life. The subjective expression of quality of life is related with the material condition of the people. An individual with better material condition would more likely to report better quality of life and *vice versa.*

Conclusion

The stress caused by personal and financial loses in the aftermath of flood results in poor quality of life among affected groups. Additionally, literacy came handy as it provides with self-control and problem-solving skill at the time of disaster. The findings are important because it provides significant relation between that of education and quality of life. Further there is a need for a detailed study in order to identify the mechanisms by which education affects psychological wellbeing. Economic needs in form of alternate employment options, restoring the social fabric by checking out migration and adequate health and educational facilities were the main concern among the respondents. Thus following a major disaster, there is a need to specifically address the problems of women, empower them and provide adequate financial and social support to enhance the overall wellbeing.

NOTES

1. Kar *et al.* studied mental health consequences of the trauma of super cyclone 1999 in Orissa.
2. Irene Van Kamp *et al.* studied physical and mental health in Enschede, The Netherlands fire work disaster in 2000.
3. Shirley Telles *et al.* studied PTSD and Depression in survivors of flood in Bihar, 2008.

REFERENCES

Adams, R.E. and J.A. Boscarino. (2005). "Stress and Well-Being in the Aftermath of the World Trade Center Attack: The Continuing Effects of a Communitywide Disaster", *J Community Psychol.* Vol. *33*(2), 175–190.

Adams, R.E., Bromet, E.J., Panina, N., Golovakha, E., Goldgaber, D. and S. Guzman. (2002). "Stress and well-being after the Chernobyl nuclear power plant accident", *Psychological Medicine. 32*:143–156.

Ardalan, A., Mazaheri, M., Vanrooyen, M., Mowafi, H., Nedjat, S., Holakouie Naieni, K. and M. Russel. (2011). "Post-disaster quality of life among older survivors five years after the Bam earthquake: implications for recovery policy", *Ageing and Society.* Vol. *31* (2), 179-196. Cambridge University Press.

Bolin, R.C. (1998). "Response to Natural Disasters", In *Mental Health Response to Mass Emergencies*. Mary Lys tad (ed.). New York. Brunner/Mazel. Inc.

Burckhardt, C.S. and Anderson, K.L. (2003). "The Quality of Life Scale (QOLS): Reliability, Validity, and Utilization", *Health and Quality of Life Outcomes*. Vol. *1*:60. doi :10.1186/1477-7525-1-60.

Carr, V.J., Lewin, T.J., Webster, R.A. and J.A. Kenardy. (1997). "A synthesis of the findings from the Quake Impact Study: A two-year investigation of the psychosocial sequelae of the 1989 Newcastle earthquake". *Soc Psychiatry Psychiatr Epidemiol*. Vol. 32. pp. 123-136.

Cornali, F. (2011). "The Strange Relationship between Literacy and Well-Being: The Results of an International Survey with Special Focus on Italy", *International Journal of Human and Social Sciences*. Vol. 6:2.

Diener, E. (1994). "Assessing Subjective Well-Being: Progress and Opportunities", *Social Indicators Research*. Vol. *31*(2), 103-157.

Diener, E. (2005). "Guidelines for National Indicators of Subjective : Well-Being and Ill-Being". Mimeo.

Erikson, K.T. (1976). *Everything in its path*. Simon and Schuster: New York.

Frankl, V.E. (1963). *Man's search for meaning*. New York: Pocket Books.

Freedy, J.R., Kilpatrick, D.G. and H.S. Resnick. (1993). "Natural disasters and mental health: Theory, assessment, and intervention", *Journal of Social Behaviour and Personality.* Vol. 8, 49–103.

Green, B.L., Lindy, J.D., Grace, M.C. and J. Titchener (1985). "Psychotherapy and Survivors of the Beverly Hills Super Club Fire", *American Journal of Psychotherapy.* Vol. *37* (4), 593-610.

Green, B.L. (1995). "Long-term consequences of disasters", In Hobfoll SE, de Vries M.W., (eds.) *Extreme stress and communities: Impact and intervention*. Kluwer Academic: Amsterdam. pp. 307–324.

Janssen Quality-of-life Studies. Retrieved 14 August (2012) from: www.gdrc.org/uem/qol-define.html

Kar, N., Jagadisha, Sharma, P.S.V.N., Murali, N. and S. Mehrotra. (2004). Mental Health Consequences of the Trauma of Super-Cyclone 1999 in Orissa. *Indian Journal of Psychiatry.* Vol. 46(3), 228-237.

Khattri, P., Wind, T.R., Komproe, I.H. and P.C. Joshi. (2009). *Anxiety, Depression, and Functioning Among a Population Struck By Recurrent Floods in Uttar Pradesh. India*. MICRODIS working paper series. Unpublished.

Khattri, P., Joshi, P.C., Wind, T.R., Komproe, I.H., Guha-Sapir, D. (2012). "Understanding mental health as a function of social vulnerabilities in a disaster situation: Evidence from recurrent flooding in Bahraich district, Uttar Pradesh", *J Anthropol Survey India*. 2012; *61*(1):109-125.

McCall, S. (1975). Quality of Life. *Social Indicators Research*. Vol. 2, pp. 229-248.

Mirowsky, J. and Catherine E. Ross. (1989). *Social Causes of Psychological Distress*. New York. Aldine de Gruyter.

Norris, F.H. (2005). Psychosocial Consequences of Natural Disasters in Developing Countries: What Does Past Research Tell Us About the Potential Effects of the 2004 Tsunami? National Center for PTSD.

Norris, F.H., Friedman, M.J., Watson, P.J., Byrne, C.M., Diaz, E. and K. Kaniasty. (2002). "60,000 disaster victims speak: Part I. An empirical review of the empirical literature. 1981-2001", *Psychiatry*. Vol. 65, pp. 207-239.

Pearlin, L.I. (1989). "The Sociological Study of Stress", *Journal of Health and Social Behaviour*. Vol. 30. pp. 241-56.

Quarantelli, E.L. (ed.). (1985). *Disasters: Theory and Research*, Beverly Hill. CA: Sage Publications.

Revicki, D.A., Osoba, D., Fairclough, D., Barofsky, I., Berzon, R., Leidy, N.K. and M. Rothman. (2000). "Recommendations on health-related quality of life research to support labeling and promotional claims in the United States", *Qual Life Res*. Vol. 9, pp. 887-900.

Ross, C.E. and M.V. Willigan (1997). "Education and the Subjective Quality of Life", *Journal of Health and Social Behaviour*, pp. 275-297.

Rotter, J.B. (1966). "Generalized Expectancies for Internal *vs.* External Control of Reinforcements", *Psychological Monographs*. Vol. 80. pp. 1-28.

Sai Ti, (2007). "Health Related Quality of Life of Myanmar Migrant Workers in Takuapa and Kuraburi Districts Phangnga Province". Thailand (Thesis). Chulalongkorn University.

Santos, P.R. (2006). "Relationship between gender and age with quality of life in chronic hemodialysis patients", *Rev Assoc Med Bras*. Vol. 52(5), pp. 356-359.

Stanley, E., Muntner, P., Richard, N. Re., Frohlich, E.D., Holt, E. and M.A. Krousel-Wood. (2011). "Quality of Life in Hypertensive Clinic Patients Following Hurricane Katrina". *Ochsner J.*, Vol., 11(3), pp. 226–231.

Telles, S., Singh, N. and M. Joshi (2009). "Risk of post-traumatic stress disorder and depression in survivors of the floods in Bihar. India", *Indian Journal of Medical Sciences,* Vol. 63(8), pp. 330-334.

Turner, R.J. and Noh, S. (1983). "Class and Psychological Vulnerability Among Women: The Significance of Social Support and Personal Control", *Journal of Health and Social Behaviour*, Vol. 24, pp. 2-15.

Ware, J.E., Kosinski, M. and S.D. Keller. (1996). "A 12-item short-form health survey: Construction of scales and preliminary tests of reliability and validity", *Medical Care,* Vol. 34, pp. 220–233.

Ware, J.E., Kosinski, M., Turner-Bowker, D. M and B. Gandek. (2002). *How to score version 2 of the SF-12 Health Survey*. Health Assessment Lab., Boston.

Wheaton, B. (1983). "Stress, Personal Coping Resources, and Psychiatric Symptoms: An Investigation of Interactive Models", *Journal of Health and Social Behaviour*. Vol. 24, pp. 208-29.

WHO, (1997). *Introducing the WHOQOL instrument.* Division of Mental Health and Prevention of Substance Abuse, World Health Organization.

Wind, T.R., Joshi, P.C., Kleber, R.J., Komproe, I.H. (2013). "The impact of recurrent disasters on mental health: A study on seasonal floods in northern India", *Prehosp Disaster Med.* 2013; *28*(3):1-7.

Wu, H.C., Chou, P., Chou, F.H., Su, C.Y., Tsai, K.Y., Ou-Yang, W.C., Su, T.T., Chao, S.S., Sun, W.J., and M.C. Chen. (2006). "Survey of quality of life and related risk factors for a Taiwanese village population 3 years post-earthquake", *Aust N Z J Psychiatry*. Vol. *40*(4), pp. 355-361.

24
A Study on Attitudes towards Menstruation in Assam

M. Kennedy Singh and *Angana Goswami*

Introduction

Menstruation has always been a debatable issue across the world as people from different cultures share different opinion about it. Though Menstruation is considered to be a natural process yet it is linked with various false perceptions. That arises mainly from the menstrual related myths and stigmatization of menstruation found in different cultures. And menstrual hygiene is achieved mainly through some traditional beliefs and restrictions imposed on women during their periods. There are still some places where the menstrual-related absenteeism is very much prevalent. In some cultures, during menstruation, a woman needs to maintain a physical seclusion in a hut or segregated area and interaction with the male members as well. Also in some culture menarche is marked with a particular puberty ritual which signifies the transition of girl into womanhood and Assam is among such place. In Assam, during menstruation a girl has to remain isolated for a period, she is not allowed to touch anything but her belongings, male members are to be avoided for a period and she is not allowed to cook or go to the temple until her menstrual cycle gets over. However, we will find very few studies focusing on cultural dimensions of menstruation. Through this study, an attempt has been made to grasp the basic cultural values and attitudes attached with the Menstruation in Assam with special reference to young adolescent girls. As in Assam, the basic idea of menstruation forms during the adolescence stage with the help of a puberty ritual called ***TuloniBiya*** which will be discussed further.

Furthermore, Menstruation Hygiene has always been an integral part of a particular culture because we can observe certain values attached to it mainly in the form of menstrual taboos. Such traditional practices strengthen negative perceptions about the whole process of menstruation. Their implications can be seen in the form of embarrassment, shame and low self-esteem among girls who have transition into womanhood, affecting not only their school attendance but their academic performance and their social interactions within the school and at home—where in many cases they are confined into segregated spaces during their menstruation (Karki and Espinosa, 2018: 111).

Assam is known as one of north-eastern states of India where we will find rich socio-cultural diversity. Interestingly, in Assam, a girl is taught about menstrual hygiene through a long puberty ritual during menarche locally called ***TuloniBiya***. The ritual involves a big ceremony and parents arrange a big feast for the relatives and for the neighbourhood. Basically, menstruation is a matter of celebration in Assam. Though, menstruation is a matter of celebration but menstrual related absenteeism and taboos are very much prevalent which will be further discussed.

Research Objective

The following are the objectives of the study:

- To study the attitude towards menstruation among the Assamese Hindu.
- To understand traditional practices related to menstruation.
- To analyze the menstrual hygiene management among adolescent girls and women.

Methodology

This study primarily draws from the auto-ethnographic research method that describes events based mostly on personal narratives. The first hand experience of the author with the puberty ritual helped in the study. Data have also been gathered from participant observation and interviews conducted with women and parents residing in the author's hometown, Darrang. Also to understand the puberty ritual, several young adolescent girls were interviewed as this ritual forms the base for the menstrual related knowledge.

Discussion

It is remarkable that the concept of Menstruation and Menstrual Hygiene Management seems to have attracted numerous discussions very recently.

These discussions have led to take some actions and it has been witnessed when the two international organizations, namely WHO and UNICHEF initiated a join programme on Menstrual Hygiene Management (MHM) which basically focuses on maintaining a hygienic environment for women. Also, the introduction of various government policies has prompted the concept of MHM in different parts of the world like in 2015, Ministry of Drinking Water and Sanitation released National Guidelines for Menstrual Hygiene Management (MHM) with the support of UNICHEF, India.

While reviewing literatures, so many definitions of Menstrual Health were found but the most widely accepted definition of menstrual hygiene management which has been taken into consideration is given by the Joint Monitoring Programme by World Health Organization (WHO) and United Nations Children's Fund (UNICEF) in 2012, is as follows:

> *"Women and adolescent girls using a clean menstrual management material to absorb or collect blood that can be changed in privacy as often as necessary for the duration of the menstruation period, using soap and water for washing the body as required, and having access to facilities to dispose of used menstrual management materials"* (Bay. 2017). This definition includes the aspects of physical necessities for hygienic, effective management of menstrual bleeding.

In general terms, "Menstrual Hygiene" can be understood as a state of an individual which includes the psychological, socio-cultural and emotional aspects of a woman while menstruating. Nonetheless, the idea of menstrual health has existed long before this programme was introduced to people. So, to uncover such ideas on menstrual health, Assam has been chosen as a study area which is considered to be among such places where menstruation is celebrated like wedding and menstrual hygiene is introduced through a puberty ritual.

Among the Hindu families, menstruation is believed to be a significant part of women's life and also an important part of the whole culture as people have laid down definite rules of behaviour. And some of these rules actually prohibit the girl from several aspects of society. In the course of menstrual cycle, a girl must follow some customs related to the menstruation. These can be associated with the term taboos which refer to those social customs that restrict or forbid an individual from many facets of social life (Young and Albert, 1965: 225).

Tuloni Biya: An Event to Celebrate Menstruation in Assam

It is believed that Assam is among such places where the onset of menstruation is celebrated like a real wedding where people arrange for big feasts when girls get their first period. Being a member of this society, it can be said that the experience of the puberty ritual called '***TuloniBiya***' was one of the life-changing moments. The author's experiences and interviews conducted among girls have helped in developing the further discussion on the subject matter.

In general, the puberty ritual continues for a long period including three days of confinement period. One of the key features of this ritual is the girl's introduction to the menstrual health and the ritual begins with the first day of menstruation and it continues for a period of four to seven days (Sangeeta Das, 2017: 243). Generally, a girl is kept in a separate room as soon as the family members find out about her periods. She would not be permitted to touch anything nor touched by anyone for four or seven days. Perhaps it was because the girl is considered as '***chua***', meaning impure (Gogoi, 1964: 33). From that day onwards she is supposed to stay in isolation for a period of four or seven days. Moreover, a girl is not permitted to see the Sun or the Moon or any other male members of the family including her father. She has to remain confined in her bed until she gets her first ritual bath. There are some societies, where a girl is married to a banana tree during the ritual bath. This particular ritual marks the transformation of an adolescent girl into a woman who is being ultimately prepared for marriage and reproduction by the other female members of the community. People have been practicing this ritual in several ways but in this study the focus has been given towards the ultimate aim of understanding on how this ritual practice is organised within their socio-cultural milieu.

What we have understood from this ritual is that it is a traditional way of informing a girl about her menstrual health in Assamese society. Moreover, she is expected to follow all those rules throughout her life such as staying in isolation, keeping distance from prayer house and kitchen, and also maintaining distance from men for the first three days of menstrual cycle. This shows how for the first time a girl gets to know about her bodily process of menstruation and through this ritual a girl is being introduced to definite set rules.

Some writers have also tried to capture the significance of this ritual. An article has been found on menstrual taboos and it was written by Mitoo Das (2008). In this article the author attempts to look into the sociological world of menstruation in the form of taboos in the life of Hindu Assamese women in *Simlitola* and how it defines the existence of women in it (Mitoo Das, 2008: 29).

Menstrual Hygiene Management (MHM) Among the Young Girls

Menstrual hygiene can be achieved through the use of sanitary pads, washing of the genital area and proper disposal of sanitary pads. Among the young girls the basic idea of menstruation and its hygiene develops during the puberty ritual. Throughout the ritual, mothers give instructions to the girl regarding the menstruation and also mothers are the only person with whom a girl comfortably talks about her periods.

In many society, a girl basically hides menstrual related matters or things from her father or other male members because a girl are taught to do so during the puberty ritual. It has been found that traditionally, in the name of menstrual hygiene girls have been maintaining distances from others and living in separate room and cooking separately so that girls do not spread dirt (menstrual blood) in other places. According to the customs, a girl should stay at her room for the first three days of her period and this way a girl missed classes for three consecutive days in every month. These restrictions tend to develop a negative attitude towards menstruation as these are hard to follow and people do not like to indulge or even talk with girls during their menstruation as she is considered to be polluted.

This study also reveals that girls living in the urban areas have improved in terms of MHM as use of sanitary pads, regular washing of genital areas and proper knowledge of disposing are well known to girls. While in rural areas we have talked with people who are still practicing unhygienic method during menstruation such as the use of old clothes and reuse of the same cloth because it is hard to get access to stuffs like sanitary pads as these items were sold in a very high cost. Therefore, people do not prefer to buy these expensive sanitary pads instead they use old clothes during menstruation. Moreover, girls living in the rural areas lack information about good hygiene and menstrual related absenteeism, food taboos, not visiting to religious places tend to have a negative impact among girls (Sonika, Neha, Wahida and Ishrat. 2019: 5125).

The above mentioned customs are mostly found in Assam particularly among the Hindu families. Now-a-days, these restrictions are hardly followed by the school going girls or working women. Though the young girls are found to be well aware of menstruation process but the misconceptions and ignorance are still prevailing among the general population. The menstrual related misconceptions could be removed by creating awareness and by providing facilities in schools, working places and in other public places.

Analysis

From the above discussion on attitudes towards menstrual hygiene in Assam, it can be analyzed that menstruation is not just a bodily phenomenon but also a psychological phenomenon. In some societies, menarche is celebrated to signify the transition of a girl into a woman. During this particular period a girl comes to know about her menstrual health along with the menstrual taboos. But then menstrual related absenteeism differs from culture to culture. For instance, a Hindu woman, during her menstruation, will refrain from going to the temple, kitchen and keeps distance from the other family members as she is considered to be impure during her menstruation. As per the Islamic Law, a menstruation woman will not be allowed to pray, fast or have sex. The woman is not allowed to touch the "Quran" unless it is a translation. According to the Bible, "when a woman has her monthly periods, she remains unclean for seven days. Any one touches her is unclean until evening. Anything on which she sits or lies during her monthly periods is unclean." So, the attitudes towards menstruation vary from culture to culture. Despite of adequate knowledge about the process, these practices tend to stigmatize menstruation.

If we talk about the attitudes found among the Assamese people towards the menstruation then we must consider their perceptions and experiences related to menstruation. As mentioned above, the perceptions regarding menstruation are mainly developed from the puberty ritual, '***TuloniBiya***'. This ritual is believed to be a traditional method adopted mainly to teach a female about her menstrual health. But, the restrictions and poor menstrual hygiene management do not help in developing a positive attitude among girls. It has been found that those girls, who have given information and awareness about menstruation prior to their menarche, develop a positive attitude and handle the first period without any panic. While the girls, whose parents shy away from talking about menstruation, tend to develop a negative attitude towards menstruation as they start panicking and feel anxious during the first period.

A paper stated that the menstrual behaviours are mostly affected by literacy status and awareness among people in Assam (Das. Tasa. 2019:3068). It has been found that most school going girls are developing a positive attitude towards the menstruation and menstrual hygiene management as most of the school are providing early education on menstruation and the impact of poor menstrual hygiene management.

Without a denial, ***TuloniBiya*** does introduce a woman about her bodily process of menstruation and works like a ban-aid for different menstrual issues but it does not address the underlying menstrual matters. If we look deep into the puberty ritual practiced in Assam we will encounter something really ironic. We can observe a big celebration during the onset of menarche while the ritual clouded with many taboos. Due to the situation, girls do not talk about the process openly to others and it is still a "hush affair" among girls. Moreover, the process is connected with some connotations like '***Chua***' means 'impure', '***Axuubidha***' means 'difficulty' and etc. These connotations have implication on young girls and women that are being neglected for years.

In spite of isolating women in a room, people need to think for an alternative of such practices or making hygienic provisions in various places including provisions for washing and access to clean toilet. We need to educate them about the correct materials to be used as absorbent to catch the blood. While, the focus remains on the impurity of the process and we need to change the narratives of the people to create a menstruation-positive atmosphere.

An Assamese Hindu woman refrains from cooking, going to temples and maintains a great distance by confining herself to her room as she is considered to be impure. Here, we would like to recall Mary Douglas's work on "Ritual Uncleanness" which was extensively discussed in her book entitled, Purity And Danger (1966). In this book, she also elaborately discussed about the symbolic interpretation of purity and impurity. She believed that people tend to comprehend their social environment into a well categorized system and when the objects or phenomena do not fall under any system they are considered as impure or phenomena that are out of the symbolic order of the society (Douglas, 1966: 7-29). This can be one of way of explaining the existing concepts of impurity and pollution in Assam. However, the great irony is that in Assam only, Hindus worship Goddess Kamakhya, and people worship as well as celebrate the menstruation of Goddess by arranging an annual fair called "AmbuvachiMela".

We have already seen that menstruation involves several taboos or stigmas and we will find a number of myths attached with it. All these stigmatization have implications on mental health such as insecurity and low self-esteem among young girls and women. It has been observed that due to the practice of isolation during menstruation girl's attendance goes on dropping (Bay, 2017).

If we analyze these factors affecting the menstrual hygiene in Assam, it happens to be the poor menstrual hygiene management and stigmatization of the menstrual cycle. Among the Assamese Hindus, it is considered to be a taboo topic in the state, people choose to hide about it and rarely talks about the menstrual hygiene management including proper use of sanitary napkins, use of clean toilet, keeping of pubic area clean and undergarments dry, wrapping of sanitary pads in a paper bag before disposing and vaginal infections. Hardly, people initiate a discussion on menstruation or menstrual hygiene as this natural phenomenon is attached with several taboos or stigmas. Hence, there is an immediate need of a menstrual-positive environment where people can discuss about menstruation freely.

A shift in attitudes of people was seen especially after the introduction of modern education and girls started going to schools during their menstrual cycle. The attitudes have also shifted when the schools have started giving information about menstruation with the help of scientific reasons. People have actually started understanding the factors which cause menstruation. Though such initiatives, many misconceptions about menstruation will fade away from the society.

Another shift has been observed especially when period products were made available as an alternative for dirty clothes. The use of period products enabled girls to go to school with confidence and without thinking of period stains. This helped girls in attaining classes regularly and eventually people have started letting go off restrictions on isolation period and on touching. People started realizing the fact that some customs like isolation were holding back girls from getting quality education.

Further changes in attitudes could be seen after the introduction of various government schemes and policies. In 2015, Ministry of Drinking Water and Sanitation released National Guidelines for Menstrual Hygiene Management (MHM) with the support of UNICEF, India, as per this guideline, "Menstrual Hygiene Management: Menstrual Hygiene is the (i) articulation, awareness, information and confidence to manage menstruation with safety and dignity using safe hygienic materials together with (ii) adequate water and agents and spaces for washing and bathing with soap, and (iii) disposal of used menstrual absorbents with privacy and dignity" (MHM National Guidelines, 2015:6).

Additionally, Swachcha Bharat Mission Guidelines has also made an effort to raise awareness on menstrual hygiene specifically amongst young girls. This Mission has guided various educational institutions to design clean toilets for girls. From such missions girls will have the opportunity to maintain their menstrual hygiene in schools and will have easy access to infrastructure for disposal of used menstrual absorbent. Also, girls will have the freedom from fear of leakage or unpleasant odour. Such programmes even help comforting school boys about menstruation and prevent them from mocking and understanding their friends. Moreover, Debadeep and Giridhar pointed about the behaviour change in communication in their article that it is to bring hygienic practices during menstruation through different stakeholders and ultimately will help in understanding menstruation related issues (Kalita and Pathak, 2019: 759). We will get several such efforts but then there are still some places where the idea of Menstrual Health is yet to be delivered. Besides, a need has been felt to encourage more and more discussion on menstrual hygiene among people. Only then, it is possible to remove false perceptions and bring in a positive attitude towards menstruation and its hygiene.

Conclusion

There is a wide scope of improving the Menstrual Hygiene and of restoring a positive attitude towards menstruation among the people of Assam. They believed that menstruation is impure in thought to have prevented young girls and women from discussing menstrual related matters that ultimately lead to poor menstrual hygiene management which does not address the underlying menstrual concerns. The stigmatization of menstruation has deep implications on female's mental health such as insecurity and low self-esteem. Such topics are very complicated to understand but hard to ignore. This study is an attempt to understand the practices related to menstruation in the state of Assam with special reference to the puberty ritual called ***TuloniBiya*** and its implication on young adolescent girls. The topic of menstruation is a very sensitive one and people do not feel comfortable while talking which could be one of the limitations that the study has faced but the study is largely based on auto-ethnography. The study reveals that though the young girls are found to be well aware of menstruation process due to the practice of ***TuloniBiya*** yet misconceptions are still prevailing among them as people tend to ignore discussion on menstruation. Therefore, it demands for more scientific discussion on this subject matter to remove misconceptions. Now it is the time to support women to face the existing challenges of menstruation in a hygienic manner.

REFERENCES

Bay, Sophia A. (2017). Moving Toward a Holistic Menstrual Hygiene Management: An Anthropological Analysis of Menstruation and Practices in Western and Non-Western Societies. M.Sc. Thesis. University of Montana Missoula, MT.

Das, Mitoo (2008). "Menstruation as Pollution: Taboos in Simlitola, Assam", *Indian Anthropologist*, Vol. 38, No. 2, pp. 29-42.

Das, Sangeeta (2017). "Declining of TuloniBiya: A Case Study", *Rupkatha Journal on Interdisciplinary Studies in Humanities*, Vol. IX, No. 1, pp. 243-249.

Department of Drinking Water and Sanitation, Ministry of Jal Shakti, Government of India, (2015). *Menstrual Hygiene Management: National Guidelines.* New Delhi.

Douglas, Mary 1966. *Purity and Danger: An Analysis of Concepts of Pollution and Taboo*, New York, Routledge and Kegan Paul.

Gogoi, N.K. (1964). *Continuity and Change Among the Ahom*, New Delhi: Concept Publishing Company.

Kalita, Debadeep and Giridhar Pathak (2019). "Study on Hygiene Practice among Adolescent girls with Special Reference to Menstrual Hygiene in Barpeta, Assam", *Internal Journal of Medical Science and Public Health*. Vol. 8, No. 9, pp. 759-764.

Karki, Richa and Cristina Espinosa (2018). *Breaking Taboos: Menstruation, Female Subordination and Reproductive Health, the Case of India.*

Sangra. Sonika, Neha Choudhary, Wahida Kouser and Ishrat Faizal (2019). "Assessment of knowledge, attitude and practice about menstruation and menstrual hygiene among adolescent girls in rural area of district Kathua, Jammu and Kashmir". *International Journal of Community Medicine and Public Health*. Vol. 6, No. 12, pp. 5215-5218.

Young, Frank W. and Albert A. Bacdayan (1965). "Menstrual Taboos and Social Rigidity", *Ethnology*, Vol. 4, No. 2, pp. 225-240.

Das, Netri and Anadi Swami Tasa (2019). "Menstrual Hygiene: Knowledge and practices during menstruation among adolescent girls in urban slums of Jorhat district, Assam", *International Journal of Community Medicine and Public Health*, Vol. 6, No. 7, pp. 3068-3075.

25

A Discourse on Gender, Health, and Sustainable Development in India

An Ecofeminist Thought

Kalindi Sharma

Introduction

The unbridled development around the globe has raised several questions on the voracious appetite of human beings especially with regard to the depleting natural resources. For scholars of gender and feminist studies, this unconstrained ability of 'development' to plunder and ravage biodiversity bears an uncanny resemblance with the oppression of women and other marginalized categories. The parallels between the vulnerability of women and the susceptibility of the environment to unmindful exploitation emphasize on the inherent power dynamics within the climate-change and environmental politics in general. The sustainable model of development seemed like a providential response that could reverse the massive anthropogenic exploitation by restoring the balance between human beings and natural resources. Sustainable development was brought into mainstream policy making commissions with the view of preserving the leftover resources and also instilling in people a mindfulness with regard to the utilization of these resources. The entire idea of sustainability was initially dominated by two paradigms, namely 'resourcism' and 'preservationism'(Callicott & Mumford, 1997). However, both 'resourcism' and 'preservationism' seemed more integrated with the needs and survival of the people rather than the needs of the environment. Scholars pointed out that both these ideologies focused on consumption of resources sooner or later by the existing or the future generation, which seemed anthropocentric and exploitative rather than environment centric. Advocates of sustainable environmental management have since avoided references to these ideologies (Noss, 1995).

The earliest reference to women's contribution towards the protection and conservation of nature was the *Chipko Movement* which was a massive non-violent and organized ecological response by indigenous communities to widespread clearing of forests in Uttarakhand, India in 1970s. The role of women in the movement became a matter of global recognition and initiated debates about representation of women in climate-change policies. In 1985, a world conference on women in Nairobi, cited *the Chipko Movement* as a major step towards introducing a shift towards inclusion of gender in policy and planning in order to protect the environment. In the Earth Summit of 1992 in Rio De Janeiro, the voices of women from the global south became more palpable and their vulnerability to sudden catastrophic events as well as long-standing environmental degradation was acknowledged by the stakeholders (Resurrección, 2013). At this time a number of ecofeminist voices had found representation at the United Nations conference on 'Environment and Development' (Lorentzen & Eaton, 2002).

It seemed like the daily realities of women and their secondary position *vis-à-vis* men, resonated on the forums for environmental management. However, there were several arguments by feminist scholars that pointed out the inherent contradiction of this belief wherein women faced a sort of quandary of being a disproportionate victim of natural resource depletion while being a repository of knowledge about its preservation, and protection. The scholars *"...also warned of the risks of positioning women in environmental projects and programmes that sidestep existing disproportionate workloads and gendered hierarchies. In short, the slogans that drew attention to women as the environment's victims and caretakers did not match more complex and daily realities of resource use, power, and negotiation"* (Resurrección, 2013:34). Such manifestation of the woman's predicament as the sole bearer of knowledge and the simultaneous position of marginality raises concerns about their inclusion in policy framing regarding environmental conservation.

Exploring Trends and Paradigms of Ecofeminism in India

The ecofeminist movement came to the forefront of environmental advocacy in 1980s following the concerted effort by feminist scholars who saw a similarity between exploitation of women and that of nature. The integration of the lived experiences of women and the widespread destruction of natural flora and fauna of the planet was not merely a metaphor for the sake of ecofeminism, instead the movement intended to convey how the entire human race was so deeply entrenched with the environment that any detrimental impact on the environment would eventually lead to adversity for the entire human race. The term 'Ecofeminism' was first used by French feminist Francoise d'Eaubonne in 1974 and it was considered a hallmark of the third wave of feminism that promoted a more action-oriented approach and intersectionality within the gamut of feminist movement. The ecofeminist theoretical paradigm has primarily been supported by three models viz. empirical, conceptual, and epistemological. The empirical model claims that women are more prone to suffer from environmental degradation than men owing to a gendered division of labour where all the domestic responsibilities are attributed to women around the world. These domestic roles lead to a greater dependence of women on natural resources and its depletion is a major cause of concern for them. The conceptual model is a more cultural/symbolic idea that promotes a maternal imagery of women who is fertile, capable of bearing children, feminine, supports, and nurtures life etc. This imagination is in stark contrast with the images of power, dominance, control, and protection beholding men. The conceptual model justifies the superiority of men over both nature and women. Finally, the epistemological structure of ecofeminism accords women the epistemological superiority over men, following their own experiences of oppression and struggle, which makes them better equipped to understand resource depletion and advocate for its conservation (Lorentzen & Eaton, 2002).

Examples of women as the nurturer and caregiver were used far too often by environmental policy stakeholders because most of the examples that were cited at international forums came from rural or tribal regions of South Asia where women bore the weight of reproductive labour and would procure various kinds of forest produce for the survival of their families. Scholar and environmentalist Vandana Shiva who championed the epistemological paradigm within the ecofeminist view in South Asia posited that patriarchy was not only responsible for subjugation of women, it also worked towards destruction of diversity of nature as it was a major roadblock in the larger project on developmental expansion. Shiva claimed that '*destruction of diversity and the creation of monocultures becomes an imperative for capitalist patriarchy*' (Shiva, 1992:205). For Shiva, women are the keepers of biodiversity. '*Women have been the custodians of biodiversity in most cultures...However, like all other aspects of women's work and knowledge, their role in development and conservation of biodiversity has been rendered as non-work and non-*

knowledge. Their labour and expertise has been defined into nature, even though it is based on sophisticated cultural and scientific practices. Women produce, reproduce, consume, and conserve biodiversity in agriculture. Women's biodiversity conservation however differs from the dominant patriarchal notions of biodiversity conservation in a number of ways. The recent concern with biodiversity at the global level has grown as a result of the erosion of diversity due to the expansion of large-scale monoculture based production in agriculture and the vulnerability associated with it (Shiva, 1992:210). Shiva's claims were further bolstered by psychoanalyst Rosemary Ruether who believed that the marginality of women and disregard for environment are essentially operationalization of a strictly hierarchical society that has legitimized such power dynamics. Reuther termed this 'transcendent dualism' which builds on separation between sexes, human and non-human species, social class etc. (Li, 2007). It is important to remember that the feminization of nature does not naturally or biologically bestow the responsibility of protecting and preserving nature on women, rather if we look at cross-cultural examples, we would be able to perceive diversity in the lived experiences of women *vis-à-vis* nature. The tendency of ecofeminists to create a monolith category of 'women' and the universalization of their oppression across the world has been proclaimed as feminist essentialism by the sceptics. Li (2007) explained that it is vital *"to examine the feminization of nature as an imported idea that has been accepted and popularized in non-Western societies in the age of globalization"* (p. 356). Furthermore, Li pointed out that this analogy between women and nature and nature as 'mother' are Western thoughts that have been imposed on the global south. "*For instance it has become common for Chinese people to employ the metaphor of "the rape of mother earth" to refer to human exploitation of nature even though traditionally they did not identify earth as a mother....Therefore, while the feminization of nature may not be the main contributing factor in today's ecological destruction, it is still critical to attend to how male hegemony facilitates the successful transplantation of gender imagery across cultural boundaries*" (p. 356). Such cultural hegemony is even more common in India and its neighbouring countries owing to a history of colonization by the Western world. Both, Maria Mies and Vandana Shiva (2014) believed that for many tribal and peasant communities in developing countries like India dependence on biodiversity for subsistence is a common phenomenon. Their methods of sustenance are often considered 'primitive' and 'backward' and the regional governments are quick to replace their slow-paced lifestyle that serves the cause of conservation of natural flora and fauna, with new age technology that is output oriented and statistically more yielding even though it is at the core of destruction of natural habitats. Shiva (1992) clearly demonstrates that the comparison between the "*low productivity of diverse, multiple dimensional systems and the high productivity of uniform, one dimensional systems of agriculture, forestry, and livestock*" is partial towards the commercial benefits of a capitalism driven world. This capitalist patriarchy is only motivated by higher yield and output by minimizing cost of production as opposed to a more balanced and simple livelihood strategies of rural and indigenous communities of South Asia.

Mies integrated Marxism and feminism together to illustrate how capitalist regimes have exploited colonized people, women, and biologically diverse regions. Additionally, it is capitalism that endorses modern scientific endeavours that have '*eroded a feminine conception of biodiversity*'. However, the 'subsistence perspective' propounded by Shiva, even though, idyllic and arcadian, does not seem feasible in contemporary times. So much so, that critics of Shiva have accused her of '*romanticizing with the poor, rural, Indian woman*' (p. 14), who supposedly did not witness a history of oppression and exploitation in times preceding colonization and technological expansion. Several critics of ecofeminism have argued that introduction of technology did overcome physical drudgery of women in sensitive and tough eco-zones hence the proclivity of ecofeminists to condemn all things Western and 'development' holds little significance (Fredell, 1996). However, the critics like Braidotti do not overlook the efforts of Shiva and Mies in bringing to light the '*subjugated knowledges of oppressed people*' and the need for integrating knowledge of culturally pluralistic societies (Mellor, 2009). Bina Agarwal (2000), who popularized 'feminist environmentalism' as a form ecofeminist thought, did not overlook the influence of intersecting elements of caste, class, religion, and power dynamics among women. As a matter of fact, Agarwal affirmed that the seemingly eternal bond which women share with nature is influenced by their class, caste, and access to resources, healthcare services, than their gender alone. For instance, a woman in urban India is less likely to be in tune with nature when compared to her rural or tribal counterpart because her survival is not entirely dependent on access to forest produce or other forms of diverse flora and fauna. Such factors are to be taken into consideration when citing examples from India or global south in general. Hence, addressing intersectionality within the purview of ecofeminist thought becomes the onus of the researchers for there are numerous social constructs that define the relationship human beings have with their natural surroundings. The utilization of intersectionality would ensure a more comprehensive understanding of a broad range of environmental issues that have a gendered connotation in South Asia (Kings, 2017).

A Critical Inquiry of Sustainable Development

In 1987 the Brundtland Commission's report *Our Common Future* described sustainable development as "*development that meets the needs of the present without compromising the ability of future generations to meet their own needs*". The report did not intend to impose strict limits on the use of resources but encouraged countries to develop strategies with the aim of confronting abject poverty in underdeveloped or developing nations and to also concentrate on the basic needs of population around the world. The report claimed that poverty would lead to severe depletion in the ecological resources and that we must aspire for redistribution of resources. Therefore, sustainability must also be instilled within the social and economic institutions of the society (World Commission on Environment and Development, 1987). In the report, the Brundtland Commission elaborated upon the delicate balance between economic growth, population expansion, and resource exploitation and it outlined a course of planned exploitation of ecology wherein there would be a scope for expansion of natural resources elsewhere. Each point in the course of action charted out by the Commission bears awareness about the exhaustion of naturally occurring resources if the pace of utilization was not curbed. At the same time the report relays the entire future of the planet in the hands of those stakeholders who are the participants of the said exploitative order. While it is reasonable to entrust the stakeholders with the responsibility of preserving and replenishing the natural resource base, it is only feasible when the stakeholders realize the importance of the objectives defined by the Brundtland Commission. The key objectives outlined in the report include —

- "reviving growth;
- changing the quality of growth;
- meeting essential needs for jobs, food, energy, water, and sanitation;
- ensuring a sustainable level of population;
- conserving and enhancing the resource base;
- reorienting technology and managing risk; and

- Merging environment and economics in decision making" (World Commission on Environment and Development, 1987; p. 46).

"*The 1992 Rio agenda was of course extravagantly ambitious, and high hopes depended on the processes that arose from it*" (Scoones, 2007: 592). The ideology propounded by the Commission was essentially conservationism that focused on the responsible choices of the developed nations and socio-economically privileged population of the world. It also acknowledged that countries with surplus resources tend to be more wasteful despite less population when compared with underdeveloped nations struggling with paucity of resources. The underlying philosophy of conservationism has ensured continuous focus on biodiversity protection and strategic efforts have been directed towards regulating the responsible use of the naturally occurring resources. International panels have been actively participating in implementation and monitoring of the environmental goals since the Rio De Janeiro Earth Summit of 1992. Despite the perseverance and accomplishment of remarkable milestones, environmental conservationists, environment monitoring and regulating agencies (like World Wildlife Fund, Intergovernmental Panel on Climate Change, International Union for Conservation of Nature, and several others) have lost sight of the long term goals of biosphere conservation. There is lack of consensus in the understanding of what constitutes 'environmental conservation' and which other species other than our own should be protected.

Furthermore, central to the vision of this sustainability programme is the vitality of the planet, not for the sake of the planet but to aid human survival. If any other species were to be protected, it would be for the role it plays in the sustenance of the human species. The concept of environmental sustainability was always narrowed down by its ability to cater to human needs. Human needs have proliferated at an alarming rate and it has become a major challenge to provide for the ever-increasing world population. Sharp decline in the natural resource base is a reality that man had to witness sooner or later. There have been other struggles of the socio-political order that the environmental community has had to face since the culmination of the environmental task force post 1992 Rio summit. It is this strategic and planned exploitation of resources that ecofeminists have vehemently opposed as it would lead to further marginalization of the vulnerable population of the region. Moreover, the destruction of habitat for non-human species is a major cause of concern for it would inevitably change the face of the natural habitat.

To an ecofeminist scholar, this ideology of sustainable development is characterized by anthropocentrism and self-serving ideals of humanity.

One cannot expect sudden curbs on the utilization of natural resources as a feasible option to revitalize the planet as there are several constraints to such an '*absurdly strong environmental sustainability*' (Goodland, 1995). Economists as well as ecologists favour a more achievable means to sustainable development, that of '*substitutability*' which outlines three crucial areas where one needs to attend to—

Foster Regeneration of Natural Capital: This approach rejects the current scale of resource exploitation and proposes strategic utilization of resources by allowing time to the resource base to replenish and strengthen before it is consumed.

Relieve Pressure on Natural Capital: This approach proposes opportunities to create alternatives to the naturally occurring resource base in an attempt to contain the exploitation of limited resources. For instance, development of alternative fuels to limit the use of fossil fuel.

Improve Efficiency in Use of Natural Capital: This aspect of substitutability focuses primarily effective usage of the resources that are already in use in order to avoid wastefulness and thereby increase the longevity of the resource. The approach also draws our attention to the durability and recyclability of products in order to provide long-term end use (Goodland, 1995:16).

There are common misconceptions regarding the scope for substitutability in reference to the present state of environmental damage. Substitutability is an effective mode of coping with limited resource base but it does not safeguard the environment from exploitation *per se.* Substitutability only provides man-made alternatives to the naturally occurring capital. Moreover, we must also acknowledge the limits of human capability in providing safe alternatives to breathable air and clean drinking water. Most of what man has acquired or conceived of as substitute to natural capital is not entirely indisputable for its impact on the human beings or the environment. *"For natural life-support systems no practical substitutes are possible, and degradation may be irreversible. In such cases (and perhaps in others as well), compensation cannot be meaningfully specified"* (Toman, 1994). It is pertinent to understand that the goals of sustainable development cannot remain selective about human progress. If we are to provide for the future generations we must include non-environmental aspects of sustainability paradigm such as focusing on the social implications of responsible resource use and spreading awareness about environmental decline (Pezzey, 2004). One of the major drawbacks in the way of sustainable development that was viewed in the twentieth century was its limited focus on socio-political dimensions of the society. The focal point of sustainable development was restricted to environmental and economic dimension. The pioneers of '*Our Common Future*' discussed about the importance of an alliance between the socio-political, economic, as well as environmental domains but it failed to impress upon the inclusion of the socio-political domain of the society as a means to facilitating sustainability through the establishment of robust governance in nation and states. Needless to say, the model has been selectively successful in fulfilling the millennium development goals and the subsequent sustainable development goals owing to its inconsistent understanding.

Negotiating Sustainable Development in the Global South

The framework of sustainability holds greater significance for the global South and not the Northern hemisphere, even though the global North can be held accountable for the rampant consumption of natural resources. With the introduction of 'sustainable development' in global environmental concerns the Western world has recognized the need for development for the Third world countries and have granted them the opportunity to utilize their resources with a long-term vision to provide for the subsequent generations. The countries in the global South have been reluctant to accept and ratify the goals of sustainability as it hampers their economic ambitions and they attribute the current environmental condition to the neglect and overexploitation of the Western world. Hence, the responsibility of being prudent with regard to the natural resource use, falls in the hands of the Western world, that has in the past consumed resources in an unhindered manner. The sustainable development approach is meant to challenge the conventional paradigms of development by imposing sanctions regarding resource use and by introducing strict protocols for biodiversity conservation. The conventional and dominant framework of development that Vandana Shiva termed as '*maldevelopment*' favours rapid industrial expansion and global trade agreements between the Northern hemisphere and the Global south. This model of development opposes the 'subsistence' economy of the third World countries that is both capable of fulfilling basic human needs and will cause least exploitation to natural resources. However, the subsistence structures of economy are proclaimed as penurious and incapable of establishing trade agreements on an international forum, for they are not inclined to exchange commodities and earn profit. Therefore, developing nations that are driven by subsistence economy, when faced with an environmental catastrophe or any other trauma, rarely find themselves being granted aid by international trade forums. In the light of this fact, the notion of sustainability has failed to lure developing nations into a more far-sighted and visionary approach to development. Furthermore, from a philosophical point of view, the idea of sustainable development has been marred with ambivalence, much like the ecofeminist thought.

Much like an oxymoron in figure of speech, the concept of sustainable development relies on terms 'sustainable' and 'development' that are in contradiction with each other in terms of their respective ideological frameworks (Sachs, 1999). The two terms claim extremely separate positions from a philosophical perspective. The central precept of the developmental paradigm aims at broadening the scope for the growth of 'human ambitions' especially with regard to technological and industrial advancements. On the contrary, the 'sustainability model' functions on the dimension of time and a cogent use of resources over this period in time. Together, the concept of 'sustainable development' imparts an antithetical understanding of growth, i.e. something on the lines of decelerating the progress of human aspirations within an environment that has finite resource base (Goodland, 1995). There are three primary aspects of sustainability, viz. environmental, social, and economic, that are interlinked and the visions of all three domains need to be in alliance with one another if the sustainable model is to succeed. However, one has to again address these factors with the inherent ambivalence of sustainable development, and it would appear that economic growth shares an inverse relationship with environmental growth. Man not woman, can develop and grow economically if he exploits the resources of the planet, for instance the availability of fossil fuel governs the global political position of oil-based countries in the world. The inclusion of a sustainable framework provides limited respite to these resources as the extraction and utilization of similar resources continues, may be not in an unrestrained and imprudent manner. Therefore *"we cannot grow into sustainability"* (Goodland, 1995:5). The concept of sustainable development has been explored from multiple vantage points which has given rise to a broad range of meanings and the associated implications of such varied understanding have given rise to some degree of ambiguity. Owing to such vague and fluid boundaries of the sustainable model and the underlying uncertainty pertaining to the long-term goals of the framework, scholars have debated over a more nuanced approach to address grave environmental concerns that plague the world today.

Gender, Health and Sustainable Development

The sustainable development goal 3 of the United Nations 2030 agenda for sustainable development provides for health and wellbeing for all at all stages of life universally. The relationship between SDG goals 3 (health and wellbeing for all), 4 (inclusive and quality education and lifelong learning), and 5 (gender equality and empowerment for women and girls) in relation to health equity is crucial and has significant impacts on the health outcomes of women.

Mary Manandhar *et al.* (2018) discussed the link between gender health and other SDGs especially in three specific domains of gender and health: "gender as a social determinant of health; gender as a driver of health behaviours; and the gendered response of health systems" (p. 644).

To understand this complex relationship, it is imperative to take a look at the role of construction of gender in society. Indeed, the social configuration of gender in a society impacts the lives of both men and women in unequal ways and often calls for gender equality at universal level. The experience of health and wellbeing is shaped by the gender construction with specific reference to the subjective and socio-cultural determinants, health beliefs, attitudes and systems. Factors such as, class, caste, gender, and socio-economic status impact the health outcomes in significant ways. Elimination of Gender inequalities is not so easy and to assume health and wellbeing, free of gendered differences is far from reality rather difficult to realize. The health inequalities must be monitored and evaluated (Hosseinpoor, Bergen and Magar, 2015) through a multi-sectoral, multi-stakeholder approach as the gender influences health and wellbeing of individuals in many significant ways (Kurruvilla *et al.*, 2018; Colbourn *et al.*, 2015). The health systems are also prone to changes brought about by social process of oppression and dissemination based on class, caste, and gender prevalent in the society (Scott *et al.*, 2017). The climate change and its concomitant consequences also widen the existing gender gap in relation to health disparities. Gender policies are needed to empower women so that they can function efficiently in their social, biological and work roles (Langer *et al.*, 2015).

The gender factor in certain sense promotes or hinders equity in the pursuit of heath for all. Both the masculinities and feminists shape the women and men's health (Wilsnack and Obot, 2005). The relationship between women and health seems to be complex as factors like environmental, epidemiological, and social also affect women and health (Ann Langer, Lancet Commission, 2015). The changes in population movement, disease, and mortality pattern are influenced by environmental factors (Costello, 2009). As a consequence of the disasters due to the environmental factors, the poor and marginal who rely primarily on environment for their livelihood suffer. Women and girls being primary contributors to the discharge of domestic responsibilities are also subject to the effects of environmental change (Dankelman, 2005). If one takes into consideration the overall disease burden, the social determinants of health contribute to an increase in the reproductive health, nutrition related infections besides non-communicable diseases. Many factors like low education level, economic vulnerability, compromised social status and gender discrimination render them vulnerable to various hazards and also affect the health outcomes of women and their access to health services (Mumtaz and Salway, 2009). In view of such compromised circumstances that women have to struggle with, the women and girls of vulnerable subpopulations given to their language and cultural barriers face specific challenges (Adanu and Johnson, 2009). Although with the opening up of economies across globe and creation of opportunities of work due to industrialization, women have come to the forefront to demand and claim equity in health, education and governance but still the gender gaps are very much prevalent across globe. The women of course have a role in being a user as well as provider of health care and for achieving sustainable development goals; there is a need for gender parity across all levels of health governance as well to ensure greater participation of women and to create better working conditions. Gender still needs to be understood as a social construct where power is associated with inequities in access to facilities of health and wellbeing. However, in this debate in the context of SDGs, the role of women is discussed mainly as mothers, care givers, and victims of violence. Indeed, to achieve health and wellbeing of all universally gender equality is of crucial significance.

Concluding Remarks

This chapter has attempted to outline how 'sustainable development' presents a quandary for most environmental scholars, social scientists, and economists as it compels them to choose between the health and well-being of humanity and the wellbeing of the planet. The task of bridging the gap between the two has been nothing less than a challenge and has ended up being a pursuit for unattainable balance. Despite the numerous controversial debates and discourses on the concept of sustainable development and SDGs per se as the most effective methodological tool, it still remains the most refined and significant step towards environmental protection. Moreover, the allocation of the entire gamut of environmental concerns under an umbrella term of 'sustainable development' has led to widespread attention on the issue of natural resource depletion. The discourse of sustainable development also has reinforced the dominance of the Western world in a manner where Western powers are using this to define the course of resource utilisation of developing nations while also according them the right to develop as a nation (environmental colonialism). This creates a counter consciousness whereby the first world with all its economic and trade negotiations in the Third World feels obligated to champion the environmental goals of sustainable development that they have inspired and insisted upon. This chapter also explores how ecofeminism studies women in relation to their ecological surrounding and comes to exclude men, who bear an irrefutable stake in environmental concerns in trying to negotiate the 'exclusion of oppressed and vulnerable voices' at large. The narratives of sustainable development as well as those of ecofeminism both have proclaimed vulnerability of women and nature as natural corollaries and symbols. The subsequent narrative is thereby of repudiation of technological advancement and other parameters of industrial capitalism. It is often forgotten that dynamism of industrial progress at times alleviates the marginal position of women, amongst many others, in terms of labour, health or education. This chapter probes into these many contradictions and explores through its critical inquiry the monoliths of sustainable development and the fables of eco-feminism that perennially negotiate the space of women at the face of changing patterns of development in India. The last section of the chapter discusses the crucial role of social construction of gender in relation to health and wellbeing of women and how gender policies are needed to empower women and enhance their capabilities to perform their biological, social and work roles. In order to achieve these goals in the agenda for gender and health, multi-sectoral, multi-stakeholder, efforts involving policy planners, civil society activists, the womenfolk themselves, the academia, and researchers are a must.

REFERENCES

Adanu, R.M., and Johnson, T.R. (2009). "Migration and women's health", *Int J Gynaecol Obstet*; *106*: 179–81.

Agarwal, B. (2000). "Conceptualising environmental collective action: Why gender matters", *Cambridge journal of economics*, *24*(3), 283-310.

Aguirre, B.E. (2002). "Sustainable Development" as a Collective Surge. *Social Science Quarterly, 83*(1), 101-118.

Buell, L. (2009). *The future of environmental criticism: Environmental crisis and literary imagination* (Vol. 52). John Wiley & Sons.

Braidotti, R., Charkiewicz, E., Hausler, S., and Wieringa, S. (1994). *Women, the environment and sustainable development: towards a theoretical synthesis*. Zed Books.

Callicott, J. Baird and Mumford, K. (1997). "Ecological Sustainability as a Conservation Concept", *Society for Conservation Biology, 11*(1), 32-40.

Colbourn, T., Gideon, J., Groce, N., Heinrich, M., Kelman, I., Kett, M.,... & Waage, J. (2015). *Human health*. London: Ubiquity Press.

Costello, A., Abbas, M., Allen, A., *et al.* (2009). "Managing the health effects of climate change: Lancet and University College London Institute for Global Health Commission", *Lancet*; *373*: 1693–733.

Dankelman I., Alam K., Ahmed W., Gueye Y., Fatema N., Mensah-Kurin R. (2005). *Gender, climate change and human security: Lessons from Bangladesh, Ghana and Senegal.* New York: Women's Environment and Development Organization.

Forstater, M. (2003). "Public Employment and Environmental Sustainability", *Journal of Post Keynesian Economics*, *25*(3), 385-406.

Fiorino, D.J. (2010). "Sustainability as a Conceptual Focus for Public Administration", *Public Administration Review*, *70*, 70-88.

Fredell, K.A. (1996). *Women and sustainable development: an empirical analysis of ecofeminism*. University of Calgary.

Goodland, R. (1995). "The Concept of Environmental Sustainability", *Annual Review of Ecology and Systematics*, *26*, 1-24.

Groenewegen, J., Schreuders, W., and Paridon, K.V. (1992). "Environment, Growth, and Sustainability", *Journal of Economic Issues*, *26*(3), 915-919.

Hosseinpoor, A.R., Harper, S., Lee, J.H., Lynch, J., Mathers, C., and Abou-Zahr, C. (2012). "Better health for everyone»". *Bulletin of the World Health Organization*, *90*: 588-594.

Husted, Brian C. (2005) "Culture and Ecology: A Cross-National Study of the Determinants of Environmental Sustainability", *Management International Review, 45*(3), 349-371.

Irving, S. and Helin, J. (2018). "A world for sale? An ecofeminist reading of sustainable development discourse", *Gender, Work and Organization*, *25*(3), 264-278.

Kings, A.E. (2017). "Intersectionality and the changing face of ecofeminism", *Ethics and the Environment, 22*(1), 63-87.

Kuruvilla, S., Sadana, R., Montesinos, E.V., Beard, J., Vasdeki, J.F., de Carvalho, I. A.,... & Bustreo, F. (2018). "A life-course approach to health: synergy with sustainable development goals", *Bulletin of the World Health Organization, 96*(1), 42.

Langer, A., Meleis, A., Knaul, F.M., Atun, R., Aran, M., Arreola-Ornelas, H., ... and Frenk, J. (2015). "Women and health: the key for sustainable development", *The Lancet, 386*(9999), 1165-1210.

Leach, M. (2007). "Earth mother myths and other ecofeminist fables: How a strategic notion rose and fell", *Development and change, 38*(1), 67-85.

Lewis, D. (2003). "NGOs, Organization Culture, and Institutional Sustainability", *The Annals of the American Academy of Political and Social Science*, 590, 212-226.

Li, H.L. (2007). "Ecofeminism as a pedagogical project: Women, nature, and education", *Educational Theory, 57*(3), 351-368.

Lorentzen, L.A. and Eaton, H. (2002). "Ecofeminism: an overview", In *The Forum on Religion and Ecology at Yale.*

Mumtaz, Z. and Salway, S. (2009). "Understanding gendered influences on women's reproductive health in Pakistan: Moving beyond the autonomy paradigm", *SocSci Med*; *68*: 1349–56.

Noss, R.F. (1995). *Maintaining Ecological Integrity in Representative Reserve Networks. World Wildlife Fund,* Canada/*World Wildlife Fund*— United States, Toronto, Ontario, and Washington D.C.

Paehlke, R. (2005). "Sustainability as a Bridging Concept", *Conservation Biology, 19*(1), 36-38.

Passerini, E. (1998). "Sustainability and Sociology", *The American Anthropologist, 29*(3), 59-70.

Perlman, B.J. (2009). "Governance & Sustainability", *State and Local Government Review, 41*(1), 37-38.

Pezzey, John C.V. (2004). "Sustainability Policy and Environmental Policy", *The Scandinavian Journal of Economics, 106*(2), 339-359.

Reid, A. and Petocz, P. (2006). "University Lecturers' Understanding of Sustainability", *Higher Education, 51*(1), 105-123.

Resurrección, B.P. (2013, September). "Persistent women and environment linkages in climate change and sustainable development agendas", In *Women's Studies International Forum* (Vol. 40, pp. 33-43). Pergamon.

Rochette, A. (2002). "Stop the rape of the world: An ecofeminist critique of sustainable development", *UNBLJ, 51*, 145.

Rosen, C.M. (2007). "Environmental Sustainability in the Twenty-First Century", *Environmental History, 12*(2), 362-364.

Ross, A. (2009). "Modern Interpretations of Sustainable Development", *Journal of Law & Society, 36*(1), 32-54.

Sachs, W. (1999). "Sustainable Development and the Crisis of Nature: On the Political Anatomy of an Oxymoron", In Fischer, F. and Hajer, M. (Eds.), *Living with Nature: Environmental Politics as Cultural Discourse.* Oxford: Oxford University Press, pp. 25-42.

Scoones, I. (2007). "Sustainability", *Development in Practice*, *17*(4/5), 589-596.

Scott, K., George, A.S., Harvey, S.A., Mondal, S., Patel, G., and Sheikh, K. (2017). Negotiating power relations, gender equality, and collective agency: are village health committees transformative social spaces in northern India? *International journal for equity in health*, *16*(1), 1-12.

Shiva, V. (1992). "Women's indigenous knowledge and biodiversity conservation", *India International Centre Quarterly*, *19*(1/2), 205-214.

Shiva, V. and Mies, M. (2014). *Ecofeminism*. London: Zed Books Ltd.

Toman, M.A. (1994). "Economics and 'sustainability': Balancing trade-offs and Imperatives", *Land Econ*. *70*(4): 399-413.

Whitford, Andrew B. and Wong, K. (2009). "Political and Social Foundations for Environmental Sustainability", *Political Research Quarterly*, *62*(1), 190-204.

Williams, C.C. and Millington, A.C. (2004). "The diverse and contested meanings of sustainable development", *Geographical Journal*, *170*(2), 99-104.

Wilsnack, R.W., Wilsnack, S.C., and Obot, I.S. (2005). "Why study gender, alcohol and culture", *Alcohol, gender and drinking problems: Perspectives from low and middle income countries.* Geneva: World Health Organization, 2005, 1-25.

World Commission on Environment and Development (1987). *Our Common Future*. Oxford University Press.

PART VI

Reflections on Corona Virus Pandemic

26

Pandemic as a Disaster

A Theoretical Montage for Exploring COVID-19

Prashant Khattri

Introduction

There has been a tendency of human mind to segregate and categorize. It tends to segregate concepts in order to understand them better. This is a kind of reductionism that is done at the level of cognition. This general tendency of separation sometimes gets converted into watertight compartmentalization of concepts and disciplines with limited or no flow between them. If one thing that this pandemic has done then it is that it has made us realize that our existence is shared. This emphasis on shared existence has also led us to believe that human knowledge cannot be categorized and must be understood in its holistic perspective. This also has an important implication for the conceptualization of the 'other' in anthropological literature. From its inception, the 'other' in anthropology was conceptualized as a distant, 'un-civilized', non-literate entity that needs to be studied and documented by a more 'superior' European administrator. During the later half of the twentieth century, the 'other' was conceptualized as the suffering subject largely residing in the Third World. They were seen as vulnerable to disease and disasters and in need of help. The pandemic, however, has forced us to re-conceptualize the entire notion of 'otherness' as it subjugated the category owing to its global prevalence. However, the orient and the occident loomed large in the public imagination of people about the ways and methods through which the pandemic was tackled globally. More specifically, the media coverage of the response of the Third World countries was seen in this light.

It happened for the first time in the history of the world and more specifically India that we are faced with the situation where compartmentalization of knowledge in the field of medicine, health, medical anthropology and sociology and that of disaster studies was challenged. In the form of the pandemic, we are faced with a situation where a health issue has taken the proportion of a disaster. This needs to be seen in the context of the management of the pandemic. It happened for the first time that the management of a medical emergency was done using the Disaster Management (DM) Act, 2005. It also follows from this that since the DM Act came into effect only in 2005, previous such situations, although qualify under disasters, like plague, cholera etc. could not be managed using the legal vocabulary of Disasters and their management especially in the Indian context. This, however, has its own problems when critically evaluated from the perspective of bio-power and bio-politics but this we will deal with later in this chapter. For now, we need to understand that there is a case for visualizing a medical emergency from the lens of disasters. This has important bearing on the theoretical perspectives from which a pandemic can be seen. But before we move on to that, we need to talk a bit more on the pandemic and the DM Act, 2005 (Mohan and Alex, 2020).

The nationwide lockdown that was imposed in the month of March 2020 was based on the provisions of the DM Act, 2005. In the act, disaster management has been conceptualized as a three-tier system in which the central authority named the National Disaster Management Authority (NDMA) is placed at the top with the Prime Minister heading it. Next in line are the various State Disaster Management Authorities (SDMA) headed by the Chief Ministers of respective states and the District Disaster Management Authorities (DDMA) headed by the District Magistrate. The NDMA formulated guidelines for the management of biological disasters in 2008 and the nationwide lockdown was imposed under the DM Act through an order of the NDMA for ensuring social distancing and preventing the spread of COVID-19. The Act, together with various state acts and the Epidemic Diseases Act, 1897, gave wide powers to the state for administering the huge population in the pandemic (Mohan and Alex, 2020).

This was at the legal and administrative front. On a more academic front, the pandemic needs to be visualized from the perspectives formulated through the studies of disasters in social science. This becomes even more important in the light of academicians getting worried about the crisis in social sciences in explaining and theorizing the pandemic (Visvanathan, 2020). This crisis to me is more about not writing about the pandemic in the language already available with the social scientists rather than a complete lack of it. It is in this context that we need to re-look at the theoretical perspectives generated in the context of extreme events. In doing so we may also realize that such perspectives are already in use and are being propagated and used by the state machinery and people at large. Policies of the state are being projected within such perspectives without realizing that they first appeared in the context of disaster studies. This chapter tries to explore the theoretical perspectives to conceptualize the pandemic.

It has been argued that labelling the pandemic as a disaster was inevitable and extremely necessary since there was no other legislation available to deal with a crisis of this magnitude. It was in this context that the DM Act was invoked and legal provisions were put in place in order to manage the crisis. The epidemic act which was already in place was considered to be archaic and not suitable to deal with the situation. However, critiques have argued that labelling pandemic as a disaster had serious consequences as it shaped the response of the state towards its citizens in a very specific way. The power and authority of the state became absolute and the state entered into a legal contract with its citizens, the breach of which was to be dealt with punishment. This led to the categorization of human movement and behaviour into normal and abnormal. Any deviation from the normal was bound to invoke punishment. Latour (2005) has argued in his Actor-Network Theory (ANT) that knowledge is not dependent on any kind of truth waiting to be discovered but is based on the perception and analysis of the interaction between various networks and actors. Thus, labelling a pandemic as a disaster is not based on any natural connection between the two or a universal truth but it is more to do with the networks and actors that will be involved in different ways in order to exercise power and authority on the people.

The field of disaster studies offer a wide range of concepts and theories to conceptualize the pandemic. Not only does it provide a lens to understand the pandemic but it also opens up the scope for critical understanding of the situation. Many formulations of the event—mostly coming from the positions of power and dominance— may sound plausible in the absence of any relevant critique. It also gives us the chance to question the state response in the light of the critique of various theoretical positions and definitional issues in disaster research. Disasters have been defined as events where the coping capacity of the affected population is challenged. The capacity to respond and overcome the event is seriously undermined and thus external support and help is the only way out of the crisis. It also calls for technological and scientific interventions in order to cope with the situation. This, however, is not the complete picture as people have their own theories and explanations of the event that in the light of the dominant modernist and scientific outlook is best labelled as the 'alternative' way of thinking. Such explanations and theories are invoked in the time of crisis to make sense of the situation. In disaster literature, these explanations are labelled as the traditional approaches to disasters.

Cosmological Explanations of Pandemic: The Realm of Moral-Political

It has been argued that the disasters are not about the dead. They are about the living. This is because the dead are gone but it is the people who are left behind have to deal with the pain and sufferings due to their loss. They have to make sense of the situation and continue living. Damaged houses, roads, drainage systems, all can be built back and compensated but loss of the loved ones leave scars that take considerable time to heal. They also require explanations that may rationalize the loss. In most common terms, the pandemic from its very inception was defined as the metaphor for *pralay*. Within the Judo-Christian religion, the same can be translated as the end of the world. This is the linear thought process. In contrast to this, within the Hindu philosophical mode of thinking, creation and dissolution are cyclical processes with no end. There is no disaster that can put the world to an end as there are only phases of creation and dissolution and not destruction. Dissolution on the other hand happen due to the imbalance of *gunas* within the *Prakriti*. When seen from this perspective, the pandemic can be visualized as an event that altered the way we live. Instead of bringing an end to this world, the pandemic led to new ways of existence. The theory of *Pralay* also rationalizes the loss. God is not held responsible for the disaster within this view. Individual and collective actions become important rallying points leading to the imbalance of the *gunas* (Kapur, 2010).

Doctrine of *Karma* becomes very important in making sense of the crisis. Human beings philosophize not to alleviate suffering but for making sense of it. In other words, we philosophize in order to make suffering sufferable. The unfolding of a disaster when viewed from this perspective implies that 'what we sow so shall we reap'. In the context of the pandemic, this perspective occupied an important place as the collective deeds of human beings were held responsible for the pandemic. In this context disasters are not seen as discrete events or chance happenings or an accident but are part of the larger plan which says that every event has a cause which may or may not be immediate but may lie at a distant past. A disaster therefore is not considered as an aberration or a purposeless happening but it is seen more as a moral judgement. This idea of morality is also sometimes used by those who are entrusted with the task of managing the disasters. It is in this context that disaster management moves into the realm of moral-political. This is to say that the issue of morality in disaster works as a from of social control. It also sometimes absolves the state of its responsibilities towards its citizens. Recovery from the disaster is an important phase in its management. Within the moral-politics, the recovery is entrusted solely upon the individual and the state absolves itself from its responsibilities. Most important outcome of the filter of *Karma* is that it absorbs anger and frustration against the authority which is so common in a disaster situation. It also averts violence of any kind and helps in maintaining social equilibrium. In other words, it restores order in a situation of chaos and disorder. A belief in *Karma* works in favour of the state. Traditionally, the bipolar conception of vice and virtue (*paap* and *punya*) were used to 'manage' disasters. Within this context the state is absolved from its duties towards its citizens. Historically, states were not responsible for the management of disasters. This happened because of two reasons— (a) states were not welfare states and were only concerned with their revenues and (b) states and state machinery were also causalities in disaster context. However, with the emergence of the conception of welfare state, state became a major stakeholder in disaster recovery and rehabilitation. Nonetheless, traditional narratives are still used to in order to deflect responsibilities (Kapur, 2010).

In contrast to the above explained principle of absorption, where the pain and sufferings are absorbed through the notion of *Karma*, the principle of 'appeal' presents another paradigm to understand disasters. Anu Kapur (2010) has labelled it as the folk paradigm to disasters. This paradigm is based on an appeal to the deity considered to be listening to cases related to disaster loss and damage. Gods that are considered to be bringing misery and disasters are appeased in order to maintain the equilibrium. Disaster is considered to be caused by angering the concerned deity. Since the cause is located in anger, solution lie in appeasement. Hymns, chants, praise, offerings, sacrifice and religious ceremonies form an integral part of the ritual. It is believed that there is a divine power that receive all these hymns and chants. There is a hope from this power that everything will be made fine and back to normal. This is a hope generating paradigm. It gives much needed psychological confidence and assurance at the time of crisis and distress. In contrast to the principle of absorption, the principle of appeal releases us from suffering and disaster. It does not only make the suffering sufferable but it also gives us hope.

Social Contract in a Pandemic: The Citizen-State Dyad

Within a democratic set-up, the citizen-state relationship emerges as an important unit of analysis in disaster context. Citizenship is asserted by the civil-society groups and downplayed by the state. Situations of crisis puts pressing demands onto the state and it becomes imperative for both the parties to win the game. This situation calls for a closer look into the concept of citizen and citizenship. Within the liberal discourse on citizenship, social element is given much importance beside political and civic elements. This is to say that beside economic welfare and security a citizen enjoys the right to live a life of a civilized being in accordance with the prevailing standards in a society. It is this social element that takes a beating during a crisis. This became even more stark and visible in the context of the pandemic in the form of social-distancing and nationwide lockdowns. It is also true that although the social element is regarded as an important part of the concept of citizenship, its full realization in most of the democracies is yet to be seen. This, however, is a generalizing statement that emerges out of a monolithic understanding of citizenship. In a more grounded approach, citizens are formed as part of the larger social and political processes. There are societies where active struggle against the authority led to the formation of 'active citizens' and there are others where citizenship is bestowed by the authority themselves making it a more passive process. However, within the post-colonial context, citizens are often 'target populations' that are dependent upon the state driven welfare programmes and activities related to larger development (Robins *et al.*, 2008). Citizens are also often part of the traditional clientele politics that ensures some kind of security in receiving and becoming beneficiaries of the welfare schemes (Siddiqi, 2019). It is in this context that a disaster situation is visualized with the lens of welfare distribution. In the context of the COVID-19 pandemic people saw their 'welfare' in getting some kind of relaxations in rules to travel despite lockdowns.

Rights and entitlements also form important components of citizens in a disaster context. Amartya Sen (1981) was of the view that crisis like famines is not the result of the decline in food availability rather they are a result of entitlement failures. In fact, the issue of rights came-up in a big way in the pandemic. People in countries like USA refused to follow government regulations as they were infringing upon their rights and entitlements. Although this might have resulted into increasing infections but in comparison to this, in India, since people were unable to assert their rights, they were subjected to all kinds of hardships in the form of large-scale urban to rural migration. Moreover, frontline workers like doctors, nurses and the paramedics were not in a position to demand their dues from the government. There were some agitations seen among some group of doctors not getting their salaries on time and long working-hours that they were subjected to but this could not get translated into any kind of right and their duty as doctors was weighted more against their rights as individuals. This also suggests that the making of a political public is actually grounded in the local and national traditions. Citizenship then is the result of the larger socio-political environment or pre-condition rather than something that is given in the context of a democratic polity.

Disasters are situations that are politically very sensitive. This is to say that these situations have all the ingredients that may challenge the incumbent regime. Disasters may bring political instability and may erode the very basis of political power-people's support. The public very critically examine the role of the state in dealing with disasters and organize to protest. However, the pandemic presented a very unique situation where protesting rights were suspended as a measure to avoid crowding during lockdowns. Studies have also suggested that vulnerabilities to disasters are more political issues rather than being technological. This is to suggest that those areas that form important vote banks of the incumbent party are given preference in dealing with disasters. It is also documented that natural disasters hit the politically peripheral regions, the hardest. Disaster situation also gives us a glimpse into the minds of people who are at the governing positions. In case of the pandemic, it was seen that it was the rural poor who was hit the hardest. They had to walk long distances in order to reach their homes. People in the urban areas however were given all the facilities to deal with the crisis. They were in their homes getting food and other stuffs delivered to their door-steps. This suggests that within the political imagination, urban India rules. This is also evident from the concentration of economic activities in the urban areas that lead to a large-scale migration towards urban areas. A lot of people were asking this question that why there are fewer opportunities to people living in rural areas and other places that are not part of the dominant development discourse. Why people need to migrate in search of livelihood to places far away from their homes. Such questions, however, were not addressed in a manner that they should have been as they question the larger narrative on development and progress (Pelling and Dill, 2008).

Disasters, therefore, have the capacity to increase the political heat. Pre-existing political struggles are fed with increased inequalities on the basis of region, class, caste, religion etc. Thus, there is a reproduction of inequalities in a disaster context. This conception, however, also has a flip side to it. More often it is observed that politics and power are sustained through generating inequalities within the populations. In this context disasters or crisis may help in sustaining and reinforcing the dominant political narrative on which the ruling elite bases their political power. In the absence of any strong opposition and a counter-narrative, the reproduction of inequality supports the incumbent regimen. Disasters happening in some of the developed countries have shown that such situations of crisis allow the citizen to talk-back with the people in power. This feature, however, is contingent upon the creation of the kind of political public in a socio-historical context. As mentioned earlier, in post-colonial societies where citizens are mostly the 'target populations', such talking-back may not be possible as the dimension of clientele politics may prevent the creation of citizen as an agent of political change. "*The disaster, while clearly seen to have political consequences, is rarely, if ever, known to push certain progressive elements of the social contract along*" (Siddiqi, 2019:32-33). Instead, they open up space for 'fundamental' political ideologies that may result into authoritarian state. One of the ways among many, in which this is done is to project the crisis in a language that is hard to counter as in the case like the nationalist discourse or patterns of war approach.

Patterns of War Approach: Discourse on Bio-Power

War has been one of the most consistent themes in disaster analysis. This is also one of the earliest ways of visualizing disasters. Hazard agent or hazardous event is seen as an external enemy that needs to be fought-back and defeated. As in the case of a war, the enemy is almost always an external agent, similarly in case of a disaster, the cause is sought outwardly. This approach visualizes a situation of conflict between the agent and the community. The agent is external to the community and is harmful and the community needs to fight back the agent in a collective manner as it is done in the context of war. The human community is also visualized as an organism or as an organic body having different parts. These parts work in tandem and work against the external agent. Within the anthropological discourse of functionalism, human society is seen as a harmonious system having different parts and function together to maintain the whole just like different parts of a body. Disasters then are events that break this harmony and therefore, a process of restoration—which in disaster literature is known as recovery-sets in (Quarantelli, 1998; Gilbert, 1998).

The patterns of war approach to disaster has its emergence in the context of the cold war and the role of United States in it. Fritz (1968, 1961) has argued that during the cold war, US funded many research projects that were aimed at knowing the reaction of people in case there is an air strike in their area. In other words, reaction of people to external threat was being recorded through such projects. They wanted to know and test that how people will behave in the context of an external threat. Disaster research became an institutional demand during the war periods. An entire market for such research funding was generated in the context of the cold war. People and areas affected by disasters like floods, hurricanes or earthquakes were supposed to resemble victims of an air raid. This approach was also instrumental in giving rise to the first kind of response to the disasters in the form of recovery and rehabilitation as is done in case of destruction caused by war. World leaders also saw the pandemic within this perspective when Donald Trump said that we need to wage a war against the 'Chinese Virus'.

It has been argued that this traditional approach to disaster is very popular among the political and public servants and scientists. They tend to see disasters in terms of war rhetoric. The most common and dominant narrative around the COVID-19 pandemic is the patterns of war approach. Within this narrative, all those fighting against the external agent, a virus in this case, become warriors. This kind of a conception leads to the militarization of the discourse. On one hand it gives a sense of urgency and utmost importance to the event and on the other it gives a lot of control in the hands of the state. Through this discourse the notion of bio-power emerges. Foucault talks about bio-power in the context of the discourses that exercise power and control over the human bodies. The war rhetoric is one such discourse.

The discourse on war tries to project an image of the state and of the administration that can resolve and tackle all kinds of human vulnerabilities. It also gives scope for the emergence of iconic figures and martyrs who are supposed to have laid down their lives in the service of the country and the motherland. Within the popular and dominant image of a nation as an incarnation of a Goddess, the discourse on war is directed towards saving the nation from an external threat. Although such a discourse might generate patriotism and nationalism among the citizens, and they may become ready to sacrifice their lives for their country but on the other hand it also stops people who are at the forefront of the fight to question the decision of their masters. Like a foot soldier never questions the General, in the same way 'warriors' never question the policies and decisions of the political elite.

Philosophers and social scientists have questioned this approach to disasters. I will discuss the critique through the work of a philosopher Albert Camus (2020, 1947) and a social scientist Quarantelli (1998). Camus was of the view that it is quite impossible to reduce all vulnerabilities to disasters. This is not a pessimistic view of disaster but a view that is more nuanced. According to him, since we cannot tackle all the vulnerabilities, therefore, human beings must not behave in a way that is heroic. Instead, we must behave in a way that is more 'descent'. Heroism will give us a false hope that we are able to conquer all vulnerabilities which is actually not the case. Life according to him can be lived in a better way by not giving too much meaning to it. Quarantelli on the other hand critiques the pattern of war approach through the concept of consensus crisis. He is of the view that there is a consensus crisis in the war approach as it is mostly propounded and held by the ruling elite. People on the ground, however, may not subscribe to the war rhetoric of the disaster. There emerges a consensus crisis that questions the war rhetoric. The pattern of war approach also assumes that there is a universal response to the crisis. A response that remains same across various groups and communities in a society. This, however, is not the case. Response to the crisis is constructed on the basis of past experiences and available resources. This way of looking at disasters is centred around the community and not around the external agent. It also tries to understand the vulnerabilities of peoples, groups and communities that are responsible for precipitating events into disasters. Thus, disasters are not seen as a result of any external factor but are to be located within the human group itself. Large scale migration of people from urban to rural areas in the pandemic points to the variable degrees of vulnerabilities people suffer from.

The 'Affective Turn' in Disaster Studies: Implications for Conceptualizing a Pandemic

Disasters are testing times. Moreover, in the context of the present pandemic, a new norm has emerged with which we are tackling in our everyday lives. Disasters are associated with a lot of personal and social suffering. Death and damage need to be tackled at the individual and community level. Individuals might experience situations in which they had never been before. Such traumatic situations had been studied under the technical and bio-medical and psychological language of the Post-Traumatic Stress Disorder (PTSD). Such bio-medical terms have led to the universalization of human emotions and pains and sufferings. However, ethnographic works have suggested that human feelings and emotions are culture-bound and have a social dimension to it. The study of trauma and disaster events underwent a paradigm shift after such ethnographic works. Suffering was now considered to be more structural rather than being universal. More than disaster events, it is the social structure that becomes the cause and a channel for expression of the suffering. Mothers who lost their sons in Latur earthquake were made to undergo recanalization (surgical operation on those women who earlier underwent tubectomy to re-conceive.) so that they can once again bear a child. The centrality of male child in Indian society led to re-medicalization of women's body within a patriarchal set-up where women cannot speak much. Similarly, Veena Das demonstrated that the 1984 anti-Sikh riots in Delhi that led to the feelings of emotional distress on people who suffered personal losses were a blend of the event and the social structure (Gupta *et al.*, 2019).

Both the example discussed above could be narrativized with the help of language. Such emotions were communicated to the ethnographer in a very specific language. In contrast to this there are feelings and emotions that cannot be structured in any language. Linguistic frameworks are not sufficient to express such emotional feelings. This happens more often in case of traumatic events. Such feelings remain at the individual level at the level of their bodies. These feelings are termed as affective. Sarbhadikary (2018) writes, "Recently, scholars have initiated new debates with what is being called the 'affective turn' in theory. Taking effective leads from the works of Deleuze and Guattari (2004) and Massumi (2002), they are trying to conceptualize sensory states at pre-linguistic levels. These non-linguistic levels of the viscera, like lightning flashes, apprehend a temporal instance which the subject does not and even cannot anticipate. These states thus overwhelm the experiencer's thought structure, and supersede their cognitive capacities.....Affect in other words, is pre-conscious, or better still, supra-conscious, and supra-subjective" (pp. 235). Emotions in contrast are sensations that have a language and can be communicated through linguistic means. Emotions exemplify relationships between language and thought. Affect on the other hand is not consciously registered and therefore, eludes linguistic explanations.

Sarbadhikary (2018) while writing on the importance of affect in ethnography emphasizes on the fact that the affective ethnography has an important methodological issue that needs to be addressed. That is actually how the ethnographer or the field worker is supposed to understand the individual embodied reactions to events that cannot be narrativized or linguistically communicated? How as an ethnographer we are supposed to write about affect? She contends that this methodological issue is probably an important reason that affect is not taken-up adequately as a theoretical tool by the ethnographers especially in the context of anthropological work in South Asia. The ethnographer needs to overcome this handicap while attempting an affective ethnography. Sarbadhikary (2018) further proposes two ways through which this handicap can be overcome, viz. self-reflexivity and auto-ethnography. In order to enter the affective world of the people whom the ethnographer is studying, he needs to experience the emotive dimensions himself. In the case of disaster then it can be said that an auto-ethnographic approach is best suited for an affective ethnography. This means experiencing the disaster by an ethnographer himself.

While I am writing this chapter the world is going through the pandemic of COVID-19. Death and destruction are in the minds of every individual. We all are directly and indirectly affected by this Corona crisis. Anthropologists are especially apprehensive about the future of anthropological field research in the context of social distancing. Anthropological field research involves participant observation and living with the community under study. In the wake of the corona crisis, however, there is a sense of suspicion and fear in the minds of people and are actively avoiding the outsiders. It needs to be seen that till what time such protocols and behavioural patterns are going to last. This may have some impact on the fieldwork of the individual and also of the team. However, I contend here that in the context of the affective turn in anthropology of disasters this corona crisis could be seen as 'every persons first-hand experience with the disasters.' I do realize, however, that this experience is not similar with all and it is affected by categories of caste, class, gender and other social groupings. But, still it can be seen as an important turning point in the 'affective' studies of disasters and doing 'affective ethnographies' of the disaster events.

Death and the Pandemic

One of the central issues concerning the COVID-19 pandemic is death. How can be make sense of dying in a pandemic? What meaning can be give to death? It is a reality and we know that it will happen to all living creatures on earth. Still human beings have ritualized and symbolized death in several ways across different cultures. Functional interpretation of death suggests that death performs a very crucial function to maintain the society as a whole. By replacing old members in the society it gives opportunities to the new members to enter into the shoes of their elders and take responsibilities of households and families (Srivastava and Srivastava, 1997). Within the French Structuralism one similarity among all cultures symbolizing death is that they all have some or the other ritual associated with it. This is the underlying similarity amidst the surface ritual differences related to death and dying. Robert Hertz (1960) has suggested that differences exist in terms of rituals and beliefs related to death in different cultures but there is a similarity in the underlying logic. This logic is patterned on a triangular principle where the dead body, the survivors and the place where the dead is supposed to have gone after death form three points of a triangle. It is this triangular model of death that seems to be disturbed in this pandemic. Although people are still quite sure about the place where their dead relatives have gone but their relations with the corpse underwent a change. People were not allowed to see their dead ones for the one last time. They got apprehensive about the COVID infection that might be transmitted from the dead to the living. This resulted in a total institutional takeover of the disposal of the dead body.

The pandemic has also altered and dented our conception about 'good death'. A 'good death' has been conceptualized in a number of ways, from a biomedical conception that envisages the age at which a person dies to a more personal conceptions of painless death. Good death has always been celebrated especially in the Indian context. This is actually an integrated conception of the biomedical and the personal. A good death is conceptualized as one where a person dies only after completing all his/her duties towards family, friends and relatives and then dies a painless death. In the pandemic, however, people died at ages when they were not supposed to and also, they died painful deaths—both physically and socially. Once diagnosed with the disease, many were hospitalized to never return again and not to be seen by any member of their families. Besides this, death has never been a subject of overt discussion in houses, especially not in front of children who are considered to be too young to grasp the whole idea. There was a certain amount of decorum maintained while talking about death and the dead—both in linguistic terms where we never say that a person died but only say that he/she passed away and in our body language (Green, 2008). However, the pandemic has brought the discussion of death and the dead in a very new and crude way to our discussions about it. A new kind of language, one which is also numerical and statistical in nature suddenly emerged in our discussions.

Death has always been a 'process' cross-culturally (Hertz, 1960). There are elaborate rituals and ritual specialists that try to rationalize death and convert it into a process sharing the grief. However, in the case of the pandemic, death has come to be known more as an event. An event that is guided from beginning till end by the biomedical and state norms and rules. Intrusion of state has never been so much as in the case of this pandemic *vis-à-vis* death and dying. Mass deaths and limited capacities of health care systems has led to a lot of confusion. Cases have been reported where people got the mortal remains of dead people not related to them in any ways. The pandemic pushed the health care systems to its limits and therefore, influenced the experience of people whose loved ones have died.

From the perspective of depth psychology of heroism, Becker (1973) has argued that "we strive to be heroic because that is the only reasonable response to the terrible truth of mortality" (Green, 2008:11). A paradoxical discourse is what we heard and saw in the context of the pandemic. There were actually two groups of people generating different discourses around death. On the one hand there were people mostly the celebrities who said that being fearful is actually being heroic and then there were people who were actually working at the ground zero—in hospitals, in ambulances, as paramedics and others labelled as frontline workers who were doing heroic deeds in the midst of the pandemic. There is actually a conflict seen between the 'cultural-hero-system (CHS)' and the 'mythical-hero-system (MHS).' Within the MHS people try to serve the humanity in order to gain cosmic specialness. Becker (1973) has seen this within the context of living in a creative illusion without knowing for sure about your permanent place in the cosmos. Again, within those religious philosophies where re-birth is an important theme, deeds in the present birth becomes important to secure a better place in the future births. Also, good deeds are believed to be leading unto salvation.

Conclusion

In this chapter I have tried to understand the single reality of a pandemic from different vantage point of views. I have largely used the theoretical premises that have been developed in the context of disasters to understand pandemic as a disaster. One of the most striking features of a disaster event is that it puts a lot of adjustive demand over the human mind. The human mind wants to make sense of all the deaths and destructions happening around it. Nonetheless, the sheer size and impact of the event is such that there sometimes occur a total loss of meaning. Immanuel Kant 2007,

(1952) has tried to grasp this dimension of extreme event through his conception of the 'Analytic of the Sublime'. He writes that sublime is a pleasure produced by the mind as soon as it reaches its own limits. The humiliation of the mind through the thoughts of destruction and loss is overcome soon by the mind itself that restores its power by reckoning its own superiority to the nature (Simpson, 2013). It is also in this context that the depth psychology of Becker and the heroic deeds in a disaster situation can be located.

This is not the exhaustive list of theoretical paradigms as many more have been suggested by social scientists who consider that the in general social sciences lack the necessary language to capture the realities in the pandemic. This chapter is also an attempt to bring to the fore, researches that are done in the field of disaster studies and that provide necessary language to understand the pandemic and other such events in future. Moreover, I have already mentioned in the section on the affective turn that not every felt emotion can be translated into the language of science. Sometimes, we need to feel it as others are doing in an ongoing social crisis.

REFERENCES

Becker, E. (1973). *The Denial of Death*. New York: Free Press.

Camus, A. 2020 (1947). *The Plague*. London: Penguin Classics.

Fritz, C. (1961). "Disasters", In R. Merton and R. Nisbet (eds.) *Contemporary Social Problems*. New York: Harcourt Brace.

Fritz, C. (1968). Disasters. *International Encyclopedia of Social Sciences*. New York: Macmillan.

Gilbert, C. (1998). "Studying Disaster: Changes in the main conceptual tools", In Quarantelli, E.L. (ed.). *What is a Disaster? Perspectives on the Question*. London: Routledge.

Green, J.W. (2008). *Beyond The Good Death: The Anthropology of Modern Dying*. Pennsylvania: University of Pennsylvania Press.

Gupta, A., Bhattacharya, P., and Priya, K.R. (2019). "Revisiting the Paradigm Shift in Trauma Studies: Twenty-Five Years of Veena Das' 'Our Work to Cry: Your Work to Listen'," *Journal of the Anthropological Survey of India*. *68*(1). 70-84.

Hertz, R. (1960). *Death and the Right Hand*. Glencoe: Free Press.

Kant, I. 2007 (1952). *Critique of Judgement*. Oxford: Oxford University Press.

Kapur, A. (2010). *Vulnerable India: A Geographical Study of Disasters*. New Delhi and Shimla: Sage and IIAS.

Latour, B. (2005). *Reassembling the Social: An Introduction to Actor-Network-Theory*. New York: Oxford University Press.

Mohan, M.P.R. and Alex, J.P. (2020, April 26). "COVID-19 and the ambit of the Disaster Management Act", *The Week Magazine*.

Pelling, M. and Dill, K. (2008). "Disaster Politics: From Social Contract to Human Security. Department of Geography", King's College, London. *Environment, Politics and Development Working Paper Series*. Paper no. 1.

Quarantelli, E.L. (ed.) (1998). *What is a Disaster? Perspectives on the Question*. London: Routledge.

Robins S.A. Cornwall and B. VonLieres. (2008). "Rethinking Citizenship in the Postcolony", *Third World Quarterly*. *29*(6). 1069-86.

Sarbadhikary, S. (2018). " 'For the Skin is Faster than the Word': Towards an Ethnography of Affect", In Maitrayee Chaudhuri and Manish Thakur (eds.) *Doing Theory: Locations, Hierarchies and Disjunctions*. Hyderabad: Orient BlackSwan.

Sen, A. (1981). *Poverty and Famines: An Essay on Entitlement and Deprivation*. New York: Oxford University Press.

Siddiqi, A. (2019). *In the Wake of Disaster: Islamists, the State and a Social Contract in Pakistan*. UK: Cambridge University Press.

Simpson, E. (2014). *The Political Biography of an Earthquake: Aftermath and Amnesia in Gujarat, India*. New Delhi: Oxford University Press.

Srivastava, K. and Srivastava, V.K. (1997). "On Anthropology of Death", *Economic and Political Weekly*, *32*(16), 827-832.

Visvanathan, S. (2020). "The COVID 19 Pandemic and the Crisis of the Social Sciences", *Economic and Political Weekly*, *55*(42): 29-33.

27

The Effects of Corona Virus Disease-19 (COVID-19) on Non-human Primates and Probable Way-out

A Review

Prakash Ranjan Mondal and *Surendra Kumar Sagar*

Introduction

The accidental arrival of the Corona Virus Disease 19, also abbreviated as COVID-19 during December 2019 inside the Wuhan City of Hubei province of China, is the cause of global pandemic situation in present days. Therefore, from the Wuhan City of Southern China this virus had spread quickly worldwide within 2-3 months. After examining the taxonomy, genetic similarities and phylogeny between the present virus and the virus which had effect on the severe acute respiratory syndrome-related coronavirus (SARS-CoV) outburst during the year 2002 and 2003, it has been decided that the new virus will be called as SARS-CoV-2 (Gorbalenya *et al.*, 2020).

Since, non-human primate models will not only help us to comprehend the viral disease biology in terms of mechanisms and pathogenesis of SARS-CoV-2, but also will assist to explain immunological, pharmacological and toxicological aspects of the candidate vaccines and therapeutic approaches or strategies (Hewitt *et al.*, 2020). The aim of this review is to highlight the effects of SARS-CoV-2 in different non-human primate models and possible remedies that can be applied to prevent this virus in the non-human primates.

Effects of Corona Virus Disease 19 (COVID-19) on the Non-Human Primates

As the non-human primates have phylogenetic proximity with humans so using those animals in bio-medical research can be very valuable for knowing the characteristics and behaviour of different viral diseases, which affect human beings (Colman, 2018; Santos *et al.*, 2020). Experimentally, non-human primates also can be contaminated by the coronavirus and can exhibit several symptoms that are visible in coronavirus affected human individuals (de Wit *et al.*, 2020; Santos *et al.*, 2020).

Experiments for studying the clinical symptoms and behaviour of coronavirus in non-human primates have primarily done worldwide on rhesus macaques (*Macaca mulatta*) and cynomolgus macaques (*Macaca fascicularis*) (Santos *et al.*, 2020). According to the basic records, these monkeys after the infection, on the first day exemplify changes in the breathing process, and also being escorted with pulmonary infiltrate, which linger for minimum one week. Therefore, during this period, pneumonia like fever occurs in human beings which is a general symptom in humans but in case of rhesus macaques, it becomes visible as a mild symptom (Munster *et al.*, 2020a; Santos *et al.*, 2020) or not yet monitored in this species (Bao *et al.*, 2020; Santos *et al.*, 2020). Thus, in some non-human primates, haematological alterations were identified, for example, neutrophilia and leukocytosis, although within a few days the values become normal (Santos *et al.*, 2020). While, experimental studies indicate that after the subsequent years of the outbreak of severe acute respiratory syndrome-related coronavirus (SARS-CoV) during 2002 and 2003, lighter forms of the symptoms were identified in the non-human primates as compared to those observed in humans (Lawler *et al.*, 2006; Santos *et al.*, 2020).

During the first days of infection, researchers have detected similar observations inside the oropharyngeal and nasal swabs of rhesus macaques like humans, while talking about the positive effects of the coronavirus RNA. This incidence directs towards the high opportunity or chance for the spread of coronavirus which can happen through the proximity existence with infected individuals or animals. It will not be possible to comment that coronavirus affected human individuals directly infect the non-human primates or *vice versa*, although the experimental research on viral cultures taking specimens from affected human individuals sturdily point towards that the SARS-CoV-2 can obviously contaminate or infect the non-human primates (Santos *et al.*, 2020).

Lu *et al.* in 2020 conducted an experiment on three non-human primate species, namely *Macaca mulatta* (n = 14), *Macaca fascicularis* (n = 6) and one New World monkey, *Callithrix jacchus* (n = 6), to identify an appropriate non-human primate model for coronavirus-19 (SARS-CoV-2). During this study, an increase in the temperature of the body, a decrease in body weight with abnormal chest radiographs were obtained from infected *Macaca mulatta* and *Macaca fascicularis* individuals. From all these animals coronavirus genomes were identified from the blood and swab samples. Within the pulmonary tissues of *Macaca mulatta* and *Macaca fascicularis* viral load was identified but this was not identified in *Callithrix jacchus*. Among these three non-human primate species, only *Macaca mulatta* proved to be evident for the most appropriate model for SARS-CoV-2 because of enhancement of pathological changes and amplified inflammatory cytokine expressions within the pulmonary tissues of this species (Lu *et al.*, 2020).

In a study conducted by Zheng *et al.* (in 2020), they focused on interstitial pneumonia and virus shedding in the rhesus macaques (n = 14) which was identical to human cases. They also detected local chemokine or cytokine changes in the respiratory tracts and T cell subsets' response in the lung tissues which can be identified as the significant parameters for evaluation of a triumphant animal model for SARS-CoV-2 (Zheng *et al.*, 2020).

Adding together, in the study of Rockx *et al.* (2020) on four cynomolgus macaques inoculated by SARS-CoV-2 strain, serous nasal discharge was emitted in one aged individual on the 14th day of post inoculation, and there was non-existence of overt clinical symptoms in all individuals. In this study, the type I and II pneumocytes were also identified, whereas there was severity in lung lesions. By the 14th day of inoculation of the virus, all remaining individuals sero-converted which were revealed by the occurrence of SARS-CoV-2 exact antibodies (Rockx *et al.*, 2020).

Gonçalves *et al.* in 2021 have shown that mild clinical symptoms were revealed in a non-human primate model when infected by SARS-CoV-2 virus. In this research they have utilized a mathematical model to exemplify in detail of the dynamics of the virus within the 31 virus infected cynomolgus macaques. In these macaques, nasopharyngeal and tracheal swabs were repeatedly measured or assessed for examining the viral load. By means of this mathematical model they could do estimate the key parameters for the pathogenesis of virus, exactly the viral infectivity rate or speed within nasopharyngeal and tracheal compartments as well as the rate of loss of infected cells within both compartments. They have recognized in this research that the infected cells had a huge rupture size (>10^4 virus) within these macaques. They have also examined that after the peak viral load; the infected cells were quickly vanished by means of a half-life of 9 hours, with no important relationship flanked by or between the elevation and clearance of the cytokine, directing towards a median time on the way to viral clearance of 10 days, reliable by inspections within mild infections in the humans (Gonçalves *et al.*, 2021). From the estimated parameters in this research, Gonçalves *et al.* (2021) expected that a prophylactic action or treatment obstructing 90 per cent of the production of virus or the infection from virus that could stop the growth of virus. In concluding remarks, their results give estimations of kinetic parameters of SARS-CoV-2 virus in a mathematical experimental model bearing mild infection, further their effort implies to calculate the effectiveness of antiviral handling or treatments which will be conducted in the future (Gonçalves *et al.*, 2021).

Angiotensin-converting enzyme 2 (ACE2), was discovered or determined as the receptor intended for SARS-CoV and as well as has established or proven to be the receptor for SARS-CoV-2 (Hewitt *et al.*, 2020; Zhou *et al.*, 2020). The phylogenetic contrasts of ACE2 proteins permitted for predictions or calculations of species which were susceptible towards SARS-CoV-2 infection (Hewitt *et al.*, 2020; Liu *et al.*, 2020; Luan *et al.*, 2020; Qiu *et al.*, 2020; Wan *et al.*, 2020), while taking about viral infectivity, ACE2 is a key or highly important determinant (Hewitt *et al.*, 2020; Liu *et al.*, 2020). Melin *et al.*, in 2020 have examined comparative ACE2 variation and COVID-19 risk or threat in the non-human primates in their study. Their study recommends that some lemurs, African and Asian monkeys and apes are possibly to be extremely susceptible towards SARS-CoV-2 rather than the American monkeys and some tarsiers, lemurs and lorisoids (Melin *et al.*, 2020).

Way-out for Corona Virus Disease 19 (COVID-19) in the Non-Human Primates

Studies on severe acute respiratory syndrome-related coronavirus (SARS-CoV) and Middle East respiratory syndrome coronavirus (MERS-CoV) depict that non-human primates can be used as good models for doing research on COVID-19 vaccines (Gao *et al.*, 2003; Xu *et al.*, 2007; Santos *et al.*, 2020).

In the study of Corbett *et al.* (2020), they have showed the assessment of mRNA-1273 Vaccine as against SARS-CoV-2 in the non-human primates which ultimately gave them positive neutralizing results against this virus (Corbett *et al.*, 2020).

For the progress of drugs and vaccines against the pandemic coronavirus, these studies can be useful to direct and guide the scientists worldwide. For maintaining the health of the non-human primates, specifically throughout the pandemic COVID-19 phase, it is essential for the veterinary doctors, zoo keepers and zoo employees as well as primatologists who deal with non-human primates, mainly in laboratories, zoos and parks where visitors come, it is better to adopt and practice protective measures, precautions and stay alert as we do not have much knowledge about SARS-CoV-2 disease in non-human primates, we will require veterinary care during the time of their infection. Additionally, there can be a chance of infection in the unaffected non-human primates from the affected ones, so the veterinary and zoo management teams must be very prompt and aware in dealing these critical issues (Santos *et al.*, 2020).

Discussion

The non-human primates are essential animal models for estimating medical opposed-assesses in opposition to infectious viral diseases (Hewitt *et al.*, 2020).

Rhesus macaques (*Macaca mulatta*) uncovered to SARS-CoV-2 show infection and exhibit a mild or placid, non-lethal peeling viral disease phenotype. This comprises little to negative clinical surveillances (Hewitt *et al.*, 2020). Thus, if clinical surveillances are accounted, they comprise mild dehydration, dyspnea, piloerection, tachypnea and reduced appetite (Hewitt *et al.*, 2020; Munster *et al.*, 2020b). The infected rhesus macaques which are accounted, exhibited mild and transient fever starting shortly subsequent to exposure and recovering in 2 or 3 days (Hewitt *et al.*, 2020; Munster *et al.*, 2020b). Though, transient or temporary neutrophilia, lymphopenia, monocytosis and leukocytosis were accounted in the infected rhesus macaques (Hewitt *et al.*, 2020; Munster *et al.*, 2020b; Singh *et al.*, 2020).

Therefore, cynomolgus macaques (*Macaca fascicularis*) have been utilized, to examine the pathogenesis of SARS-CoV where elderly animals were more prone to extend the viral infections. When the cynomolgus macaques are exposed or uncovered to SARS-CoV-2, they came about infected, although display no evident clinical symptoms of infectious disease (Hewitt *et al.*, 2020; Rockx *et al.*, 2020). In several studies, it has been reported that the infected cynomolgus macaques have a fever taking place on the day 2 to 3 of infection (Hewitt *et al.*, 2020; Johnston *et al.*, 2020; Lu *et al.*, 2020). Therefore, advanced levels of virus peeling or shedding were calculated in elderly or aged cynomolgus macaques than the young ones (Hewitt *et al.*, 2020; Rockx *et al.*, 2020). The infected cynomolgus macaques produce mild to moderate or reasonable lung abnormalities as well as macroscopic lesions within the lungs counting alveolar edema, alveolar and bronchiolar epithelial necrosis, accumulation or gathering of immune cells and hyaline membrane construction or formation (Finch *et al.*, 2020; Hewitt *et al.*, 2020; Johnston *et al.*, 2020).

The African green monkeys (AGMs) uncovered to SARS-Cov-2 as young adult monkeys exhibit a mild and non-lethal shedding or peeling infectious disease phenotype which comprises little to negative clinical manifestations (Hartman *et al.*, 2020; Hewitt *et al.*, 2020). Thus, if clinical surveillances, like fever, are accounted, they are normally temporary or transient and placid or mild with no severe expressions or manifestations (Hartman *et al.*, 2020; Hewitt *et al.*, 2020; Woolsey *et al.*, 2020). Infected African green monkeys expose transient and mild changes within leukocyte populations, selected or certain liver enzymes and mild thrombocytopenia (Hewitt *et al.*, 2020; Woolsey *et al.*, 2020). During the early stage of infection in African green monkeys acute or severe inflammation occurs with raised or elevated CRP (Hewitt *et al.*, 2020; Woolsey *et al.*, 2020).

However, limited or inadequate data is obtainable on unfolding viral disease appearance following SARS-Cov-2 disclosure or exposure in marmosets, pig-tailed macaques and baboons. According to the data accumulation it can be revealed that these monkeys can be infected by SARS-CoV-2, although they are not as extensively utilized in medical research (Hewitt *et al.*, 2020). While infected by virus, marmosets did not display fever and did not mount or raise an immune reaction or response yet while positively affected by the SARS-CoV-2 detected *via* nasal swabs (Hewitt *et al.*, 2020; Lu *et al.*, 2020). Therefore, the pig-tailed macaques have simply been utilized for immunogenicity research (Erasmus *et al.*, 2020; Hewitt *et al.*, 2020). Thus, baboons had additionally rigorous or severe viral pathology and shed SARS-CoV-2 extensively or longer than macaque populations and the baboons may be an excellent animal model for diabetic and cardiovascular comorbidities (Hewitt *et al.*, 2020; Singh *et al.*, 2020). The baboons can be subsequently utilized for immunogenicity research (Hewitt *et al.*, 2020; Tian *et al.*, 2020).

The global increase or spread of the new SARS-CoV-2 and their recent mutants, quick transmission and severity or harshness of the viral disease have made the development or expansion of vaccines and therapeutics which are the urgent priorities in the current world scenario (Hewitt *et al.*, 2020). Hence, COVID-19 is a multi-factorial, multi-faceted, multi-systemic and a highly infectious viral disease which reminds us widespread or extensive reactions or responses in the human beings. Therefore, no single non-human primate model is sufficient or can be summarized to understand the complete pathogenesis of SARS-CoV-2 like in humans. With the response or reaction to other rising or emerging viral infections, non-human primate models can be utilized for playing key role or responsibility, even when candidate vaccines and therapeutics have emerged globally at a record level (Hewitt *et al.*, 2020).

REFERENCES

Bao, L., Deng, W., Gao, H., Xiao C., Liu J., *et al.* (2020) Reinfection could not occur in SARS-CoV-2 infected rhesus macaques. bioRxiv. https://doi.org/10.1101/2020.03.13.990226

Colman, R.J. (2018). "Non-human primates as a model for aging", *Biochimica et Biophysica Acta, Molecular Basis of Disease 1864* (9 Pt A): 2733–2741. https://doi.org/10.1016/j.bbadis.2017.07.008

Corbett, K.S., Flynn B., Foulds, K.E., Francica, J.R., Boyoglu-Barnum, S., *et al.* (2020). "Evaluation of the mRNA-1273 Vaccine against SARS-CoV-2 in nonhuman primates", *N Engl J Med 383*: 1544-55. https://doi.org/10.1056/NEJMoa2024671

de Wit, E., Feldmann, F., Cronin, J., Jordan, R., Okumura, A., *et al.* (2020). "Prophylactic and therapeutic remdesivir (GS-5734) treatment in the rhesus macaque model of MERS-CoV infection", *Proceedings of the National Academy of Sciences of the United States of America, 117*(12): 6771–6776. https://doi.org/10.1073/pnas.1922083117

Erasmus, J.H., Khandhar, A.P., O'Connor, M.A., Walls, A.C., Hemann, E.A., Murapa, P., Archer, J., Leventhal, S., Fuller, J.T., Lewis, T.B., *et al.* (2020). An <em>Alphavirus</em>-derived replicon RNA vaccine induces SARSCoV-2 neutralizing antibody and T cell responses in mice and nonhuman primates. *Science Translational Medicine 12*, eabc9396.

Finch, C.L., Crozier, I., Lee, J.H., Byrum, R., Cooper, T.K., Liang, J., Sharer, K., Solomon, J., Sayre, P.J., Kocher, G., *et al.* (2020). Characteristic and quantifiable COVID-19-like abnormalities in CT- and PET/CT-imaged lungs of SARSCoV-2-infected crab-eating macaques (<em>Macaca fascicularis</em>). bioRxiv, 2020.2005.2014.096727.

Gao, W., Tamin, A., Soloff, A., D'Aiuto, L., Nwanegbo, E., *et al.* (2003). Effects of a SARS-associated coronavirus vaccine in monkeys. *Lancet* 362(9399): 1895–1896. https://doi.org/10.1016/S0140-6736(03)14962-8

Gonçalves, A., Maisonnasse, P., Donati, F., Albert, M., Behillil, S., Contreras, V., *et al.* (2021). SARS-CoV-2 viral dynamics in non-human primates. *PLoS Comput Biol* 17(3): e1008785. https://doi.org/10.1371/journal.pcbi.1008785

Gorbalenya, A.E., Baker, S.C., Baric, R.S., de Groot, R.J., Drosten, C., *et al.* (2020). Coronaviridae Study Group of the International Committee on Taxonomy of Viruses, *The species severe acute respiratory syndrome-related coronavirus*: classifying 2019-nCoV and naming it SARS-CoV-2. Nat Microbiol 5: 536–544. https://doi.org/10.1038/s41564-020-0695-z

Hartman, A.L., Nambulli, S., McMillen, C.M., White, A.G., Tilston-Lunel, N.L., Albe, J.R., Cottle, E., Dunn, M., Frye, L.J., Gilliland, T.H., *et al.* (2020). SARSCoV-2 infection of African green monkeys results in mild respiratory disease discernible by PET/CT imaging and prolonged shedding of infectious virus from both respiratory and gastrointestinal tracts. *bioRxiv*, 2020. 2006.2020.137687.

Hewitt, J.A., Lutz, C., Florence, W.C., Pitt, M.L.M., Rao, S., Rappaport, J., and Haigwood, N.L. (2020). ACTIVating Resources for the COVID-19 Pandemic: In Vivo Models for Vaccines and Therapeutics. *Cell Host and Microbe 28*, 646–659. https://doi.org/10.1016/j.chom.2020.09.016

Johnston, S.C., Jay, A., Raymond, J.L., Rossi, F., Zeng, X., Scruggs, J., Dyer, D., Frick, O., Moore, J., Berrier, K., *et al.* (2020). Development of a Coronavirus Disease 2019 Nonhuman Primate Model Using Airborne Exposure. bioRxiv, 2020.2006.2026.174128.

Lawler, J.V., Endy, T.P., Hensley, L.E., Garrison, A., Fritz, E.A. *et al.* (2006). Cynomolgus macaque as an animal model for severe acute respiratory syndrome. *PLoS Medicine 3*(5): e149. https://doi.org/10.1371/journal.pmed.0030149

Liu, Y., Hu, G., Wang, Y., Zhao, X., Ji, F., Ren, W., Gong, M., Ju, X., Li, C., Hong, J., *et al.* (2020). Functional and Genetic Analysis of Viral Receptor ACE2 Orthologs Reveals a Broad Potential Host Range of SARS-CoV-2. bioRxiv, 2020.2004.2022.046565.

Lu ,S., Zhao, Y., Yu, W., Yang, Y., Gao, J. *et al.* (2020). *Comparison of nonhuman primates identified the suitable model for COVID-19*. Signal Transduction and Targeted Therapy 5: 157. https://doi.org/10.1038/s41392-020-00269-6

Lu, S., Zhao, Y., Yu, W., Yang, Y., Gao, J., Wang, J., Kuang, D., Yang, M., Yang, J., Ma, C. *et al.* (2020). Comparison of SARS-CoV-2 infections among 3 species of non-human primates. *bioRxiv*, 2020.2004.2008.031807.

Luan, J., Lu, Y., Jin, X., and Zhang, L. (2020). Spike protein recognition of mammalian ACE2 predicts the host range and an optimized ACE2 for SARSCoV-2 infection. Biochem. *Biophys. Res. Commun.* 526, 165–169.

Melin, A.D., Janiak, M.C., Frank, Marrone, III F., Arora, P.S., and Higham, J.P. (2020). Comparative ACE2 variation and primate COVID-19 risk. *Communications Biology 3*, 641 https://doi.org/10.1038/s42003-020-01370-w

Munster, V.J., Feldmann, F., Williamson, B.N., van Doremalen, N., Pérez-Pérez. L. *et al.* (2020a). Respiratory disease and virus shedding in rhesus macaques inoculated with SARS-CoV-2. *bioRxiv*. https://doi.org/10.1101/2020.03.21.001628

Munster, V.J., Feldmann, F., Williamson, B.N., van Doremalen, N., Pérez-Pérez, L., Schulz, J., Meade-White, K., Okumura, A., Callison, J., Brumbaugh, B., *et al.* (2020b). Respiratory disease in rhesus macaques inoculated with SARS-CoV-2. *Nature 585*, 268–272. https://doi.org/10.1038/s41586-020-2324-7

Qiu, Y., Zhao, Y.B., Wang, Q., Li, J.Y., Zhou, Z.J., Liao, C.H., and Ge, X.Y. (2020). Predicting the angiotensin converting enzyme 2 (ACE2) utilizing capability as the receptor of SARS-CoV-2. *Microbes Infect.* 22, 221–225.

Rockx, B., Kuiken, T., Herfst, S., Bestebroer, T., Lamers, M.M., Oude Munnink, B.B., de Meulder, D., van Amerongen, G., van den Brand, J., Okba, N.M.A., *et al.* (2020). Comparative pathogenesis of COVID-19, MERS, and SARS in a nonhuman primate model. *Science 368*, 1012–1015. https://doi.org/10.1126/science.abb7314

Santos, W.J., Guiraldi, L.M., Lucheis, S.B. (2020). "Should we be concerned about COVID-19 with nonhuman primates?", *Am J Primatol* 82: e23158. https://doi.org/10.1002/ajp.23158

Singh, D.K., Ganatra, S.R., Singh, B., Cole, J., Alfson, K.J., Clemmons, E., Gazi, M., Gonzalez, O., Escobedo, R., Lee, T.-H., *et al.* (2020). "SARS-CoV-2 infection leads to acute infection with dynamic cellular and inflammatory flux in the lung that varies across nonhuman primate species", *bioRxiv*, 2020.2006.2005.136481.

Tian, J.-H., Patel, N., Haupt, R., Zhou, H., Weston, S., Hammond, H., Lague, J., Portnoff, A.D., Norton, J., Guebre-Xabier, M., *et al.* (2020). "SARS-CoV-2 spike glycoprotein vaccine candidate NVX-CoV2373 elicits immunogenicity in baboons and protection in mice", *bioRxiv*, 2020.2006.2029.178509.

Wan, Y., Shang, J., Graham, R., Baric, R.S., and Li, F. (2020). "Receptor Recognition by the Novel Coronavirus from Wuhan: An Analysis Based on Decade-Long Structural Studies of SARS Coronavirus", *J. Virol.* 94, e00120–e00127.

Woolsey, C., Borisevich, V., Prasad, A.N., Agans, K.N., Deer, D.J., Dobias, N.S., Heymann, J.C., Foster, S.L., Levine, C.B., Medina, L., *et al.* (2020). "Establishment of an African green monkey model for COVID-19". *bioRxiv*, 2020.2005.2017.100289.

Xu ,Y., Jia Z., Zhou, L., Wang, L., Li, J. *et al.* (2007). "Evaluation of the safety, immunogenicity and pharmacokinetics of equine anti-SARS-CoV F(ab') (2) in macaque", *International Immunopharmacology* 7(13): 1834–1840. https://doi.org/10.1016/j.intimp.2007.09.011

Zheng, H., Li, H., Guo, L., Liang, Y., Li, J., *et al.* (2020). "Virulence and pathogenesis of SARS-CoV-2 infection in rhesus macaques: A nonhuman primate model of COVID-19 progression", *PLoS Pathogens 16*(11): e1008949. https://doi.org/10.1371/journal.ppat.1008949

Zhou, P., Yang, X.L., Wang, X.G., Hu, B., Zhang, L., Zhang, W., Si, H.R., Zhu, Y., Li, B., Huang, C.L. *et al.* (2020). "A pneumonia outbreak associated with a new coronavirus of probable bat origin", *Nature, 579*, 270–273.

28

COVID-19 and Maternal Health

Short and Long Term Implications

Naorem Kiranmala Devi and *Vineet Chaudhary*

Introduction

COVID-19 pandemic is arguably the worst pandemic that humankind has seen in the last one hundred years. No wonder a major share of funds and health care resources have been directed towards containment, treatment and research pertaining to COVID-19. Although no one can contest the rationale behind the diversion of funds and resource, however due to this, other public health and welfare issues have taken a hit. Such an unprecedented situation is particularly critical for those who are already at an immune-compromised state and require healthcare intervention at regular intervals. They are not just more vulnerable to COVID-19, the pandemic is making the access to healthcare facilities and healthy lifestyle extremely constrained. One of such groups is pregnant women.

Immune system of a pregnant woman is supposed to create an immune tolerant environment for the foetus (Giri, 2021). This unique 'immunological' condition during pregnancy increases the risk of bacterial and viral infections (Mor and Cardenas, 2010). As reported by Dashraath *et al.* (2020) pregnant women are disproportionately affected by respiratory illnesses leading to increased infectious morbidity and high maternal mortality rate. Hence comes the question—are pregnant women at greater risk of COVID-19?

Apart from those who are infected with COVID-19, even those who are not infected are facing psychosocial adversities like fear, anxiety, depression etc. (Chakraborty, 2020), as well as financial losses due to both the gruesome circumstances engendered by the pandemic and the containment measures, like quarantine and lockdown etc., enforced by the states (Nicola *et al.*, 2020). These conditions are neither ideal for the pregnant women nor for the newborn babies to say the least. Furthermore, restricted availability of healthcare facilities (as a result of rising COVID-19 cases) for maternal and child care is making the situation grimmer.

In this chapter we have tried to investigate the impact (both direct, i.e. due to incidence of COVID-19 during pregnancy and indirect, i.e. due to psychological and socio-economic stresses) of COVID-19 on maternal and child health. We have also tried to understand this impact through the prism of 'Developmental Origins of Health and Disease (DOHaD)' hypothesis and underlying epigenetic mechanisms.

Coronavirus and Maternal and Child Health

Since this is not the first coronavirus to infect human beings, this gives us an opportunity to study the impact of SARS-CoV-2 in comparison with other coronaviruses on maternal health.

Several coronavirus species belonging to the genus Alpha corona virus like (HCoV-229E and HCoV-NL63); and genus Beta corona virus (like HCoV-OC43, HCoV-HKU1, MERS-CoV, and SARS-CoV), have produced human infection before December 2019 (Schwartz, 2020). While most of these cause mild infections, two zoonotic coronaviruses—SARS-CoV and MERS-CoV can produce severe lower respiratory tract infection (Schwartz, 2020).

The outbreak of SARS-CoV (causing SARS) happened during 2002-03 and by the end of the epidemic, in June 2003, the global cumulative total was 8422 cases with 916 deaths (case fatality rate of 11%) (Chan-Yeung and Xu, 2003).

Literature recounting the impact of SARS on pregnancy outcomes reveals that severe maternal illness, maternal death, and spontaneous abortion could be attributed to SARS. Maternal mortality rate due to SARS was reported to be around 25 per cent to 30 per cent (Wong *et al.,* 2004; Di Mascio, 2020). Most common symptoms were fever, chills and rigour, headache, malaise, myalgia and cough (Lam *et al.*, 2004). Pregnancy related complications included first trimester miscarriage, preterm birth, preterm premature rupture of membranes (PPROM) and fetal growth restriction (FGR). According to a meta-analysis pooled proportion of first trimester miscarriage for SARS infection was 64.7 per cent, preterm birth before 37 weeks and 34 weeks were 15 per cent and 28.9 per cent respectively, PPROM occurred in 50 per cent and FGR in 18.5 per cent cases respectively, although no perinatal death was recorded (Di Mascio *et al.*, 2020). Lam *et al.* (2004) conducted a case control study on 10 pregnant and 40 non-pregnant women who all had SARS, and reported that pregnancy appears to have no effect on clinical symptoms of SARS, however, complications or adverse outcomes were more common in pregnant women, for example 40 per cent of pregnant women required ventilation compared to 13 per cent of non-pregnant women.

Outbreak of another coronavirus, MERS-CoV causing MERS, started in September 2012 in Saudi Arabia (Hui, 2017). Since then, more than 2494 confirmed cases of MERS resulting in 858 deaths globally have been recorded (case fatality rate 37%) (Peng *et al.*, 2020; Schwartz, 2020; WHO, 2020a).

Till 2020, very few MERS cases (n = 11) in pregnant women have been documented, with 91 per cent of them having adverse clinical outcomes (Schwartz, 2020). Maternal mortality rate due to MERS has been reported to be around 30 per cent to 35 per cent (Al-Tawfiq, 2020). Other complications included premature delivery, perinatal death and newborn babies requiring intensive care treatments (Al-Tawfiq,2020).

In a meta-analysis by Di Mascio *et al.* (2020), there was no data on miscarriages during first trimester due to MERS infection, preterm birth (all occurring before 34 weeks of gestation) was observed in 32.1 per cent cases, preeclampsia in 19.1 per cent and perinatal death in 33.2 per cent (including 2 stillbirths and 1 neonatal death) cases. No case of PPROM or FGR was reported. According to de Souza Silva *et al.* (2020), "MERS-CoV can be the most dangerous for newborns and complications may include high blood pressure, pre-eclampsia, pneumonia, acute renal failure, and multiple organ failure in mother."

Direct Impact of COVID-19 on Maternal Health and Child Health

Clinical features of COVID-19 in the general public appear to be similar to SARS but it has a case fatality rate lower than that of SARS and much lower than that of MERS (Petrosillo, 2020). Multiple studies have reported the case fatality rate of COVID-19 between 0.68-4 per cent (Meyerowitz-Katz and Merone, 2020; Petrosillo, 2020; Mahase, 2020; Singhal, 2020; WHO, 2020b). To understand the effect of incidence of COVID-19 on maternal and child health, we carried out a narrative review and findings have been summarized in subsequent paragraphs.

Maternal mortality rate due to COVID-19 has been reported between 0-3 per cent (Zaigham and Andersson, 2020, Gajbhiye *et al.*, 2020,

Schwartz, 2020). Most of the pregnant women with COVID-19, who were otherwise healthy, showed only mild respiratory symptoms (Schwartz, 2020; Li *et al.*, 2020). Some of the most common symptoms are fever, cough, myalgia, dyspnea and diarrhoea; pneumonia can be diagnosed in majority of cases by CT scan (Gajbhiye *et al.*, 2020). Zhang *et al.* (2020) in their study (retrospective comparison of pregnancy outcomes of 16 women with COVID-19 and 45 women without COVID-19) reported that 15 women had mild symptoms, whereas one had moderate symptoms, but none of them developed critical pneumonia.

Pregnant women with COVID-19 infection do not show severe maternal and neonatal complications (Li *et al.*, 2020). Gajbhiye *et al.* (2020) in their systematic review (n = 441) observed that pregnancy complications included delivery by cesarean section in 80 per cent cases, preterm labor in 26 per cent, fetal distress in 8 per cent, premature rupture of membranes in 9 per cent and still births in 2 per cent cases. Chen *et al.*, (2020) in their study (a retrospective review of clinical records, lab results and chest CT scans of 9 pregnant women with COVID-19), reported that all 9 patients had cesarean section in the third trimester. None of the patients developed severe pneumonia or died, 9 live births were recorded and no complications observed in newborn babies (Chen *et al.*, 2020). They also reported that samples like amniotic fluid, cord blood, neonatal throat swab and breast milk were tested negative for SARS-CoV-2 (Chen *et al.*, 2020).

Reports on vertical transmission of SARS-CoV-2 are inconsistent with some suggesting lack of evidences *vis-à-vis* vertical transmission (Karimi-Zarchi *et al.*, 2020; Chen *et al.*, 2020), while others have not ruled out mother to child transmission of COVID-19 (Gajbhiye *et al.*, 2020, Zaigham and Andersson, 2020).

The situation is still evolving; however current data do not appear to suggest an increased risk of miscarriage or early pregnancy loss in pregnancies with COVID-19 (López *et al.*, 2020, Yan *et al.*, 2020). As observed by López *et al.* (2020) "the mother and fetus do not seem to be at particularly high risk."

It can be concluded that the impact of incidence of COVID-19 during pregnancy is less severe (reflected by lower maternal case fertility rate and milder symptoms) than SARS and MERS. This conclusion is in sync with the observation that overall case fertility rate in the general public due to COVID-19 is lesser than SARS and MERS. In fact none of these three coronavirus diseases appear to be particularly affecting pregnant women with prognosis similar to (or not much worse than) the general public.

However, thc number of COVID-19 cases is far greater than other two diseases meaning that secondary or indirect impact of COVID-19 on maternal and child health can be far worse.

Indirect Impact of COVID-19 Pandemic on Maternal and Child Health

A Pandemic as big as COVID-19 does not affect only those who are infected or their kin, rather psychological and socio-economic repercussions are felt by one and all. Pregnant women and in utero or new born babies are no exceptions. Let's look at socio-economic implications of COVID-19 on Maternal and Child Health.

Fore (2020) highlights that children are at risk not only of infection, but also of losing caregivers, Mothers and children are affected by the disruption of essential support and supplies, constrained access to clinics, schools, social workers, water, and sanitation (Fore, 2020).

As reported by Akseer *et al.* (2020) sectors like food systems, incomes, and social protection, health care services for women and children, and access to clean water and sanitation are at particular risk of collapse or reduced efficiency due to COVID-19. This may lead to increased maternal and child under-nutrition (Akseer *et al.*, 2020). Hostile circumstances like insecure economic conditions, restricted travel and access to health care services, delayed vaccination schedules, and shuttering of educational facilities fostered by COVID-19 will further deteriorate health conditions for young children, especially in low- and middle-income countries (LMICs) (Akseer *et al.*, 2020; UNICEF, 2020).

Roberton *et al.* (2020) used Lives Saved Tool (LiST) to estimate additional maternal and child deaths due to reduced coverage of maternal and child health interventions, and increased prevalence of wasting, under three scenarios and for three time periods. They reported that in case of the least severe scenario (coverage reductions of 9·8–18·5% and wasting increase of 10%) there can be 253500 additional child deaths and 12200 additional maternal deaths over 6 months (Roberton *et al.*, 2020). However, in case of most severe scenario (coverage reductions of 39·3–51·9% and wasting increase of 50%) there would be 1157000 additional child deaths and 56700 additional maternal deaths over 6 months (Roberton *et al.*, 2020). Due to these additional deaths around 9·8 to 44·7 per cent increase in under-5 child deaths and around 8·3 to 38·6 per cent increase in maternal deaths per month could be seen across the 118 countries (Roberton *et al.*, 2020).

Furthermore, let's also look at the psychological implications of COVID-19 on maternal health. Due to COVID-19 some pregnant women may suffer from psychological stressors like depression and anxiety (Thapa *et al.*, 2020). According to Davenport *et al.* (2020) during the perinatal period, depression and anxiety can affect one in seven women. However, studies show an increase in both number of depressed pregnant females as well as the severity of depression during COVID-19 pandemic (Davenport *et al.*, 2020; Saccone *et al.*, 2020). These mental stressors are associated with "increased risk of preterm delivery, reduced mother-infant bonding, and delays in cognitive/emotional development of the infant, which may persist into childhood" (Davenport *et al.*, 2020).

Thus, it can be concluded that the indirect (socio-economic and psychological) impact of COVID-19 on maternal and child health can be more widespread as well as critical in both short and long run than the direct impact. Also, since the outbreaks of SARS and MERS were not as big as that of COVID-19, the indirect impact of those two on maternal health was far less severe than of COVID-19.

COVID-19, DOHaD and Future

Apart from direct and indirect impacts on maternal health, it appears appropriate to discuss DOHaD Hypothesis and epigenetics in reference with COVID-19.

Characteristics of the early environment (in utero or even before), can represent major risk factors for a lifetime of physical and mental health problems for the individual (Van den Bergh *et al.*, 2017). According to Developmental Origins of Health and Disease (DOHaD) hypothesis proposed by Barker, the environment in which the individual finds himself during his early development (pre-conceptional, in utero and early post-natal periods) may have important consequences for his health, during his adult life (Safi-Stibler and Gabory, 2020). Early embryos and/or the gametes before fertilization can pick up several types of environmental cue that can lead to permanent changes in the developmental programme culminating in an altered postnatal phenotype associated with increased disease risk (Fleming *et al.*, 2015). Fleming *et al.* (2015) elucidates "the early embryo and periconceptional period is a window during which environmental factors may cause permanent change in the pattern and characteristics of development leading to risk of adult onset disease."

Various studies are increasingly identifying links between diverse stressors during pregnancy and NCD risk to offspring (Goldstein *et al.*,

2017). Not just this, prenatal exposure to maternal stress can also increase the risk for behavioural and mental health problems later in life. Examples of stressors during pregnancy include nutritional stress (both under and overnutrition), exposure to environmental toxicants, and maternal immune activation (MIA) provoked by infectious diseases (Goldstein *et al.*, 2017). New evidences are also showing that maternal psychological distress, as well as stress from exposure to life events and natural disasters during pregnancy gives rise to behaviour and mental health problems (Van den Bergh *et al.*, 2017).

According to DOHaD disturbance in environmental factors has an organizational effect on biological systems (including the central nervous system, autonomic nervous system, neuroendocrine, cardiovascular, and immune systems) with a long development and/or intrinsic plasticity to react and adapt to environmental influences (Van den Bergh *et al.*, 2017). Exposure to prenatal stressors induce changes in foetus such as an altered set-point in HPA-axis, changes in glucocorticoid receptor sensitivity, changes in proteins and neurotransmitters involved in neuronal development and function in the CNS (Matthews, 2002; Wyrwoll and Holmes, 2012), which leads to enhanced susceptibility to somatic diseases and mental health problems (Van den Bergh *et al.*, 2017).

As discussed in previous sections, COVID-19 Pandemic has created such a situation that can cause maternal immune activation in infected females and nutritional and psychological stress in both infected and non-infected females. Therefore, there is a very high probability that these factors may have long term implications on the physical and mental health of infants born during or immediately after the pandemic.

Accounts of 'Dutch Hunger Winter' and 'Holocaust' also point in this direction. Studies on the survivors of 'Dutch Hunger Winter' and 'Holocaust' and their offspring across generations have revealed the range of physical and mental health consequences that may be associated with the exposure (Lumey *et al.*, 2007; Bowers and Yehuda, 2020).

The winters of 1944 to 45 (a period of six months) is known as Dutch Hunger Winter in the Netherlands, during which German occupiers imposed a food restriction that resulted in severe and widespread famine among Dutch citizens (Lumey *et al.*, 2007). Dutch adults who were in utero during the famine exhibited increased prevalence of type II diabetes, cardiovascular disease, and age-associated cognitive decline (Tobi *et al.*, 2014; Bowers and Yehuda, 2020).

Poorer health outcomes among offspring who were famine-exposed in utero, regardless of socio-economic status, lent evidence to the developmental origins of health and disease (DOHaD) hypothesis (Hoy and Nicol, 2018; Bowers and Yehuda, 2020).

Similarly, empirical data show that offspring of Holocaust survivors are at greater risk for developing post-traumatic stress disorder (PTSD) if one or both parents had PTSD (Bergmann and Jucovy, 1982; Solomon *et al.*, 1988; Yehuda *et al.*, 2008; Bowers and Yehuda, 2020). As reported in multiple studies, children of Holocaust survivors have been at a greater risk for health conditions like hypertension and type II diabetes, as well as mental health conditions like depression and anxiety disorders (Flory *et al.*, 2011; Gangi *et al.*, 2009; Yehuda *et al.*, 1998, 2001, 2008; Bowers and Yehuda, 2020).

These examples clearly show that COVID-19 and the stressful environment that it has created across the world may affect the overall health status of the next generation in the long term.

DOHaD and Underlying Epigenetics

Epigenetics include heritable changes other than those in the DNA sequence like DNA methylation, histone modification, acetylation, phosphorylation etc. (Callinan and Feinberg, 2006). Epigenetic modifications are a critical part of normal development, helping to activate or silence specific genes during cell differentiation (Barrett, 2017). However, not all changes are benign, as epigenetic alterations may lead to disorders including cancer, neuro-degeneration, and diseases of the cardiovascular and immune systems (Barrett, 2017). Epigenetic mechanisms allow organisms to respond to rapid changes in their environment (Herrel *et al.*, 2020). But, exposure to a stressful environment may lead to adverse phenotypic outcomes in the individuals experiencing the environmental stress as well as in the next generation through epigenetic transmission. Parental environment, during the development of the individual from gametogenesis to weaning and beyond, can shape the adult and the elderly person's susceptibility to her/his own environment and diseases (Safi-Stibler and Gabory, 2019). Preconception stress can be transmitted by both mothers and fathers through epigenetic changes in gametes (Bowers & Yehuda, 2020).

Epigenetics carries with it the notion of memory of a developmental event, even when the initial stimulus has disappeared, therefore, it must obviously be considered as one of the key mechanisms underlying DOHaD (Safi-Stibler and Gabory, 2019). Animal studies too have provided strong evidences supporting epigenetic basis for the DOHaD model of disease pathogenesis (Wadhwa *et al.,* 2009; Gluckman and Hanson, 2006). It has been observed that minor alterations in the diet of the mother during pregnancy can produce long-term changes in the physiology and metabolism of the child (Wadhwa *et al.,* 2009; Gluckman and Hanson, 2006). In their review study, Bianco-Miotto *et al.* (2017) concluded that "increasing evidence also points to the involvement of epigenetic mechanisms in mediating the effects of early life exposures on later life obesity and T2DM risk." Various other reviews too have invoked epigenetic principles to understand the DOHaD hypothesis (Wadhwa *et al.,* 2009; Waterland and Michels, 2007).

This epigenetic impact of COVID-19 is not yet being discussed widely, but in the light of the DOHaD hypothesis and underlying epigenetic mechanisms, it appears that COVID-19 may have widespread intergenerational consequences. Having said that, it is also important to point out that epigenetic changes are modifiable as well as reversible (Schuebel *et al.*, 2016). Thus, there is a need to undertake researches to understand the epigenetic impact of COVID-19 on maternal and child health (in particular and humankind in general) and hence to find out the approaches to reverse or at least reduce the alleged impact.

Conclusion

Our review suggests that unlike hypertension, diabetes and many other health conditions, pregnancy does not make a woman more vulnerable to COVID-19 infection in most of the cases. It is more likely that a pregnant woman who develops COVID-19 will sail through the infection with no or mild complications (although adverse outcomes too have been reported in a some cases). However, increasing number COVID-19 cases has the potential to overwhelm the medical infrastructure, especially in low and middle income countries. This may lead to an extreme shortage of maternal and child health facilities. Poor socio-economic conditions coupled with constrained medical facilities may result in additional maternal and child deaths. Furthermore, a much less discussed aspect of this pandemic is its intergenerational epigenetic consequences. If we scrutinize the implications of COVID-19 on pregnancy through the lens of DOHaD hypothesis and underlying epigenetic mechanisms, it appears that COVID-19 may have intergenerational long term physical and mental health consequences. We shall have to closely monitor the evolving circumstances and undertake more researches to say anything conclusive on the long term epigenetic implications of COVID-19.

REFERENCES

Akseer, N., Kandru, G., Keats, E.C., and Bhutta, Z.A. (2020). "COVID-19 pandemic and mitigation strategies: Implications for maternal and child health and nutrition", *The American journal of clinical nutrition, 112*(2), 251-256.

Al-Tawfiq, J.A. (2020). Middle east respiratory syndrome coronavirus (MERS-CoV) and COVID-19 infection during pregnancy.

Barrett, J.R. (2017). Programming the future: Epigenetics in the context of DOHaD.

Bergmann, M.S., and Jucovy, M.E. (1982). *Generations of the Holocaust*. Columbia University Press.

Bianco-Miotto, T., Craig, J.M., Gasser, Y.P., van Dijk, S.J., and Ozanne, S. (2017). *Epigenetics and DOHaD: From basics to birth and beyond.*

Bowers, M.E., and Yehuda, R. (2020). "Intergenerational transmission of stress vulnerability and resilience", In *Stress Resilience* (pp. 257-267). Academic Press.

Branch, D.W. (1992). "Physiologic adaptations of pregnancy", *American Journal of Reproductive Immunology, 28*(3-4), 120-122.

Callinan, P.A. and Feinberg, A.P. (2006). The emerging science of epigenomics. *Human molecular genetics, 15*(suppl_1), R95-R101.

Chakraborty, Nandini. "The COVID-19 pandemic and its impact on mental health," *Progress in Neurology and Psychiatry 24*, no. 2 (2020): 21-24.

Chan-Yeung, M., and Xu, R.H. (2003). "SARS: epidemiology", *Respirology*, 8, S9-S14.

Chen, H., Guo, J., Wang, C., Luo, F., Yu, X., Zhang, W.,...and Zhang, Y. (2020). Clinical characteristics and intrauterine vertical transmission potential of COVID-19 infection in nine pregnant women: A retrospective review of medical records. *The lancet, 395*(10226), 809-815.

Dashraath, P., Wong, J.L.J., Lim, M.X.K., Lim, L.M., Li, S., Biswas, A.,... and Su, L.L. (2020). "Coronavirus disease 2019 (COVID-19) pandemic and pregnancy", *American journal of obstetrics and gynecology, 222*(6), 521-531.

Davenport, M.H., Meyer, S., Meah, V.L., Strynadka, M.C., and Khurana, R. (2020). Moms are not ok: COVID-19 and maternal mental health. Frontiers in Global Women's Health, 1, 1.

de Souza Silva, G.A., da Silva, S.P., da Costa, M.A.S., da Silva, A.R., de Vasconcelos Alves, R.R., Tenório, F.D.C.Â.M.,... and de Melo, C.M.L. (2020). SARS-CoV, MERS-CoV and SARS-CoV-2 infections in pregnancy and fetal development. Journal of Gynecology Obstetrics and Human Reproduction, 101846.

Di Mascio, D., Khalil, A., Saccone, G., Rizzo, G., Buca, D., Liberati, M.,...and D'Antonio, F. (2020). "Outcome of coronavirus spectrum infections (SARS, MERS, COVID-19) during pregnancy: A systematic review and meta-analysis", *American journal of obstetrics and gynecology MFM, 2*(2), 100107.

Fleming, T.P., Velazquez, M.A., and Eckert, J.J. (2015). "Embryos, DOHaD and david barker", *Journal of developmental origins of health and disease, 6*(5), 377-383.

Flory, J.D., Bierer, L.M., and Yehuda, R. (2011). "Maternal exposure to the holocaust and health complaints in offspring", *Disease markers*, *30*(2, 3), 133-139.

Fore, H.H. (2020). "A wake-up call: COVID-19 and its impact on children's health and wellbeing", *The Lancet Global Health*, *8*(7), e861-e862.

Gajbhiye, R.K., Modi, D.N., and Mahale, S.D. (2020). "Pregnancy outcomes, newborn complications and maternal-fetal transmission of SARS-CoV-2 in women with COVID-19: A systematic review of 441 cases". *MedRxiv*.

Gangi, S., Talamo, A., and Ferracuti, S. (2009). "The long-term effects of extreme war-related trauma on the second generation of Holocaust survivors", *Violence and Victims*, *24*(5), 687-700.

Giri, T.K. (2021). "Severity of Maternal Illness in Pregnancy during COVID-19 Pandemic", *Journal of Advanced Research in Medical Science and Technology*, *8*(1), 3-6.

Gluckman, P.D., and Hanson, M.A. (2006). "The developmental origins of health and disease", In *Early life origins of health and disease,* pp. 1-7. Springer, Boston, MA.

Goldstein, J.A., Norris, S.A., and Aronoff, D.M. (2017). "DOHaD at the intersection of maternal immune activation and maternal metabolic stress: a scoping review", *Journal of developmental origins of health and disease*, *8*(3), 273-283.

Herrel, A., Joly, D., and Danchin, E. (2020). *Epigenetics in ecology and evolution*.

Hoy, W.E. and Nicol, J.L. (2019). "The Barker hypothesis confirmed: association of low birth weight with all-cause natural deaths in young adult life in a remote Australian Aboriginal community", *Journal of developmental origins of health and disease*, *10*(1), 55-62.

Hui, D.S. (2017). "Epidemic and emerging coronaviruses (severe acute respiratory syndrome and Middle East respiratory syndrome)". *Clinics in chest medicine, 38*(1), 71-86.

Karimi-Zarchi, M., Neamatzadeh, H., Dastgheib, S.A., Abbasi, H., Mirjalili, S.R., Behforouz, A.,...and Bahrami, R. (2020). "Vertical transmission of coronavirus disease 19 (COVID-19) from infected pregnant mothers to neonates: A review", *Fetal and pediatric pathology*, *39*(3), 246-250.

Lam, C.M., Wong, S.F., Leung, T.N., Chow, K.M., Yu, W.C., Wong, T.Y.,... and Ho, L.C. (2004). "A case-controlled study comparing clinical course and outcomes of pregnant and non-pregnant women with severe acute respiratory syndrome", *BJOG: An International Journal of Obstetrics and Gynaecology*, *111*(8), 771-774.

Li, N., Han, L., Peng, M., Lv, Y., Ouyang, Y., Liu, K.,...and Yang, L. (2020). "Maternal and neonatal outcomes of pregnant women with coronavirus disease 2019 (COVID-19) pneumonia: A case-control study. Clinical infectious diseases", *71*(16), 2035-2041.

López, M., Gonce, A., Meler, E., Plaza, A., Hernández, S., Martinez-Portilla, R.J.,... and Figueras, F. (2020). "Coronavirus disease 2019 in pregnancy: a clinical management protocol and considerations for practice", *Fetal diagnosis and therapy*, *47*(7), 519-528.

Lumey, L.H., Stein, A.D., Kahn, H.S., Van der Pal-de Bruin, K.M., Blauw, G.J., Zybert, P.A., and Susser, E.S. (2007). "Cohort profile: the Dutch Hunger Winter families study", *International journal of epidemiology, 36*(6), 1196-1204.

Mahase, E. (2020). *Coronavirus: Covid-19 has killed more people than SARS and MERS combined, despite lower case fatality rate.*

Matthews, S.G. (2002). "Early programming of the hypothalamo–pituitary–adrenal axis", *Trends in Endocrinology and Metabolism, 13*(9), 373-380.

Meyerowitz-Katz, G., and Merone, L. (2020). "A systematic review and meta-analysis of published research data on COVID-19 infection-fatality rates", *International Journal of Infectious Diseases.*

Mor, G. and Cardenas, I. (2010). "The immune system in pregnancy: a unique complexity", *American journal of reproductive immunology, 63*(6), 425-433.

Nicola, M., Alsafi, Z., Sohrabi, C., Kerwan, A., Al-Jabir, A., Iosifidis, C.,...and Agha, R. (2020). "The socio-economic implications of the coronavirus and COVID-19 pandemic: A review", *International journal of surgery.*

Peng, P.W., Ho, P.L., and Hota, S.S. (2020). "Outbreak of a new coronavirus: What anaesthetists should know", *BJA: British Journal of Anaesthesia, 124*(5), 497.

Petrosillo, N., Viceconte, G., Ergonul, O., Ippolito, G., and Petersen, E. (2020). "COVID-19, SARS and MERS: Are they closely related?", *Clinical Microbiology and Infection, 26*(6), 729-734.

Roberton, T., Carter, E.D., Chou, V.B., Stegmuller, A.R., Jackson, B.D., Tam, Y.,... and Walker, N. (2020). "Early estimates of the indirect effects of the COVID-19 pandemic on maternal and child mortality in low-income and middle-income countries: A modelling study", *The Lancet Global Health, 8*(7), e901-e908.

Saccone, G., Florio, A., Aiello, F., Venturella, R., De Angelis, M.C., Locci, M.,...and Sardo, A.D.S. (2020). "Psychological impact of coronavirus disease 2019 in pregnant women", *American Journal of Obstetrics and Gynecology, 223*(2), 293-295.

Safi-Stibler, S., and Gabory, A. (2020, January). "Epigenetics and the Developmental Origins of Health and Disease: Parental environment signalling to the epigenome, critical time windows and sculpting the adult phenotype", In *Seminars in cell and developmental biology* (Vol. 97, pp. 172-180). Academic Press.

Schuebel, K., Gitik, M., Domschke, K., and Goldman, D. (2016). "Making sense of epigenetics", *International Journal of Neuropsychopharmacology, 19*(11), pyw058.

Schwartz, D.A. (2020). "An analysis of 38 pregnant women with COVID-19, their newborn infants, and maternal-fetal transmission of SARS-CoV-2: Maternal coronavirus infections and pregnancy outcomes", *Archives of pathology and laboratory medicine, 144*(7), 799-805.

Singhal, T. (2020). "A review of coronavirus disease-2019 (COVID-19)". *The Indian Journal of Pediatrics*, 1-6.

Solomon, Z., Kotler, M., and Mikulincer, M. (1988). "Combat-related posttraumatic stress disorder among second-generation Holocaust survivors: Preliminary findings", *The American Journal of Psychiatry*.

Thapa, S.B., Mainali, A., Schwank, S.E., and Acharya, G. (2020). *Maternal mental health in the time of the COVID-19 pandemic.*

Tobi, E.W., Goeman, J.J., Monajemi, R., Gu, H., Putter, H., Zhang, Y.,...and Heijmans, B.T. (2014). "DNA methylation signatures link prenatal famine exposure to growth and metabolism", *Nature communications*, *5*(1), 1-14.

UNICEF. (2020). *Don't let children be the hidden victims of COVID-19 pandemic.*

Van den Bergh, B.R., van den Heuvel, M.I., Lahti, M., Braeken, M., de Rooij, S.R., Entringer, S.,... and Schwab, M. (2017). "Prenatal developmental origins of behaviour and mental health: The influence of maternal stress in pregnancy", *Neuroscience and Biobehavioural Reviews*.

Wadhwa, P.D., Buss, C., Entringer, S., and Swanson, J.M. (2009). "Developmental origins of health and disease: Brief history of the approach and current focus on epigenetic mechanisms". *Seminars in reproductive medicine*, *27*(5), 358–368. https://doi.org/10.1055/s-0029-1237424

Waterland, R.A., and Michels, K.B. (2007). "Epigenetic epidemiology of the developmental origins hypothesis", *Annu. Rev. Nutr.*, *27*, 363-388.

WHO (2020a). *Middle East respiratory syndrome coronavirus (MERS-CoV).* https://www.who.int/emergencies/mers-cov/en/. [Accessed 10 February 2021]

WHO (2020). *Coronavirus disease 2019 (COVID-19): situation report, 46.* World Health Organization. https://apps.who.int/iris/handle/10665/331443

Wong, S.F., Chow, K.M., Leung, T.N., Ng, W.F., Ng, T.K., Shek, C.C.,...and Tan, P.Y. (2004). "Pregnancy and perinatal outcomes of women with severe acute respiratory syndrome", *American journal of obstetrics and gynecology*, *191*(1), 292-297.

Wyrwoll, C.S., and Holmes, M.C. (2012). "Prenatal excess glucocorticoid exposure and adult affective disorders: A role for serotonergic and catecholamine pathways", *Neuroendocrinology*, *95*(1), 47-55.

Yan, J., Guo, J., Fan, C., Juan, J., Yu, X., Li, J.,...and Yang, H. (2020). "Coronavirus disease 2019 in pregnant women: A report based on 116 cases", *American journal of obstetrics and gynecology*, *223*(1), 111-e1.

Yehuda, R., Bell, A., Bierer, L.M., and Schmeidler, J. (2008). "Maternal, not paternal, PTSD is related to increased risk for PTSD in offspring of Holocaust survivors", *Journal of psychiatric research*, *42*(13), 1104-1111.

Yehuda, R., Halligan, S.L., and Bierer, L.M. (2001). "Relationship of parental trauma exposure and PTSD to PTSD, depressive and anxiety disorders in offspring", *Journal of psychiatric research*, *35*(5), 261-270.

Yehuda, R., Schmeidler, J., Wainberg, M., Binder-Brynes, K., and Duvdevani, T. (1998). "Vulnerability to posttraumatic stress disorder in adult offspring of Holocaust survivors", *American Journal of Psychiatry*, *155*(9), 1163-1171.

Zaigham, M., and Andersson, O. (2020). "Maternal and perinatal outcomes with COVID-19: A systematic review of 108 pregnancies", *Actaobstetriciaetgynecologica Scandinavica, 99*(7), 823-829.

Zhang, L., Jiang, Y., Wei, M., Cheng, B. H., Zhou, X. C., Li, J., & Hu, R. H. (2020). *Analysis of the pregnancy outcomes in pregnant women with COVID-19 in Hubei Province*. Zhonghuafuchankezazhi, 166-171.

29

Covid-19 Pandora Box

The Current Scenario, Science and Social Science of Vaccine Uptake

Suniti Yadav and *Vijay Hadda*

Background

The emergence of Severe Acute Respiratory Syndrome-Coronavirus-2 (SARS-CoV-2), also known as 'novel Coronavirus' was first reported as 'pneumonia of unknown etiology' from the Wuhan city of China during late December 2020. On March 11, 2020, the Coronavirus Disease-2019 (COVID-19) pandemic was declared as a public health emergency by World Health Organization (WHO) (Hussain *et al.*, 2020). Since then, the world has been under a constant threat of this pandemic due to the rapid spread and resulting mortality. Despite numerous efforts from the public health experts, clinicians and epidemiologists across the world, many countries have failed to produce an effective response commensurate to the extent of COVID-19 threat. As on 10 April, 2021, almost 137 million cumulative cases and almost 29 lakh cumulative deaths due to COVID-19 have been reported across the world. Currently, as on April 10, 2021, India stands second in the total number of cases across the world with almost 14 million cumulative cases and almost 1.7 lakh deaths since the first reported case [WHO coronavirus disease (COVID-19) dashboard]. The unprecedented 'in-field' challenges set by COVID-19 have exposed the health system preparedness of all the countries owing to an 'uncertainty' of the vaccines to provide 'herd immunity'. Till date, no vaccine has been reported to provide absolute immunity against COVID-19 and the degree to which vaccines can protect has not been defined precisely (COVID-19 vaccines, WHO). Until the 'uncertain' vaccine provides the herd immunity against COVID-19, the time-tested measures of public health during pandemic outbreak such as containment of source, blocking or breaking the channels of transmission, practice of adequate measures to stop the spread of infection. Nevertheless, these measures require an active engagement from the communities irrespective of the country and ethnicity. The present chapter gives insights into COVID-19 epidemiology, challenges, vaccine hesitancy and community engagement to tackle COVID-19 pandemic. It also deals with the possible role of anthropologists in bridging the gap between communities and healthcare providers, vaccine confidence and acceptance in Indian settings, where the world's largest vaccine rollout plan is active.

Epidemiology of COVID-19: Surfing the Waves in India

The Phases

WHO specifies a six-phase alert level of any influenza-like pandemic. Generally, influenza like viruses circulate among animals, specifically birds, continuously and that may turn into pandemic viruses.

In the *Phase-1* of the pandemic, no viruses are reported to cause human-infections in the initial *Phase-1*. The *Phase-2* is characterized by human infections transmitted from animal or bird virus and hence it is considered as a potential threat of pandemic. During the *Phase-3*, an animal or now human-animal virus causes disease in small clusters of people or sporadic cases. No human-to-human transmissions that can cause community-level outbreaks are reported in this phase. However, under certain circumstances such as close contact of an infected person with an unprotected care-provider, limited human-to-human transmission may occur. Despite this, in these limited circumstances there is no indication that the virus reaches the state of transmissibility to cause a pandemic among humans. The *Phase-4* is defined by the confirmed human-to human transmission of the virus that has the ability to cause outbreaks at "community level". The considerable rising shift in the risk for a pandemic signifies the virus's ability to cause continuous disease outbreaks at community level. At this stage, WHO needs to be consulted by any country that suspects or verifies such an incident, to assess the situation jointly and the affected country may decide on implementing a rapid pandemic containment exercise. A significant increase in pandemic risk is warranted but not necessarily to indicate that the pandemic is inevitable. *Phase-5* includes human-to-human spread in atleast two countries in 'one WHO' region. The announcement of *Phase-5* is a robust signal that a pandemic is forthcoming despite the fact that not many countries would be affected at this stage. This also suggests that the countries need to work on organizing, systemizing, communicating and implementing strategies to culminate the plausible pandemic. The real pandemic phase, i.e. *Phase-6* is distinguished by community level outbreaks in 'at least one of the countries in a different WHO region' along with the existence of *Phase-5*. *Phase-6* is indicative of a pandemic that would affect the entire globe (About Pandemic Phases, WHO).

The Transmission

With the massive spread of COVID-19, the world entered into the Phase-6 on March 11, 2020 as declared by WHO (WHO Director-general Speeches). Different countries were affected at different times during the spread. Two hundred twenty-four countries/provinces are reported to have COVID-19 cases till April 10, 2021. The transmission of cases has been classified into three categories by WHO — sporadic cases, cluster of cases and community transmission. Sporadic cases have been reported in 13 countries, 42 countries with cluster of cases and 149 countries with community transmission while a few have not been updated. India has been classified into country with 'cluster of cases' as on April 10, 2021 [WHO coronavirus disease (COVID-19) dashboard].

The Waves

An influenza-like epidemic follows a predefined manner of spread and decline. An epidemic wave traces the development of an infection that spreads at an epidemic scale over time and space (Fontaine, 2019). The two defining characteristics of a "wave" include — (1) the wave/development graph constitutes peaks (upwards) and/or valleys (downward) periods; (2) the peaks or valleys are sustained significantly over a period of time clearly demarcating it from other vague reporting errors, random ups and downs or volatile reporting of new cases. The initiation of a wave is characterized when people get infected easily and the spread from person-to-person is sustained. Public health actions during the acceleration of the pandemic wave include 'pharmaceutical' interventions, i.e. medications and vaccines (if available) along with 'non-pharmaceutical interventions' such as physical distancing, use of mask, washing hands, avoiding overcrowding etc., at community level. These protective non-pharmaceutical interventions slow down the progress of the disease spread and thereby reduce the extent of burden on healthcare systems. The deceleration of the peak is characterized by gradual reduction in the number of reported cases and increased vaccination (Fig. 29.1) (Zhang *et al.*, 2021).

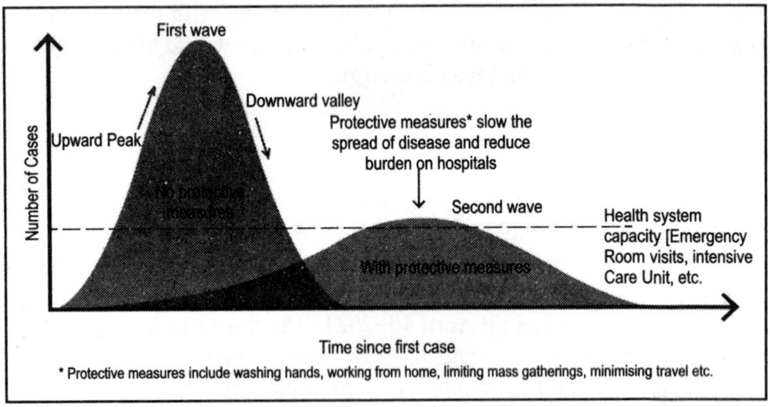

Fig. 29.1: Characteristic epidemic wave sustained over time
Source: Adapted from Fang *et al.*, 2020. Available at https://wwwnc.cdc.gov/eid/article/26/5/19-0995-f1.89

Every epidemic has an infection rate (IR) and case fatality rate (CFR) and has effects on the spread over time in normal circumstances. A few pandemics such as influenza, Spanish flu, plague etc., have reported two or multiple waves (Zheng *et al.*, 2018). The first wave generally presents with lower mortality while the second wave presents with higher incidence and mortality than the first wave. The Pandemic Intervals Framework (PIF) by Centres for Disease Control and Prevention states that the second pandemic wave may have a higher severity than the first wave. The pandemic is declared to be ended when the number of infected cases, spread of the virus and the severity of the illness caused by the virus are similar to a seasonal influenza virus (Pandemic Intervals Framework, Centres for Disease Control and Prevention) (*see* Fig. 29.2)

The fascinating scenario with COVID-19 waves is yet to be witnessed. However, the world seems to have crossed the 'first wave' of the COVID-19 pandemic and entered the second wave, with different nations/continents steering through it at different times (Salyer *et al.*, 2021).

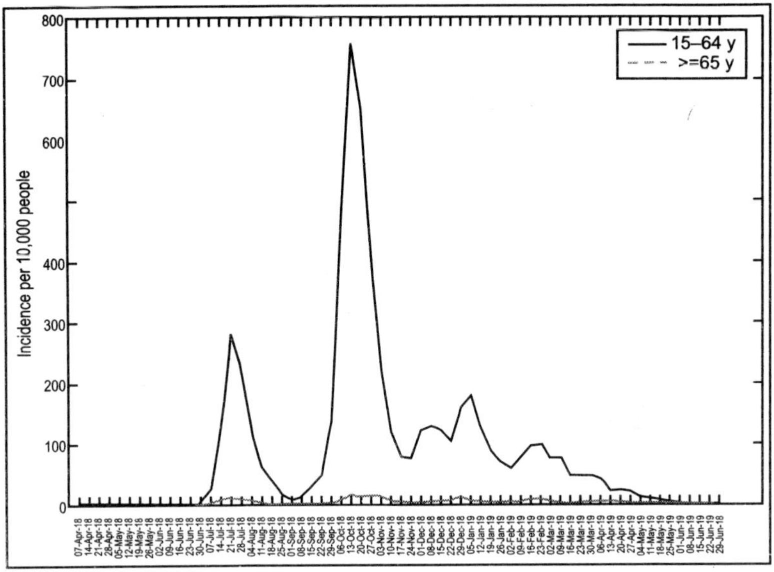

Fig. 29.2: Multiple Peaks or Waves of a Pandemic

Source: Simsonsen *et al.*, 2018.

The Indian Scenario

The first active case of COVID-19 was reported on January 30, 2020 from the State of Kerala in India. Since then, the cases rose exponentially until mid-September 2020, when the number of active cases was almost 97,000 in a single day. The results from the first national level sero-positivity rate in India showed that 0.73 per cent of Indians had been infected already with SARS-CoV2 by May 2020. Thereafter, a decline in the number of cases was seen in India and the number of active cases remained below 20,000 since January 2, 2021. The daily cases witnessed a fall of over 80 per cent, with several theories being suggested for the 'first wave' of COVID-19 in India despite its fully reopened economy, festivities and huge social mobility. It has also been suggested that the reduction in number of cases could also be because of 'localized herd immunity' achieved by Indian population. However, this respite from the effect of first wave was short-lived only until the end of March 2021. A rapid surge in the number of cases was seen in India and India was considered as a global hotspot for COVID-19. Currently in April 2021, the number of active cases are rising rapidly high and India waits to reach the next peak or the peak of the second wave.

Vaccine Effectiveness: A Multidisciplinary Approach in Indian Context

Ever since the vaccines have been introduced and their use has proliferated, the health at population level has improved and, mortalities have reduced (WHO GIVS). Polio and small pox have been eradicated from India (John and Vashishtha, 2013) and childhood diseases such as rubella, diphtheria and measles are now uncommon (Bavdekar and Karande, 2017, Murhekar, 2017). It took enormous community engagement activities, widespread acceptance of vaccines and reduction in the vaccine hesitancy due to vaccine confidence to reach this stage. Currently for this global pandemic, vaccines have been considered critical against COVID-19 by all stake-holders including the scientists, public health experts, clinicians and everyone else involved in combating this disease. However, despite the vaccines, COVID-appropriate behaviour or the 'social medicine', i.e. handwashing, mask use and adequate physical distance are considered to be the best practices to keep this disease at bay, unless otherwise exposed by chance. The important context here remains the key terms — vaccine hesitancy, vaccine confidence, vaccine acceptance and vaccine uptake.

India launched the world's largest vaccination drive in middle of the month of January for the selected age-groups and the administration plans to expand it to the 3.2 billion people in a phased manner to control COVID-19 spread. The first phase included vaccination among the frontline workers and the second phase covered elderly people in the age group 60 years and above or above 45 years of age with co-morbidities such as cancer, diabetes, hypertension, cardiovascular disease etc. The third phase is currently ongoing and covers all people above 45 years of age. Despite a huge vaccination drive, enormous awareness about the protection from vaccines, the vaccine uptake among Indians has not been as high as was expected initially. The latest data shows that approximately 7 per cent of the population in India has been given at least one dose while approximately 1 per cent of the population has been inoculated with both the doses (Ministry of Health and Family Welfare updates). As per the media reports, the vaccination centres in tribal areas and rural areas remain deserted due to vaccine hesitancy. Additional efforts are being taken up by the administration and healthcare providers to encourage people to uptake vaccine in these areas. However, these efforts may not be sufficient enough to improve the drive as they are not mandatory.

The widespread vaccine acceptance is becoming an important aspect about the disease upsurge. As an increasing number of people are making decisions about vaccine uptake, an increasing number are opting to not get vaccinated. Though no vaccine is thought to provide absolute immunity against COVID-19 currently, it is still thought to provide roughly 30 per cent immunity against the disease. At this stage, if the widespread vaccine acceptance, herd immunity may never be achieved sooner and the unvaccinated 'at-risk' group may be compromised and decline in cases may further not be expected in near time.

The vaccine uptake is based on knowledge, attitude and beliefs about the vaccine (Poland and Brunson, 2015). The vaccination programmes may be 'self-destructive' in the context that as the extent of uptake increase, perception about the risk and impact of the disease might have a direct consequence on the upatake, i.e. decrease. Now that a lot of people have been fully vaccinated with both the doses, cases have been reported that they have also been infected with COVID-19. Adverse effects on the health such as blood clots (a few random cases reported among recipients of AstraZeneca vaccine in United States) that may be an occurrence by chance or due to vaccination; however, may become more familiar and fearful to the community than the disease itself.

Researchers, clinicians and other healthcare providers have shown support for changes in health policy, health communication, and awareness among the non-vaccinated people to reduce the risk of the disease and increase vaccine confidence. However, the focus on an array of socio-behavioural factors that create vaccine hesitancy and affect uptake has not been understood. In addition to an absolute medical context, it is not just socio-behavioural issue but also a cultural phenomenon, all that may encompass religious beliefs, family-choice or kin-choice belief systems or community beliefs (Carlson *et al.*, 2019).

The population characters such as age, gender, socio-economic status, cultural beliefs, ethnicity, socio-political systems are important for the application of science beyond laboratory and clinic. Thus, there is a need for multi-disciplinary approach to tackle this complex pandemic. While the epidemic wave has a strong component of 'time' and 'space', the involvement of 'anthropology' is important for to bridge the gaps between the communities and healthcare providers.

Vaccine uptake enhancement requires a coordinated approach between the healthcare providers and communities. An important aspect is to shift or channelize people's risk assessment towards a better understanding of science behind vaccines and beyond. This continuum comprises education about the health threat, availability, accessibility and acceptability of the vaccines.

Awareness of the plausible threat to health involves educating the target population to disseminate the information about the severity of the disease, risks involved, and effectiveness of vaccine uptake to ultimately lower the risk of COVID-19. Information, education and communication means need to be effectively used through mass media, religious leaders, community health workers, public figures to disseminate about the health threat. As stated by WHO, the mis(communication) about the information or the 'infodemic' curve needs to be flattened and the correct information needs to be circulated in the community.

The availability of 'vaccine for all' is an important domain to actually provide herd immunity to the population. Equitable distribution of vaccine to all those who need it is also a challenge due to various reasons such transportation, cold chain maintenance, and few unknown factors. Vaccine procurement and distribution at the grassroots level holds the key owing to increasing demand eventually and expansion of the vaccination drive.

Easy accessibility of vaccine requires careful planning regarding dispensing vaccines even to the inaccessible and outreached populations. In rural and tribal areas, the vaccination centre, specifically the sub-centre, is located at a distance. These places are not easily accessible to the tribal people and this reduces vaccine uptake. Selection of appropriate ways such as mobile ambulances for COVID-19 vaccination may help increase the uptake. Optimization of reach and ease of access by community members may also add to enhanced uptake.

Anthropology of Vaccine: Barriers, Confidence and Uptake

The discipline of anthropology remains one of the most holistic discipline in science that generalizes, compares and understand the human diversity in time and space. Anthropologists indulge in empirical research based on the theories, methods and techniques that require understanding based on the cultural and societal settings. The macro-and micro-level understanding of a phenomenon is conducted within the framework of a community or the context of the study.

In terms of vaccine spectrum of hesitancy, rejection, acceptance and uptake, anthropology tries to understand different drivers of health behaviour in the actual cultural, social and political settings. Understanding of the acceptability of vaccine at community level may be vital for successful vaccination drive, specifically when acceptability is not homogenously governed by a single factor but multiple factors. Vaccine hesitancy is an important issue and the causes may be rooted in the belief systems — religious, natural, personal or familial.

In context of Polio Eradication Programme, anthropologist Heidi Larson at UNICEF states "Communications can not fix a problem you do not understand" (Larson and Fleck, 2014). In general, during vaccine hesitancy and uptake, policy makers tend to explain the risks and benefits of the vaccine. However, the lack in vaccine confidence is not juts limited to the science behind vaccines or information dissemination, it also involves vaccine delivery issues and belief systems etc. To understand these, 'participant observation', i.e. immersion into the community to understand the 'emic' response or human behaviour, is required. Detailed understanding of community behaviour, beliefs and insecurities may help in revealing the issues concerning the problem. For example, during the oral polio vaccination drive in Uttar Pradesh, North India, certain areas were identified where resistance towards oral polio vaccine was observed. Medi reports stated that fear of becoming 'sterile' created vaccine hesitancy (Polio Elimination in Uttar Pradesh, Cases in Global Health Delivery, 2011). However, an understanding by anthropologists among the women in these areas revealed that the community did not want the children to be vaccinated by members belonging 'outside' the community, i.e. from other regions or State. The mere fact here is that this notion was not due to any bias or hatred towards any section of people but for the fear that in case of any upcoming adversity or contra-indication, they did not know whom to report to or with whom they may need to discuss their concerns with. In addition, the women did not want their children to be vaccinated by men owing to the same reason that they would not be able to discuss the issues with men without any hesitation. A community tends to build its own notions and has its own health seeking behaviour and approach to healthcare system and during a mass-vaccination roll-out, the system is displaced (Larson *et al.*, 2018). Therefore, in such circumstances, understanding human behaviour in a particular setting is important to address such challenges of vaccine uptake.

Another important aspect of vaccine hesitancy and uptake is religion. Some communities such as the Muslim communities hesitate to take vaccine because of the presence of gelatin. According to their faith, gelatin is not '*halal*' or pure as it is derived from pork. Despite this, the community still believes that vaccines are important and given the current situation where no alternative is available, small amount of gelatin in some vaccines may be accepted (Vaccine Confidence Project). Thus, religious groups may also be involved in reducing vaccine hesitancy by disseminating the correct information about the 'layman's science' behind the vaccine and building their faith in the delivery system. These religious groups may serve as social networks and help in spreading the correct information in the community. Since these members or representatives are well-heard, they can be the stakeholders in the tight-knit communities that are generally opposed to the concept of vaccine.

Anthropologists play an important role in bridging the gap between healthcare providers and community with respect to the current need of the hour — vaccination. Huge costs are involved at the government level and the government is making best efforts to provide free of cost vaccination at its centres. The beliefs of the community, the hesitancy towards the acceptance and uptake of vaccines can best be addressed by an insider's view. Anthropologists and other social scientists need to quickly pitch into the drive and reduce the plausible bottlenecks and barriers. A holistic understanding of vaccines may be developed and disseminated to the public by anthropologists after addressing their concerns and fears. Anthropologists can bridge between the communities and ministries to develop methods on how best to communicate 'the need for vaccine' and strategize reduction in vaccine wastage. The important methods of building vaccine confidence may include —(i) listen (listen to the beliefs, concerns, perceptions and experiences of the community in previous vaccine drives), (ii) understand (understand the reasons for their concerns and hesitancy for the uptake), (iii) indulge (indulge in a dialogue between the community and various stakeholders to address the concerns of the community), (iv) create (create methods of intervention and dissemination of correct information) and (v) recognize (recognize the effort of the community, various stakeholders in successful vaccine uptake).

In conclusion, the Coronavirus Disease-2019 (COVID-19) pandemic has unfolded the unpreparedness of the health systems and much political, economical and social insecurity. The pandemic has set unprecedented challenges for the health infrastructure development for all the countries. The world seems to have crossed the first wave but the countries are surfing the second wave of this pandemic. India is going through the second wave and there is a massive burden on the healthcare systems. This pandemic created a dire need for development of vaccines and a few vaccine candidates effective to certain against SARS-CoV-2 have been launched. The Indian vaccine roll-out that includes two vaccines (Covaxin and Covishield) is one of the largest vaccination drive in the world. Despite a dire need, massive media campaigns and dissemination of information for the vaccines, the uptake has been slow. The effects of vaccine hesitancy and the vaccine wastage loom over the achievement of herd immunity against COVID-19. Hence, anthropologists need to understand the community behaviour towards vaccine uptake and bridge the gap between the community and healthcare systems. The dissemination of correct information about the disease threat, risks involved by anthropologists are required. Rapid assessment of qualitative studies to understand the dilemma, fears and hesitancy along with health system research need to be undertaken by social scientists including the anthropologists. Broadening the agendas from vaccine coverage for immunity to the end of pandemic is the need of the hour and hence a multi-disciplinary approach to tackle this pandemic is warranted.

REFERENCES

About Phases, WHO. Available from: https://www.euro.who.int/en/health-topics/communicable-diseases/influenza/data-and-statistics/pandemic-influenza/about-pandemic-phases (Last accessed on 09 April, 2021).

Bavdekar, S.B. and Karande, S. (2017). "Elimination of measles from India: Challenges ahead and the way forward", *Journal of postgraduate medicine*, *63*(2), 75.

Carlson, A., Riethman, M., Gastañaduy, P., Lee, A., Leung, J., Holshue, M.,... and Melnick, A. (2019). "Notes from the field: Community outbreak of measles—Clark County, Washington, 2018–2019", *Morbidity and Mortality Weekly Report*, *68*(19), 446.

Centers for Disease Control and Prevention (1918). "Pandemic Influenza: Three Waves", Retrived on April, 10, 2020.

COVID-19 Vaccines, WHO. Available from: https://www.who.int/emergencies/diseases/novel-coronavirus-2019/covid-19-vaccines (Last accessed on 09 April, 2021).

Fong, M.W., Gao, H., Wong, J.Y., Xiao, J., Shiu, E., Ryu, S.... Cowling, B.J. (2020). "Nonpharmaceutical Measures for Pandemic Influenza in Nonhealthcare Settings—Social Distancing Measures" *Emerging Infectious Diseases*, *26*(5), 976-984. https://doi.org/10.3201/eid2605.190995.

Fontaine, R.E. (2019). "Describing epidemiologic data", In *The CDC Field Epidemiology Manual* (pp. 105-134). Oxford University Press.

https://github.com/owid/covid-19-data/blob/master/public/data/vaccinations/country_data/ India.csv

Hussain, A., Yadav, S., Hadda, V., Suri, T.M., Tiwari, P., Mittal, S.,... and Mohan,

A. (2020). "Covid-19: A comprehensive review of a formidable foe and the road ahead", *Expert review of respiratory medicine*, *14*(9), 869-879.

John, T.J., and Vashishtha, V.M. (2013). "Eradicating poliomyelitis: India's journey from hyperendemic to polio-free status", *The Indian journal of medical research*, *137*(5), 881.

Larson, H.J., Clarke, R.M., Jarrett, C., Eckersberger, E., Levine, Z., Schulz, W.S., and Paterson, P. (2018). "Measuring trust in vaccination: A systematic review. Human vaccines and immunotherapeutics", *14*(7), 1599-1609.

Larson, H., and Fleck, F. (2014). Underlying issues are key to dispelling vaccine doubts. *Bulletin of the World Health Organisation*, *92*(2), 84-85.

Ministry of Health and Family Welfare. Available from: http://mohfw.gov.in/pdf/CumulativeCOVIDVaccinationCoverageReport12April2021.pdf (accessed on April 13, 2021).

Murhekar, M. (2017). "Epidemiology of diphtheria in India, 1996–2016: implications for prevention and control", *The American journal of tropical medicine and hygiene*, *97*(2), 313-318.

Pandemic Intervals Framework (PIF), Centers for Disease Control and Prevention. Available from: https://www.cdc.gov/flu/pandemic-resources/national-strategy/intervals-framework.html. Accessed on 26 April, 2021.

Polio Elimination in Uttar Pradesh, Cases in Global Health Delivery, 2011. Available from: https://www.globalhealthdelivery.org/files/ghd/files/ghd-005_polio_elimination_in_uttar_pradesh_x6m58r6.pdf. (Accessed on 26 April, 2021)

Salyer, S.J., Maeda, J., Sembuche, S., Kebede, Y., Tshangela, A., Moussif, M.,... and Nkengasong, J. (2021). "The first and second waves of the COVID-19 pandemic in Africa: A cross-sectional study", *The Lancet*.

Simonsen, L., Chowell, G., Andreasen, V., Gaffey, R., Barry, J., Olson, D., and Viboud, C. (2018). "A review of the 1918 herald pandemic wave: importance for contemporary pandemic response strategies", *Annals of epidemiology*, *28*(5), 281-288.

Vaccine Confidence Project. Available from: https://www.vaccineconfidence.org/blog/value-of-vaccines-vaccine-confidence-project?rq = vaccine%20confidence%20project (Accessed on 26 April, 2021).

WHO coronavirus disease (COVID-19) dashboard. Available from: https://covid19whoint/?gclid=CjwKCAjwztL2BRATEiwAvnALchxnJmzQWfM4H1VHfJh-ctOvHdzjxKN5ehDRmFtf5BxWB7-W68C3jxoCIBoQAvD_BwE. (Last accessed on 10 April, 2021).

WHO Director-General Speeches. WHO Director-General's opening remarks at the media briefing on COVID-19—11 March, 2020. Available from: https://www.who.int/director-general/speeches/detail/who-director-general-s-opening-remarks-at-the-media-briefing-on-covid-19---11-march-2020.

WHO GIVS. Global immunization vision and strategy 2006–2015. Geneva: WHO (2014). Available from: http://www.who.int/immunization/givs/en/ (Accessed on 09 April, 2021).

Zhang, S.X., Marioli, F.A., and Gao, R. (2021). "A Second Wave? What Do People Mean By COVID Waves?: A Working Definition of Epidemic Waves", *medRxiv*.

Zheng, M., Wang, W., Tang, M., Zhou, J., Boccaletti, S., and Liu, Z. (2018). "Multiple peaks patterns of epidemic spreading in multi-layer networks", *Chaos, Solitons and Fractals*, *107*, 135-142.

APPENDIX
Publications of Prof. P.C. Joshi

Books: 10

1. Explorations in Indian Medical Anthropology (Volume II): Disease, Health and Culture. (H.K. Bhat, **P.C. Joshi** and B.R. Vijayendra edited). Concept Publishing Company, New Delhi, (2013).
2. Explorations in Indian Medical Anthropology (Volume I): Illness, Health and Culture. (H.K. Bhat, **P.C. Joshi** and B.R. Vijayendra edited). Concept Publishing Company, New Delhi, (2013).
3. **Joshi, P.C.** The Gujarat Earthquake Recovery 2001 – Recovery Status Report. (2013). International Recovery Platform, Kobe, Japan.
4. **P.C. Joshi**. Relevance of Traditional Medicines in Global Era Icon Publications Pvt. Ltd., New Delhi, (2013).
5. Stress among Sunni Muslims of Delhi with special reference to Psychosociobiogenetic Correlates (Astha Bansal and **P.C. Joshi**). LAP Lambert Academic Publishing, Saarbrucken, Germany, (2012). (https://www.lap-publishing.com/catalog/details//store/gb/book/978-3-659-29474-7/stressamong-sunni-muslims-of-delhi)
6. N.K. Ganguly, R. Lakshminarayan **P.C. Joshi** *et al.* Situational Analysis: Antibiotic Use and Resistance in India. Global Antibiotic Resistance Partnership. The Centre for Disease Dynamics, Economics and Policy, Washington DC, New Delhi, (2011).
7. **P.C. Joshi**, Sonia Kaushal, Prashant Khattri and Supriya Akerkar. Impact of Floods in context of Bahraich. Microdis, Department of Anthropology, University of Delhi. (2009) (In Hindi).
8. Debarati Guha-Sapir, Lian Parry, Olivier Degomme, **P.C. Joshi** and J.P. Saulina Arnold. Risk factors for Mortality and Injury : Post-Tsunami Epidemiological findings from Tamil Nadu. WHO Centre for Research on Epidemiology of Disaster, Brussels, 2006. [Translated in Hindi and Tamil].
9. A.K. Kalla and **P.C. Joshi**. Tribal Health and Medicines (ed). Concept Publishing Company, New Delhi, 2004.
10. **P.C. Joshi** and Anil Mahajan. Studies in Medical Anthropology, Reliance Publishers, Delhi, 1990.

Reports (14)

1. **P.C. Joshi,** B. Murry, Avitoli Zhimo. Bio-anthropological study of Sirmour, Himachal Pradesh, UGCSAP Report, Department of Anthropology, Delhi University, Delhi, (2011).
2. **P.C. Joshi**, K.N. Saraswathy, R. Kumar, R. Samtani, R. Joy, M. Dhall and P.K. Ghosh. Bio-cultural Diversity in a Village of Hamirpur District in Himachal Pradesh, UGCSAP Report, Department of Anthropology, Delhi University, Delhi, (2010).
3. **P.C. Joshi,** Sonia Kaushal, B.S. Aribam and Prashant Khattri. Medical Anthropology and Disaster Management. Working Paper Series, Microdis. Department of Anthropology, University of Delhi, (2010).
4. **P.C. Joshi**. Working Paper Series, Microdis. Department of Anthropology, Delhi University, Delhi (2009).
5. **P.C. Joshi**. Impact of Economy, Culture and Environment on Health Status of Meitie Women in Manipur. Project report submitted to ICSSR, New Delhi, 2008.
6. **P.C. Joshi**. Emergence of PTSD and impact of conflict situation on the role performance of adolescents in Jammu and Kashmir, Project Report submitted to ICSSR, New Delhi, 2001.
7. V.K. Srivastava and **P.C. Joshi**. Biocultural Diversity of Kiyana: A village in Himachal Pradesh, UGC SAP report, Department of Anthropology, Delhi University, Delhi, 2008.
8. V.K. Srivastava and **P.C. Joshi**. Society and Culture in Junga of Himachal Pradesh, UGC SAP report, Department of Anthropology, Delhi University, Delhi, 2008.
9. K. Thimasarn, S. Singh, **P.C. Joshi**, R.C. Dhiman and C.P. Batra. Report of Joint Monitoring Mission on Urban Malaria and Dengue, Delhi State, National Vector Born Disease Control Programme, Delhi, 2007.
10. **P. C. Joshi**. Study of Rites and Rituals of Garhwal, 1995.
11. **P.C. Joshi**. Health Need Assessment: A Report on Soung Valley, Himgravika, Himalayan Hospital Trust, Dehradun, 1994.
12. **P.C. Joshi**. Health Need Assessment: A Report on Jolly Grant, Himgravika, Himalayan Hospital Trust, Dehradun, 1992.
13. **P.C. Joshi**. Friends of Trees: Experience and Messages, Dalyun Ka Dagriya, Srinagar. 1991.
14. **P.C. Joshi**. Anthropology and Development, Department of Anthropology, Garhwal University, Srinagar, 1985.

Research Articles (126)

2020 (2)

Joshi, P.C. (2020). Subir Kumar Dutta and Mitu De (Eds.), Understanding Autism:

Through the Lens of Parents and Professionals. *Journal of the Anthropological Survey of India*, *69*(1), 179–181.

Joshi, P.C. (2020). H.K. Kumbnani (1935–2019). *Journal of the Anthropological Survey of India*, *69*(1), 177–178.

2019 (7)

Joshi, P.C., and Khattri, P. (2019). On Gandhi and Sanitation. *Journal of the Anthropological Survey of India*, *68*(2), 210-224.

Joshi, P. C. (2019). Ethnomedical Practices and Indian Scheduled Tribes. *Romanian Journal of Sociological Studies*, (2), 111-124.

Rawat, S., Rajkumari, S., **Joshi, P.C.**, Khan, M.A., & Saraswathy, K.N. (2019). Who dies and who survives? Investigating the difference between suicide decedents and suicide attempters. *Egyptian Journal of Forensic Sciences*, *9*(1), 1-7.

Barooah, M., **Joshi, P.C.**, & Deb, R. (2019). Cultural Factors Affecting the Spread of HIV/AIDS among the Women in Jaintia Hills, Meghalaya. *Indian Journal of Public Health Research & Development*, *10*(12).

Rawat, S., Rajkumari, S., **Joshi, P. C.**, Khan, M. A., & Saraswathy, K.N. (2019). Risk factors for suicide attempt: A population-based-genetic study from Telangana, India. *Current Psychology*, 1-10.

Saraswathy, K.N., Ansari, S.N., Kaur, G., **Joshi, P.C.**, & Chandel, S. (2019). Association of vitamin B_{12} mediated hyperhomocysteinemia with depression and anxiety disorder: A cross-sectional study among Bhil indigenous population of India. *Clinical nutrition ESPEN*, *30*, 199-203.

Mishra, D., Chandel, S., Kiranmala, N., **Joshi, P.C.**, & Saraswathy, K.N. (2019). Adiposity indicators in blood pressure: A study among Bhil tribal population of India. *Applied Biological Research,* 21(2), 184-191

2018 (3)

Joshi, P.C. and Vashist, N. (2018). Illness, Health and Culture: Anthropological Perspectives on Ethno-Medicine in India. In *Psychosocial interventions for health and well-being* (pp. 227-240). Springer, New Delhi.

Rawat, S., **Joshi, P.C**., Khan, M.A., & Saraswathy, K.N. (2018). Trends and determinants of suicide in Warangal District, Telangana, India: six years retrospective study based on secondary data. *Egyptian Journal of Forensic Sciences*, *8*(1), 1-8.

Joshi, P.C. and Srivastava, V. K. (2018). Culture, Mythology, and Religion. *Social Psychiatry: Principles & Clinical Perspectives*, 130.

2017(7)

Bandooni, S.K., A.M. Hasija, M.L. Devi and **P.C. Joshi**. (2017). The Participation of Local Communities and NGOs: A Step Towards Sustainable Development in Garhwal Himalaya. *World Focus*. No 450:111-117.

Minakshi, Rahul Kumar and **P.C. Joshi.** (2017). Sustainable Development and Environment: Challenges and Responsibilities. *World Focus*. No. 450:106-110.

Sharma, K. and **P.C. Joshi.** (2017). Reinterpreting 'Sustainable Development' in Environmental Management. *World Focus*. No. 450:58-61.

Joshi, P.C. (2017). Emerging Challenges in Sustainable Development and Indian. Experiments. *World Focus*. No. 450:12-15.

Joshi, P.C. (2017). Guest Editor, Special Issue on Environment and Sustainable Development: Emerging Challenges. *World Focus*, No. 450.

Bansal, A. and **P.C. Joshi**. (2017). Assessment of Cardiovascular Risk Factors among Sunni Muslims of Delhi, India. *Eurasian Journal of Anthropology*. 7, 2: 37-50. (DOI: 10.12973/eja.2017.0055a)

Joshi, P.C. (2017). Human Rights, Wild Life and Environmental Protection. *Social Change*. 47, 1: 1-10. (DOI:10.1177/0049085716681900)

2016(16)

Joshi, P.C. (2016). Negotiating Rapport and Shades of Participant Observation: Notes from Fieldwork in Jaunsar-Bawar. *Journal of Indian Anthropological Society*. 51, 3:117-127.

Joshi, P.C. Book Review. (2016). S.K. Gupta and V.K. Srivastava (eds.), Exploring Indian Society: Essays in Honour of Yogesh Atal. *The Eastern Anthropologist*. 69, 3&4:521-522.

Joshi, P. C. Book Review. (2016).A. N. Nayak, Burden of Lymphatic Filariasis in Rural Odisha: A Study in Medical Anthropology. *The Eastern Anthropologist*. 69, 3&4:522-524.

Joshi, P.C., Prashant Khattri and Kalindi Sharma. (2016). Social Response to Extreme Weather Events: Some Empirical Evidences from India. *The Eastern Anthropologist*. 69, 3&4:489-508.

Bansal, Ashtha and **P.C. Joshi**. (2016). Association of Cardiovascular Disease risk variables with Depression in Urban population of Delhi, India. *Delhi Psychiatry Journal*. 19, 2:45-53.

Joshi, P.C. Guest Editor. Special Issue, *World Focus*, 442, October, (2016).

Joshi, P.C. (2016). Antiquity and Novelty of Climate Change. *World Focus*. 442: 5-8.

Kotwani, Anita, Chand Wattal, **P.C. Joshi** and Kathleen Holloway. (2016). Knowledge and Perception on antibiotic use and resistance among high school students and teachers in New Delhi, India: A qualitative study. *Indian Journal of Pharmacology*. 48:365-371. (DOI: 10.4103/0253-7613.186208)

Joshi, P.C. (2016). Emergence of Medical Anthropology in India. *The Eastern Anthropologist.* 69, 1:1-11.

Akerkar, Supriya, **P.C. Joshi** and Maureen Fordham. (2016). Culture of Entitlement and Social protection: Evidence from Flood Prone Bahraich, Uttar Pradesh, India. *World Development. 86:46-58.* (http://dx.doi.org/10.1016/j.worlddev.(2016).06.004)

Lamkang, S.A., **P.C. Joshi**, M.M. Singh. (2016). A Study on Knowledge, Attitude, Behaviour and Practice (KABP) towards HIV/AIDS in Manipur, India. *International Journal of AIDS Research.* 3(4):59-67.

Joshi, P.C. (2016). Forwarding Note. B.M. Mukherjee and Farhad Mollick (eds.) Tribal Unrest in Central India: Discusses, Challenges and Possibilities, New Delhi: K.K. Publications. pp. i-iv.

Joshi, P.C. (2016). Extreme Weather Events and the Himalayas: Learning from the Recent Flood Disasters. *World Focus*, 437:12-16.

Sharma, Kalindi and **P.C. Joshi**. (2016). Locating Gender within the Realm of Natural Disasters. *World Focus*, 437:83-87.

Minakshi and **P.C. Joshi**. (2016). Vulnerability of Women in Disasters: A Glance at Kosi Floods. *World Focus*, 437:92-95.

Joshi, P.C. Guest Editor. Special Issue, *World Focus*, 437, May, (2016).

2015 (10)

Joshi, P.C. (2015). Symposium on People of India. *The Eastern Anthropologist.* 68, 2&3:410-474.

Joshi, P.C. and Prashant Khattri (2015). Climate Change: Locating Diplomacy in History and Culture. *World Focus.* Vol. 430:14-22.

Joshi, P.C. (2015). Advent of Anthropology and Birth of Social Anthropology in Delhi University. *The Eastern Anthropologist.* 68, 1:35-41.

Joshi, P.C. (2015). Book Review: Sunita Reddy, Clash of Waves: Post-Tsunami Relief and Rehabilitation in Andaman and Nicobar Islands. *The Eastern Anthropologist*, 68, 1:163-164.

Joshi, P.C. (2015). Editorial, Special Issue on Climate Change and the Himalayas. *Nam Today: An International Journal of New Age Mind.* Vol. 48, 6.

Bansal, A. and **P.C. Joshi**. (2015). Predictor of Metabolic Syndrome: A Community Study from Urban Delhi, India. *International Journal of Human Sciences.* 12, 1: 1451-1462. (doi:10.14687/ijhs.v12i1.3289)

Aribam, B.S., **P.C. Joshi** and S. Sharma. (2015). Management of Acute Respiratory Tract Infections in a Slum Cluster of Delhi. *International Journal of Scientific Research*, 4, 6:642-644(doi:10.15373/22778179)

Joshi, P.C. (2015). Book Review: Manish Thakur, Indian Village: A Conceptual History. *Social Change.* 45(1):172-173. (doi:10.1177/0049085714561849)

Khattri, P. and **P.C. Joshi**. (2015). Bio-medicalization and Gandhi's vision of Health: Observations from Sevagram. *Economic and Political Weekly*, Vol. 50, No. 10: 53-58.

Joshi, P.C. (2015). Gandhi, Gita and the Idea of Sustainable Development. *World Focus*. Vol. 422:9-13.

2014 (07)

Bansal, A. and **P.C. Joshi**. (2014). Estimation of Waist and Hip Circumference using Body Mass Index in Delhi School Girls (6-11Years). *Journal of Biosocial Science*. pp. 1-5 (doi:10.1017/S002193014000273)

Kaushal, S., **P.C. Joshi**, V.D. Yengkhom, M. Srivastava and A.K. Sinha. (2011) (Published in 2014). Housing Reconstruction: A Case Study on Gujarat Earthquake (2001) Rehabilitation. *Journal of South Asian Disaster Studies*. 4, 2:123-134.

Joshi, P.C. and Prashant Khattri, (2014). Importance of Disaster Risk Reduction. *World Focus*. Vol. 15:10-14.

Krishnakumari, P., **P.C. Joshi**, M.C. Arun Kumar and M. Meghachandra Singh. (2014). Women's Perception of Reproductive Illness in Manipur, India. *Journal of Anthropology*. Article ID 321480, 9 pages.http://dx.doi.org/10.1155/(2014)/321480)

Joshi, P.C. and Prashant Khattri. (2014). India and the Climate Change Negotiations. *World Focus*. Vol.410:9-13.

Wind, T.R., **P.C. Joshi**, R.J. Kleber and I.H. Komproe. (2014). The Effect of Post-disaster Context on the Assessment of Individual Mental Health Scores. *American Journal of Orthopsychiatry*. 84, 2: 134-141. (doi: 10.1037/h0099385)

Devi, N.B. and **P.C. Joshi**. (2014). Life Experience of People in Insurgency Affected Area. *European Academic Research*. 1, 10:3170-3179. (http://www.euacademic.org/UploadArticle/231.pdf)

2013(07)

Joshi, P.C. (2013). Sustaining Recovery and Rehabilitation. *Know Disaster*, 7, 1:22-26.

Bansal, A. and **P.C. Joshi**. (2013). Physical Health of Sunni Muslim Girls of Delhi (6-12 years). *The Asian Man*. 7, 1 &2:91-94.

Krishnakumari, P., **P.C. Joshi** and M.M. Singh. (2013). Beliefs and Practices on Reproductive Health among Andro of Manipur. *South Asian Anthropologist*, 13, 2:111-119.

Sharma, K., **P.C. Joshi** and Anil. K. Sinha. (2013). Gender and Governance in Context of Post-earthquake Gujarat. *The Eastern Anthropologist*. 66, 1:61-74.

P.C. Joshi and Kalindi Sharma. (2013). Sustainability and Future of Yamuna River. *World Focus*. No. 401:26-31. (ISSN2230-8458)

Wind, T.R., **P.C. Joshi,** R.J. Kleber and I.H. Kamproe. (2013). The impact of recurrent disasters on mental health: A study on seasonal floods in Northern India. *Prehospital and Disaster Medicine*. 28(3):1-7.

Bansal, A. and **P.C. Joshi**. (2013). Manifestation of malnutrition among Sunni Muslim girls of Delhi. *International Journal of Human Science*. 10(1):1128-1134. (ISSN:1303-5134)

2012(08)

Minakshi and **P.C. Joshi.** (2012). Disaster and Domestic Violence: The Alcohol Connection. *Man In India.* 92, 3&4:551-560. (ISSN:0025-1569)

Khundongbam, G., **P.C. Joshi** and M.M. Singh. (2012). Perception of Childhood Diarrhoea in Langmeidong Village, Manipur. *South Asian Anthropologist.* 12, 2:135-140. (ISSN:0257-7348)

Khattri, P., **P.C. Joshi**, Minakshi and D. Guha-Sapir. (2012). Projection of Disaster: Investigations into Visual and Textual Images of Flood in Badaun, Uttar Pradesh. *Anukriti.* 2, 5:163-168. (ISSN:2250-1193)

Khattri, P. and **P.C. Joshi**. (2012). People's perception and State's Response during Floods: Evidence from Bahraich District of Uttar Pradesh. *The Asian Man.* 6, 1:8. ISSN:0974-6366.

Khattri, P., **P.C. Joshi**, T. Wind, I. Komproe and D. Guha-Sapir. (2012). Understanding Mental Health as a function of Social Vulnerabilities in a Disaster Situation: Evidence from recurrent flooding in Bahraich District, Uttar Pradesh. *Journal of the Anthropological Survey of India.* 61, 1:109-124.

Bansal, A., K.N. Saraswathy and **P.C. Joshi**. (2012). Psycho-social risk factors of cardiovascular disease among the female Sunni Muslims of Delhi Pilot Study. *Voice of Intellectual Man.* 2, 1:89-94. (ISSN:2231-6914)

Minakshi and **P.C. Joshi**. (2012). Contextualising Domestic Violence in Post-Disaster Situation: Qualitative and Quantitative Analysis. *South Asian Anthropologist.* 12, 1:37-44. (ISSN: 0257-7348)

Khattri, P., **Joshi, P.C.**, Minakshi, Guha-Sapir, D., (2012). Importance of Past Memories in Disaster Research. *The Journalist.* Vol. 1. No. 5. pp. 32-40 (ISSN-2231-2943)

2011(07)

Khattri, P. and **P.C. Joshi**. (2011). Anthropological Methodology and Disaster Research. *The Eastern Anthropologist.* 64, 2&3:145-152. (ISSN-0012-8686)

Ganguly, N.K., Arora, N.K., Chandy, S.J., Fairoze, M.N., Gill, J.P.S., Gupta, U., Hossain, S., Joglekar, S., **Joshi, P.C.**, Kakkar, M., Kotwani, A., Thomas, K., Wattal, C., Easton, A., Laxminarayan, R. (2011). Rationalizing antibiotic use to limit antibiotic resistance in India. *Indian Journal of Medical Research,* 134:281-294.

Minakshi, **P.C. Joshi** and D. Guha-Sapir. (2011). Health and Violence Against Women in Disaster: Preliminary Findings. *International Journal of Management and Social Sciences* (IJMSS). Volume1 (1).

A. Kotwani, C. Wattal, **P.C. Joshi** and K. Holloway. (2011). Irrational use of antibiotics and role of the pharmacist: An insight from a qualitative study in New Delhi, India. *Journal of Clinical Pharmacy and Therapeutics*. doi:10.1111/j.1365-2710. (2011).01293.x

A. Kotwani, C. Wattal. **P.C. Joshi** and K. Holloway. May (2011). PHP 86. Irrational Use of antibiotics and role of pharmacists : An insight from a qualitative study in New Delhi, India. *Value in Health.* 14, 3: A27.

Joshi, P.C., S. Kaushal, B.S. Aribam, P. Khattri, O. D'Oust, M. Marx and D. Guha-Sapir. (2011). Recurrent floods and prevalence of diarrhoea among under five children: Observations from Bahraich District, Uttar Pradesh, India. *Global Health Action***,** 4: 6335. doi: 10.3402/gha.v4i0.6355.

Joshi, P.C. (2011). Emerging Challenges for Disaster Management. *World Focus* Special Issue. N0. 375:131-133.

2010(04)

Joshi, P.C., Debarati Guha-Sapir and V.K. Srivastava. (2010). A Qualitative Account of the Impact of Disaster: The Case of Flooding in Bahraich, Uttar Pradesh. *The Eastern Anthropologist.* 63, 3-4:479-492. (ISSN-0012-8686)

Joshi, P.C. (2010) Psychotherapeutic Elements in Shamanistic Healing in the Context of Himalayan Traditions. *Delhi Psychiatry Journal*. 13, 2:254257. (http://medind.nic.in/daa/t10/i2/daat10i2p254.pdf)

A. Kotwani, C. Wattal, S. Katewa, **P.C. Joshi** and K. Holloway. (2010). Factors influencing primary care physicians to prescribe antibiotics in Delhi India. *Family Practice*. 27:684-690.

Joshi, P.C. and K. Sharma (2010). Climate Çhange Issues Beyond Copenhagen. *World Focus*. 31, 3:85-89. *(http://www.cnfWorld Focus.org/index_files/363. htm)*

2009(04)

Lamkang, A.S., **Joshi, P.C**., Singh. M.M. (2009). Assessing the Quality of life and Needs of HIV/AIDS Patients in Manipur : A Preliminary Study. *Journal of Communicable Diseases*. 41(4); 221-227.

Joshi, P.C., Singh, M. Meghachandra, Guha-Sapir, D. and Marx, Michael (2009). Social Contours of Mental Illness in a Peri-Urban Resettlement Delhi. *The Eastern Anthropologist***.** Vol. 62, No. 3 : 345-359. (ISSN-0012-8686)

Joshi, P. C. (2009). Involving Community, Civil Society and NGOs in Disaster Management. *Southasiadisasters.net.* Issue 67. p. 15.

Joshi, P.C. (2009). Culture and Nature. *World Focus*. 30, 9:351-357.

2007(03)

Kaushal, S. and **Joshi, P.C**. (2007). Ethnomedical Practices in a High Altitude Vashist village in Himachal Pradesh. *South Asian Anthropologist*, 7, 1:37-46. (ISSN:0257-7348)

Chadda, R.K., **Joshi, P.C**.. (2007). Gusain, S.S. Students' awareness about psychiatric illnesses: A study from a Hillstate. *Journal of Mental Health and Human Behaviour*, 12:26-30.

Joshi, P.C. (2007). Book Review. Anthropology, New Global Order and Other Essays by K.K. Misra, P.V. Rao, Siva Prasad and B.V. Sharma. *The Eastern Anthropologist*. 2007. 60, 1 :124-125. (ISSN-0012-8686)

2005-2006(04)

P.C. Joshi, S. Kausal. S. Katewa and O. Hemlata Devi. (2006). Witchcraft Beliefs and Practices among the Oraons. *Studies of Tribes and Tribals,* 4(2):145-149.

P.C. Joshi and U.A. Mir. (2006). Shattered Homes and Suffering Bodies: An Interpretation of Disaster in the Context of Yamuna Pushta Fire, *The Eastern Anthropologist*, 59, 2 : 195-206. (ISSN-0012-8686)

P. C. Joshi and A.K. Kalla. (2005). Counterpoint on Tribal Health and Medicines, *The Applied Anthropologist*, 25(2):180-181.

Suman Gusain. M.M.C. Singh and **P.C. Joshi**. (2005). Nutritional Status of Pre-School Children in a Remote Village of Uttaranchal in Central Himalaya. *South Asian Anthropologist*, 5(1):117-122. (ISSN: 0257-7348)

2001 and earlier (37)

M.M. Singh and **P.C. Joshi**, Pundit (Priest) as a link in improving the health of the women: An Alternative Strategy, *The National Medical Journal of India*, 2001, 14, 5:314-315, (Also see: http://mountaindiary.netfirms.com/New_Folder/temple.htm)

Joshi, P.C. and S.N. Sengupta, Health Issues of the Elderly, *Seminar,* 2000, 488:40-43.

Joshi, P.C. Relevance and Utility of Traditional Medical Systems, *Psychology and Developing Societies*, 2000, 12, 1:5-30.

Joshi, P.C. Whose Forest is it Anyway? *Mountain and People*. 1999, 1, 1:7-10.

Joshi, P.C. No Aging in India: Alzeimer's, Bad Family and other modern things (Review Article). *Social Change*. 1999, 29, 1&2:237-240.

Joshi, P.C. Heaps of Health, Metaphysical Fitness, Ayurveda and the Ontology of Good Health in Medical Anthropology (Comment), *Current Anthropology*, 1999, 40: S60-61.

Surinder Nath, Suminder Kaur, Preeti Jain & **P.C. Joshi**, Reconstruction of Stature among Rajputs and Brahmins of Srinagar, Garhwal (U.P.), *South Asian Anthropologist*, 1999, 20, 2 : 63-66. (ISSN:0257-7348)

Joshi, P.C. Health Seeking Behaviour in Tribal Population of the Himalayas. *Current Opinion in Psychiatry*. 1999, 12, 1:331.

Joshi, P.C. Technological Innovations in the Garhwal Himalayas: The HESCO Case Study. *Anthropologist,* 1999, 1, 1: 81-85.

Joshi, P.C. Book Review. Perception and Interactions in a Medical Setting: A Sociological Study of a Women's Hospital By Aneeta A. Minocha, *Sociological Bulletin*: 1998, 47, 2:271-273.

Joshi, P.C. Don't Let Me Down: Place of Worms in Culture and Reflections on Ethnophysiology in a Central Himalayan Tribe, *J. Indian Anthropological Society*, 1995, 30:253-258.

Joshi, P. C. From Territory to Caste : Process of Social Transformation in Central Himalayas, In *From Tribe to Caste*, Ed. Dev Nathan, Shimla, Indian Institute of Advanced Studies, 1995.

Joshi, P.C. In Persuit of Protein : On Meat Eating in Garhwal, *Indian Anthropologist*, 1994, 24, 2:39-44.

Joshi, P.C. Tribal Medicine in Indian Context, *Vanyajati,* 1994, 42, 1-8.

Joshi, P.C. In the Hands of Gods: Chhinga and Social Order in Khos Himalayas. In *The Indian Families*, K.K. Chakraborty (ed.), Bhopal, Rashtriya Manav Sangrahalaya, 1994:58-67.

Joshi, P.C. and B.S. Patwal. Ecological significance of Hariyali Devi. *Manav*, 1993, 21, 2: 127-131.

Joshi, P.C. Culture, Health and Illness : Aspects of Ethnomedicine in Jaunsar Bawar, In *The Central Himalayan Panorama*, Ed. S.K. Biswas, 1991, Calcutta : Institute of Social Research and Applied Anthropology, 253-380.

Joshi, P.C. Reprinted in Himalayan Economy and People, S.C. Singh edited. 1990-1991.

Joshi, P.C. and V.K. Srivastava. Dialogue and Interpretation of Illness (Review Article), *Indian Anthropologist*, 1995.

Joshi, P.C. and V.K. Srivastava Afforestation, Development and Religion. *Mainstream*, 1989.

Joshi, P.C. Some reflections on the use of traditional medicines, In *Tribal Demography and Development*, Ed. Ashish Bose *et al.* 1990, New Delhi : B.R. Publishing Corp., 155-159.

Joshi, P.C. Cultural Resources: A Case from Khos Himalayas, In *Himalayan Environment and Culture*, N.K. Rustomji and Charles Ramble (ed.), New Delhi, Indus Publishers, 1990:110-114.

Joshi, P.C. Shaman, Mystics and Doctors (Review Article), *SIMA Bulletin*, 1988.

Joshi, P.C. Traditional Medical Systems in Central Himalayas, *The Eastern Anthropologist*, 1988, 41, 1:78-86. (ISSN-0012-8686)

Joshi, P.C. Health and Healing in the Himalayas, *Journal of Himalayan Studies and Regional Development*, 1986, 10:111-117.

Lapoint, E.C. and **Joshi, P.C.** Economy of Respect, *Lambda Alfa Journal of Man,* 1985-86, 1&2:41-52. (http://soar.wichita.edu/dspace/bitstream/

handle/10057/1773/LAJ_v17_p4757..pdf;jsessionid=2 047047C83C5744E 9FB0264A6D50BDC4?sequence=1)

Joshi, P.C. Medical Anthropology: NewAreas of Researches in Anthropology, *Spectra of Anthropological Progress,* 1986, 8 : 9-14.

Joshi, P.C. and Bhattacharya, D.K. Paleoliths of Delhi, *The Eastern Anthropologist,* 1985, 4:341-345. (ISSN-0012-8686)

Joshi, P.C. Effective Elements in the Medical Culture in Jaunsar Bawar, *Research Proceedings*, 1982.

Joshi, P.C. Illness and Social Control : A Study in Ethnomedicine, *Research Proceedings*, 1981, 8, 1&2 : 9-16.

Joshi, P.C. Identity Crisis in Anthropology, *Spectra of Anthropological Progress***,** 1981.

Joshi, P.C. Marital Stability among the Khasa Tribals of Dehradun, *Spectra of Anthropological Progress,* 1981.

Joshi, P.C. Perception and Classification of Illness among the Khasa Tribals of Dehradun, *Tribe,* 1981, 23, 1:16-26.

Joshi, P.C. Concept and Causation: Ethnomedicine in Jaunsar Bawar, *Journal of Social Research*, 1981, 23, 2:16-26.

Joshi, P.C. Current Contents in Anthropological Periodicals, *Research Proceedings*, 1978.

Joshi, P.C. Ethnomedical Choice Pattern in Rural Kashmir, *Manav***,** 1978.

Joshi, P.C. Ethnomedicine: Exploration of some Folk Concepts in Jaunsar Bawar, *Research Proceedings,* 1978.

Reports Submitted to Government of India (06)

Khattri P., **P.C. Joshi,** and D. Guha-Sapir. 2013. *People's Perception and State's Response during Floods: Evidence from Bahraich district of Uttar Pradesh. First Session of National Platform for Disaster Risk Reduction.* Ministry of Home Affairs, Government of India, New Delhi. pp. 260-261.

Joshi, P.C. and Anuj Tiwari. 2013. *Mainstreaming DRR in BCP: Corporate Sufferings vis-à-vis Disaster Mitigation. First Session of National Platform for Disaster Risk Reduction.* Ministry of Home Affairs, Government of India, New Delhi. pp. 223-224.

Minakshi and **P.C. Joshi**. 2013. *Mental Health Problems among Women: Post Kosi Flood Scenario. First Session of National Platform for Disaster Risk Reduction.* Ministry of Home Affairs, Government of India, New Delhi. pp. 207-208.

Joshi, P.C., Kalindi Sharma and D. Guha-Sapir. 2013. *Impact of Cyclone Aila on the Livelihoods of the People of Sundarbans, West Bengal. First Session of National Platform for Disaster Risk Reduction.* Ministry of Home Affairs, Government of India, New Delhi. pp. 185-186.

Sharma, K. and **P.C. Joshi**. 2013. *Overcoming Disasters: Issues in Long term Recovery in Gujarat. First Session of National Platform for Disaster Risk Reduction.* Ministry of Home Affairs, Government of India, New Delhi. pp. 166-168.

Desai, N.G., Gupta, D. K., **Joshi, P. C**., Singh, R.A., Singh, T. B., Lal, Manu and Kumar, A. Mental Health Service Needs and Service Delivery Models in the Earthquake Disaster Affected Population in Gujarat : A Pilot Phase Study. *Indian Council of Medical Research.* New Delhi.

Section and Chapters in Book etc. (55)

Joshi, P.C. Obituary. 2016. Prof. I. P. Singh. *The Eastern Anthropologist.* 69, 3&4: 525-527.

Joshi, P.C. Obituary. 2016. Prof. R.S. Negi. *The Eastern Anthropologist.* 69, 3&4:529-530.

Gupta, S. and **P. C. Joshi**. 2015. Critical View on Globalization and Development with special Reference to India. In A. Matin, M. Akram and S. Nasir (eds.) *Development, Health and Globalization.* Academic Publications, Delhi. pp. 44-64.

Joshi, P.C. 2014. Anthropological Perspective on Traditional Healing Practices among Indian Scheduled Tribes. In *Health in the Context of Tribal culture* Ed. by D.K. Behera, pp. 18-31. Concept Publishing Company Ltd., New Delhi.

Joshi, P.C. 2014. Challenges of Health Care in Central Indian Tribal Areas. In B.M. Mukherjee and Farhad Mollick (eds.) *Tribal People of Central India—Problems and Prospects.* New Delhi, K.K. Publications. pp. 286-300.

Joshi, P.C. 2013. Biological Factors and Health. In *Explorations in Indian Medical Anthropology Volume II: Disease, Health and Culture,* Ed. H.K. Bhat, **P.C. Joshi** and B.R. Vijayendra, Concept Publishing Company, New Delhi. pp. 246-250.

Lamkang, A.S., **P.C. Joshi** and M.M. Singh. 2013. A Cross-Sectional Study on the Quality of Life among HIV/AIDS Patients in Manipur. In *Explorations in Indian Medical Anthropology* Volume II: *Disease, Health and Culture,* Ed. H.K. Bhat, **P.C. Joshi** and B.R. Vijayendra, Concept Publishing Company, New Delhi. pp. 211-235.

Joshi, P.C. 2013. Anthropology and HIV/AIDS. In *Explorations in Indian Medical Anthropology* Volume II: *Disease, Health and Culture,* Ed. H.K. Bhat, P.C. Joshi and B.R. Vijayendra, Concept Publishing Company, New Delhi. pp. 209-210.

Minakshi, **P.C. Joshi**, Prashant Khattri and D. Guha-Sapir. 2013. Emerging Issues in Violence against Women in Post Disaster Context. In *Explorations in Indian Medical Anthropology,* Volume II: *Disease, Health and Culture,* Ed. H.K. Bhat, **P.C. Joshi** and B.R. Vijayendra, Concept Publishing Company, New Delhi. pp. 193-207.

Joshi, P.C., P. Khattri, B.S. Aribam, S. Kaushal and D. Guha-Sapir. 2013. Association of the Long Term Flood Impacts with the Prevalence of Vitamin-A Deficiency in Bahraich district, Uttar Pradesh. In *Explorations in Indian Medical Anthropology,* Volume II: *Disease, Health and Culture,* Ed. H.K. Bhat, **P.C. Joshi** and B.R. Vijayendra, Concept Publishing Company, New Delhi. pp. 175-192.

Joshi, P.C. 2013. Anthropology and Disaster. In *Explorations in Indian Medical Anthropology,* Volume II: *Disease, Health and Culture,* Ed. H.K. Bhat, P.C. Joshi and B.R. Vijayendra, Concept Publishing Company, New Delhi pp. 171-173.

Joshi, P.C. 2013. Women and Child Health. In *Explorations in Indian Medical Anthropology,* Volume II: *Disease, Health and Culture,* Ed. H.K. Bhat, **P.C. Joshi** and B.R. Vijayendra, Concept Publishing Company, New Delhi. pp. 85-86.

Bhat, H.K., **P.C. Joshi** and B.R. Vijayendra. 2013. Introduction. In *Explorations in Indian Medical Anthropology,* Volume- II: *Disease, Health and Culture,* Ed. H.K. Bhat, **P.C. Joshi** and B.R. Vijayendra, Concept Publishing Company, New Delhi. pp. vii-xi.

Joshi, P.C. 2013. Healthcare Drives. In *"Explorations in Indian Medical Anthropology,* Volume I: *Illness, Health and Culture",* Ed. H.K. Bhat, **P.C. Joshi** and B.R. Vijayendra. Concept Publishing Company, New Delhi. pp. 297-98.

Joshi, P. C. 2013. Society, Culture and Health. In *"Explorations in Indian Medical Anthropology,* Volume I: *Illness, Health and Culture"* Ed. H.K. Bhat, **P.C. Joshi** and B.R. Vijayendra. Concept Publishing Company, New Delhi. p. 210.

Joshi P.C. 2013. Medical Anthropology and Health Sciences. In *"Explorations in Indian Medical Anthropology,* Volume II: *Illness, Health and Culture"* Ed. H.K. Bhat, **P.C. Joshi** and B.R. Vijayendra, Concept Publishing Company, New Delhi. pp. 1-2.

Bhat, H.K., **P. C. Joshi** and B.R. Vijayendra. 2013. Introduction. In *"Explorations in Indian Medical Anthropology,* Volume II: *Illness, Health and Culture"* Ed. H.K. Bhat, **P.C. Joshi** and B. R. Vijayendra, Concept Publishing Company, New Delhi. pp: ix-xiii.

Joshi, P.C. 2012. Challenges of Health Care in Central Indian Tribal Areas. In *The Other Side of Development.* Ed. A.K. Ghosh and R.D. Munda, pp. 275-290. Konark Publishers Pvt. Ltd., New Delhi.

Joshi, P.C. 2012. Ethics, Health Care and Disasters. In *Ethics, Health and Medicine: Anthropological Perspectives,* ed. U. Kalpagam, pp 395-405. Manak Publications Pvt. Ltd., New Delhi.

Mir, U.A. and **P.C. Joshi,** 2012. Dealing with Dilemma: Role of ethics and subjectivity in doing fieldwork on violence in one's own culture. In *Ethics, Health and Medicine: Anthropological Perspectives,* ed. U. Kalpagam, 152-172. Manak Publications Pvt. Ltd., New Delhi.

Joshi, P.C., 2011. *Preface.* Bio-anthropological study of Sirmour, Himachal Pradesh, *UGC SAP Report*, Department of Anthropology, Delhi University, Delhi.

Joshi, P. C. 2011. *Preface.* Anthropological Study of Sawrakot Village in Jubbal, Himachal Pradesh, *UGC SAP Report,* Department of Anthropology, Delhi University, Delhi.

Joshi, P.C. 2010. Traditional Healing Practices of Scheduled Tribes: Status, Challenges and Future. In *Tribal Health: Status, Challenges and Possibilities.* Tribal Research and Development Institute, Bhopal. pp. 79-82.

P.C. Joshi (Quoted in), 2010. Assessing the Impact of Disaster. *International Innovation: Disseminating Science, Research and Technology.* March 2010. p. 40

Joshi, P.C. and Kaushal, S. 2010. Medical Anthropology and Disaster Management. Microdis Working Papers Series. Delhi. pp. 7-11.

Joshi, P.C., Aribam, B.S., Kaushal, S. and Guha-Sapir, D. 2010. Flood Impact on Cough and Cold among under five Children in Bahraich district, Uttar Pradesh, India. *Working Papers Series.* Delhi. pp. 12-28.

Kaushal, S., **Joshi, P.C.** and Khattri, P. 2010. Health Impact of Floods in Bahraich district of Uttar Pradesh. *WorkingPapers Series. Delhi.* pp. 29-37.

Minakshi and **Joshi, P.C.** 2010. Health and Violence against Women in disaster: Case study of Kosi flood in Bihar. *Working Papers Series.* Delhi. pp. 38-48.

Mir, U.A. and **Joshi, P.C.** 2010. Trauma suffering and Medical Anthropology: some reflections in the context of findings from Jammu and Kashmir. *Working Papers Series.* Delhi. pp. 50-87.

Kumar, S. and **Joshi, P.C.** 2010. Microfinnce, women health and empowerment: A case study of self-employed women association (SEWA), Bikaner, Rajasthan. *Working Papers Series.* Delhi. pp. 88-98.

Joshi, P.C. 2009. Cultural Profile of Central Himalayas. In *Bio-cultural Profile of Central and Western Himalayas.* Ed. M.B. Sharma, V. Kaul, V. Sarkar and V. Joardar, Serials Publication. pp. 68-93.

Joshi, P.C. 2009. Contributor in Infant and Young Children Feeding in Emergencies. Solution Exchange-UN. August, 2009.

Joshi, P.C. Contributor. In *Indigenous Knowledge for Disaster Risk Reduction in South Asia.* Ed. Chakrabarti, P.G. Dhar, Srivastava, Sanjay and Shakya, Binod. 2009. New Delhi: Macmillan Publishers India Ltd.

Joshi, P.C., Singh, M.M. and Khattri, P. 2009. Social Impacts on Extreme Events: Conceptual Framework. *Microdis Working Papers Series.* Delhi. pp. 6-13.

Joshi, P.C., Khattri, P. and Singh, M.M. 2009. Social Impacts on Natural Disasters. *Microdis Working Papers Series.* Delhi. pp. 29-41.

Khattri, P., **Joshi, P.C.,** Minakshi and Guha-Sapir, D. 2009. Importance of Past Memories in disaster Research. *Microdis Working Papers Series.* Delhi. pp. 42-47.

Minakshi, **Joshi, P.C**., Khattri, P. and Guha-Sapir, D. 2009. Emerging Issues in Violence against Women in Post Disaster Context. *Microdis Working Papers Series*. Delhi. pp. 48-59.

Khattri, P., **Joshi, P.C.**, Minakshi, Singh, M.M. and Guha-Sapir, D. 2009. Projections of Disaster: Investigations into Visual and Textual Images of Floods in Badaun, Uttar Pradesh. *Microdis Working Papers Series*. Delhi. pp. 60-67.

Minakshi, **Joshi, P.C**., Kaushal, S., Khattri, P. and Guha-Sapir, D. 2009. Disaster and Domestic Violence: the Alcohol Connection. *Microdis Working Papers Series*. Delhi. pp. 68-77.

Minakshi, **Joshi, P.C**. and Guha-Sapir, D. 2009. Women in Disasters: A Case Study of Kosi Flood in Bihar. *Microdis Working Papers Series*. Delhi. pp. 78-86.

Sharma, K., **Joshi, P.C.**, Kaushal, S., Khattri, P. and Guha-Sapir, D. 2009. Stakeholder's Perception on flood Impacts: Qualitative Analysis. *Microdis Working Papers Series*. Delhi. pp. 87-93.

Joshi, P.C. 2008**.** Discussant. Can Disasters help to improve a Country's Economy? *E-Conference Summary. International Centre for Integrated Mountain Development, ICIMOD. Kathmandu, Nepal*, 2008.

Joshi, P.C. and Khattri, P. 2008. Traditional Medical System of the Bhils: Characteristics, Function and Change. In *Bio-Social Health Issues*. Ed. R.K. Pathak, A.K. Sinha, R.N. Vasishat, B.G. Banerjee and C.J. Edwin), 471-486. Northern Book Centre, New Delhi.

Joshi, P.C. Indigenous Knowledge for Disaster Risk Reduction in South Asia (contributor in P.G. Dhar Chakrabarti *et al.*). SAARC Disaster Management Centre, New Delhi, 2008.

Joshi, P.C. Culture and Risk: Socio-cultural Settings that Influence Risk from Natural Hazards. (Contributor in Kenneth Hewitt). International Centre for Integrated Mountain Development, ICIMOD. Kathmandu, Nepal, 2008.

P.C. Joshi, Main Contributor, *Mountain to Mountain Cooperation: Sustainable Use of Biodiversity, including geneticre sources, in the Himal-Andes–e-conference report*. Ranjana Sinha (Eds.). 2006. pp. 13-15. Mountain Forum Secretariat. Kathmandu, Nepal.

O. Hemlata Devi, Sonia Kaushal, Shashi Katewa and **P.C. Joshi**. Dynamics of Health and Ecology—A Study of Indigenous Medicines among the Karang Fisherman of Manipur. In *Culture Ecology and Sustainable Development*, Ed. S.K. Chaudhury, 2006. pp. 137-152. New Delhi, Mittal Publication.

P.C. Joshi. People and Culture—Himalayan Eco-system and its future. In *Culture Ecology and Sustainable Development*, Ed. S.K. Chaudhury, 2006. pp. 159-168. New Delhi, Mittal Publication.

P.C. Joshi,. S. Sharma and J.S. Bapna, Sports and Drug Abuse : An Overview. In *Issues and Themes in Anthropology*, Ed. V.K. Srivastava and M.K. Singh, Palaka Prakashan, Delhi, 2004, pp. 471-502.

Joshi, P.C., Issues in Tribal Health and Medicines, In *Tribal Health and Medicines,* Ed. A.K. Kalla and P.C. Joshi, Concept Publishing Company, New Delhi, 2004, pp. 403-407.

Chao, D., Chadha, N.K. and **Joshi P.C.**, Psychosocial Wellbeing of the Elderly among Nagas, In *Tribal Health and Medicines,* Ed. A.K. Kalla and P. C. Joshi, Concept Publishing Company, New Delhi, 2004, pp. 247-275.

Joshi, P.C., The World of Tribal Healers, In *Tribal Health and Medicines,* Ed. A.K. Kalla and P. C. Joshi, Concept Publishing Company, New Delhi, 2004, pp. 202-241.

P.C. Joshi. 2003. An Idea for a New Museum. In *Restoring Human Culture and Biospheric Environment.* Ed. KK Chakravarty, K.V. Sundaram and M. Moni, Northern Book Centre, New Delhi. pp. 115-118.

Joshi, P.C. and U.A. Mir, 2002. Psychosocial consequences of traumatic events on adolescents : A study in context of Jammu and Kashmir. In *Adolescent Mental Health : Current Status and Challenges* Ed. Uday K. Sinha (ed). 2002. Delhi, Institute of Human Behaviour and Allied Sciences, pp. 30-41.

Joshi, P.C. and U.A. Mir, Medical Anthropology and Traumatic Reactions : Emerging concerns in Medical Anthropology, *The Eastern Anthropologist,* 2002, 55, 1:71-80. (ISSN-0012-8686)

International and National Proceeding (14)

A. Kotwani, C. Wattal, **P.C. Joshi** and K. Holloway. 2011. Irrational Use of Antibiotics and Role of Pharmacists: An Insight from a Qualitative Study in New Delhi, India. *Proceedings of 16th Annual International ISPOR Meet. Baltimore, MD, USA. (ID30664)*

Kotwani, A., Wattal, C., Katewa, S., **Joshi, P.C.** and Holloway, K. 2011. Factors influencing antibiotic prescribing by Primary Care Doctors in Delhi, India: A Qualitative Study. *Proceedings of Third International Conference for Improving Use of Medicines–Informed Strategies, Effective Policies, Lasting Solutions. Alexandria, Egypt. (ID584).*

P.C. Joshi, B.S. Aribam, M.M. Singh and D. Guha-Sapir. 2010. Association of Long Term Flood Impacts with the Prevalence of Vitamin A Deficiency in Bahraich district, Uttar Pradesh. 2010. *Proceedings of Asian Symposium on Disaster Impact and Its Assessment. Hue City, Vietnam.* pp. 188-197.

S. Akerkar, M. Fordham and **P.C. Joshi**. 2010. Reciprocity, Local Entitlements and Disaster Recovery. *Proceedings of Asian Symposium on Disaster Impact and Its Assessment. Hue City, Vietnam.* pp. 311-325.

Joshi, P.C. 2010. Disaster Impact and Its Assessment in Asia. 2010. *Proceedings of Asian Symposium on Disaster Impact and Its Assessment. Hue city, Vietnam.* pp. 4-6.

K. Sharma, **P.C. Joshi**, S. Kaushal, B. S. Aribam, H. Kataria and D. Guha-Sapir. 2010. Impact of Cyclone Aila on the Livelihood of the People of West Bengal.

Proceedings of Asian Symposium on Disaster Impact and Its Assessment. Hue city, Vietnam. pp. 83-106.

P. Khattri, **P.C. Joshi**, T. Wind, I.H. Komproe and D. Guha-Sapir. 2010. Mental Health Impacts as a function of Stressors: Evidence from Recurrent Flooding in Bahraich district, Uttar Pradesh. *Proceedings of Asian Symposium on Disaster Impact and Its Assessment. Hue City, Vietnam.* pp. 171-187.

Joshi, P.C., A toolkit for studying the social and psychological effects of Disaster. *Report on Improving data quality for natural disasters and complex emergencies in Southeast Asia. 2003 Brussels, CRED, Catholic University of Louvain,* pp. 7-9.

P.C. Joshi, S. Kaushal, S. Ranjan Das, J.M. Rodriguez-Llanes, O. D'Ouost, B. Van den Oever, B.S. Aribam, L. Irvine, A. Mukhopadhyay and D. Guha-Sapir. The Nutritional and Health Status of the children in flood and non-flood exposed areas in two districts of India. *Poster Presentation at 20th IUHPE World Conference on Health Promotion.* 11-15 July, 2010, Geneva, Switzerland.

Joshi, P.C. and Guha-Sapir, D. 2009. Social Impact of Disaster in Holistic Perspective. *Proceedings of the European Sociological Association, 2009,* Lisbon, Portugal.

Joshi, P.C. Medical Anthropology and Psychiatry: Areas of common concern in Indian context. *Proceeding of the XVIth Conference of Indian Association of Social Psychiatry,* p. 59, AIIMS, New Delhi, November28-30, 2008.

Valérie Louis, Michael Marx, Mondastri Korib Sudaryo, **P.C. Joshi**, Maureen Fordham, Kristin Magnussen, Alexandre Borde, Terry Cannon, Debarati Guha-Sapir. Micromanagement of disasters and the MICRODIS project: An integrated approach to measure health social and economic impact of extreme events in Europe and Asia. *Proceedings of GHUP, Society for Hygiene, Environmental and Prevention Medicine Conference:* Bielefeld, Germany, November 22-24, 2007.

Joshi, P.C., Khatter, P., Singh, M.M., Fordham, M., Guha-Sapir. Flood: Trends and Social Impacts in Indian Context. *Proceedings of International Conference on Shift in Thinking: Perspectives of Vulnerability and hazard Assessment. Potsdam, Germany*, October 4-5, 2007.

Joshi, P.C., Singh, M.M. and Khattri, P. Social Impact of Extreme Events, *Proceedings of the EU 6th Framework International Meet on Integrated Health, Social and Economic Impact of Extreme Events : Evidence, Methods and Tools*. 18-19 April, 2007, Brussels, Belgium.

INDEX